THE CANADIAN TYPE 2 DIABETES SOURCEBOOK

M. Sara Rosenthal

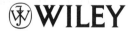WILEY

John Wiley & Sons Canada, Ltd.

First published in Canada in 2002 by
Macmillan Canada, an imprint of John Wiley & Sons Canada, Ltd.

National Library of Canada Cataloguing in Publication Data

Rosenthal, M. Sara
   The Canadian type 2 diabetes sourcebook

Includes bibliographical references and index.
ISBN 1-55335-000-6

Non-insulin-dependent diabetes—Popular works. I. Title

RC662.18.R667 2002   616.4'62   C2001-903532-2

Portions of this book were previously published as *Managing Your Diabetes* (0-7715-7560-2, 1998) and *Managing Your Diabetes for Women* (0-7715-7627-7, 1999). All such material has been reviewed and updated.

Although every effort has been made to ensure that permissions for all material were obtained, those sources not formally acknowledged should contact the publisher for inclusion in future editions of this book.

3 4 5 TRI 06 05 04 03

Cover design by Susan Thomas/Digital Zone
Text design and typesetting by Heidy Lawrance Associates
Author photo by Greg Edward

This book is available for bulk purchases by your group or organizations for sales promotions, premiums, fundraising, and seminars. For details, contact: John Wiley & Sons Canada, Ltd., 22 Worcester Road, Etobicoke, ON M9W 1L1. Tel: 416-236-4433. Toll Free 1-800-567-4797. Fax: 416-236-4448. Web site: www.wiley.ca

Macmillan Canada
An imprint of John Wiley & Sons Canada, Ltd.
Toronto

Printed in Canada

OTHER BOOKS BY M. SARA ROSENTHAL

The Thyroid Sourcebook (4th edition, 2000)

The Gynecological Sourcebook (3rd edition, 1999)

The Pregnancy Sourcebook (3rd edition, 1999)

The Fertility Sourcebook (3rd edition, 1999)

The Breastfeeding Sourcebook (2nd edition, 1998)

The Breast Sourcebook (2nd edition, 1999)

The Gastrointestinal Sourcebook (1997; 1998)

The Thyroid Sourcebook for Women (1999)

Women and Depression (2000)

Women of the '60s Turning 50 (Canada only; 2000)

Women and Passion (2000)

Managing PMS Naturally (2001)

Women Managing Stress (2001)

The Hypothyroid Sourcebook (2002)

50 Ways Series

50 Ways to Prevent Colon Cancer (2000)

50 Ways Women Can Prevent Heart Disease (2000)

50 Ways to Manage Heartburn, Reflux, and Ulcer (2001)

50 Ways to Manage Type 2 Diabetes (U.S. only; 2001)

50 Ways to Prevent and Manage Stress (2001)

50 Ways to Fight Depression Without Drugs (2002)

SarahealthGuides

These are M. Sara Rosenthal's own line of health books dedicated to rare, controversial or stigmatizing health topics you won't find in regular bookstores. SarahealthGuides are available only at on-line bookstores such as amazon.com. Visit sarahealth.com for upcoming titles.

Stopping Cancer at the Source (2001)

Women and Unwanted Hair (2001)

ACKNOWLEDGEMENTS

● ● ● ● ● ● ● ● ●

I wish to thank the following people (listed alphabetically) for their commitment, hard work and guidance on *Managing Your Diabetes*, which helped to frame so much of the content of this book:

Irwin Antone, M.D., C.C.F.P., Assistant Professor, Department of Family Medicine, University of Western Ontario; Brenda Cook, R.D., University of Alberta Hospitals; Karen Faye, L.P.N., A.F.F.A. (U.S.), Fitness Practitioner; Tasha Hamilton, Ba.Sc., R.D., Diabetes Educator-Dietitian, Tri-Hospital Diabetes Education Centre (TRIDEC); Stuart Harris, M.D., M.P.H., C.C.F.P., A.B.P.M., Assistant Professor, Departments of Family Medicine and Epidemiology and Biostatistics, University of Western Ontario, and Former Medical Director, University of Toronto Sioux Lookout Program; Anne Levin, B.Sc.P.T., M.C.P.A., Physiotherapist and Certified Hydrotherapist, Baycrest Centre for Geriatric Care, Coordinator, Arthritis Education and Exercise Program, and Lecturer, Physical Therapy, Faculty of Medicine, University of Toronto; Barbara McIntosh, R.N., B.Sc.N., C.D.E., Nurse Coordinator, Adult Diabetes Education Program, Grand River Hospital, Kitchener, Ontario; James McSherry, M.B., Ch.B, F.C.F.P., F.R.C.G.P., F.A.A.F.P., F.A.B.M.P., Medical Director, Victoria Family Medical Centre, Chief of Family Medicine, The London Health Sciences Centre; David Michaels, D.D.S; Robert Panchyson, B.Sc.N., R.N., Nurse Clinician, Diabetes Educator, Hamilton Civic Hospitals, Hamilton General Division; Diana Phayre, Clinical Nurse Specialist, Diabetes Education Centre, The Doctor's Hospital; Robert Silver, M.D., F.R.C.P.C., Endocrinologist, Division of Endocrinology and Metabolism, The Toronto Hospital. Special thanks to Gary May, M.D., F.R.C.P., Clinical Assistant Professor of Medicine, Department of Medicine, Division of

Gastroenterology, University of Calgary and William Warren Rudd, M.D., Colon and Rectal Surgeon and Founder and Director of The Rudd Clinic for Diseases of the Colon and Rectum (Toronto), who both provided some of the groundwork for this text through their roles as medical advisors on past works. Special thanks to Mark Nesbitt, Regional Coordinator (Ontario), Canadian MedicAlert Foundation and Diabetes Patient Advocate, and Judy Nesbitt, Diabetes Patient Advocate. Endocrinologists at TRIDEC as well as several diabetes educators within the Canadian diabetes community provided their time and comments.

Gillian Arsenault, M.D., C.C.F.P., I.B.C.L.C., F.R.C.P., Simon Fraser Health Unit, served as a past advisor on two works, and has never stopped advising and sending me valuable information. Irving Rootman, Ph.D., Director, Centre for Health Promotion, University of Toronto, put me in touch with several experts, and always encourages my interest in primary prevention and health promotion issues.

CONTENTS

● ● ● ● ● ● ● ● ● ● ●

FOREWORD

● ● ● ● ● ● ● ● ● ●

When I started to examine Type 2 diabetes it all seemed so simple; all you had to do was control your blood sugar. You could do this by losing some weight or taking one or two pills. I was certain that this would make sense to patients and they would comply. Now, after a few years of delving into what happens in the "real world," I have a very different view.

I think the medical community's usual approach to people with diabetes, or for that matter with any chronic disease, is somewhat flawed. The typical model is the following: the doctor diagnoses, the doctor prescribes and the patient then complies. This can work for acute medicine but not for chronic diseases. For chronic diseases, there should be an exchange of roles. Instead of the doctor or clinic being the central character in diabetes care, it should be you, the health care consumer—with clinic, nurse, doctor, pharmacist, nutritionist, etc., as the supporting actors. We need to shift from the doctor-management approach to one of self-management. Books like this one play a vital role in a self-management approach.

Some of the themes of this new pathway are as follows:

We need to move from a fixed "table d'hôte" menu to an "à la carte" menu of information, knowledge and solutions. We tend not to individualize information but rather to send out generic information that is often overwhelming or not specific enough for an individual's health care needs. The Internet has helped to change some of these problems, but the quality of that information remains a concern.

We need to consider barriers to care beyond basic information. We all know we should eat well and exercise, but how do I help you identify your unique barriers and the characteristics that enable you to actually do it? Do I bring in your partner? Put the information on your handheld computer? Talk to your peers?

We need to reframe the risks and benefits, putting them in the consumer's perspective. As health care professionals, we spend a lot of time looking at long-term trials that show "significant" gains in risk reduction. These gains may be evident in the literature but are often cold comfort to patients. For example, when I see patients for arthritis or asthma and I give them pills or puffers they usually feel better immediately. However, people with diabetes are often taking many medications but do not actually feel better—in fact they often feel worse—and the incentives for good control are very different and certainly less obvious.

We need to redefine our conception of diabetes. Diabetes is not a disease as much as it is a risk factor. Heart disease is our most common foe and diabetes is a major risk factor for heart problems. Treating diabetes is like making a contribution to your RRSP; you don't get the benefit until much farther down the road. The contribution can take many forms: lowering blood pressure and/or cholesterol, stopping smoking, maintaining good glucose control and getting active.

We need to remember the basics. In medicine we have come up with many fancy interventions, but at the end of the day, good health still rests on a few core principles: healthy eating, being active and having a positive attitude. For people who suffer from a chronic condition such as diabetes, I would add self-empowerment to the list. When an individual takes charge of their lifestyle, emotional well-being, and role as health care consumer, there is greater opportunity to improve their health.

Enabling self-management is what Sara Rosenthal's *Canadian Type 2 Diabetes Sourcebook* is all about. This book is not meant to be read all at one sitting. It is not meant to convert you from a fast food junkie to a never-make-a-mistake eater. Rather, it is meant to be a comprehensive resource that is there for you when you need the right information at the right time. There is no perfect pathway to optimum diabetes care—only *your* pathway. Health care professionals and diabetes experts can only try to make it easier for you to do the right thing. Certainly, this book gives you all the information you need to make those choices. The next step is up to you. Good luck!

Michael Evans, MD, CCFP
Principal Investigator
   Knowledge Translation Program, Continuing Education
Research Scholar, Family Healthcare Research Unit
Assistant Professor, Department of Family and Community Medicine,
   University of Toronto
Staff Physician, Toronto Western Hospital,
   University Health Network

INTRODUCTION

• • • • • • • • • • •

ALL IN THE FAMILY

Let me tell you a little bit about my family, which will tell you *why* I'm interested in the subject of Type 2 diabetes.

In 1978, my grandmother, obese and physically inactive, who had Type 2 diabetes, dropped dead from a massive heart attack at the age of 62. She was survived by her own mother by a full decade. I have still never quite recovered from the loss because it was such an untimely death. To this day, I dream of her. In a recurring dream, she is alive and well, but I know that her heart will give out at any moment. The feeling that she will "die again" always interferes with my dream visits; even in the dream world, my time with her is limited. My grandfather, a family physician who died in 1989, used to say that my grandmother "ate herself to death." And the more I research Type 2 diabetes, the more I understand what he meant by this comment.

Roughly 85 percent of those diagnosed with Type 2 diabetes are obese. My grandmother was a textbook case. In her mid-40s, she developed "late-onset diabetes mellitus," known today as Type 2 diabetes. (I explain all the labels of this disease in Chapter 1.) My grandmother was an out-of-control diabetic who outlived her baby sister, who also died from complications of Type 2 diabetes. (My aunt, too, was obese.) Despite the fate of her little sister, my grandmother never made any effort to adjust her own eating habits. My mother, who has spent most of her adult life battling obesity, used to be coaxed into eating rich desserts by my grandmother with comments such as "It's a *sin* not to eat it."

Indeed, my grandmother's great character flaw was her appetite. She could never pass up rich and tasty foods. And part of the reason is attributed to the hard times she experienced coming of age in the Prairies during the Depression. She went on to develop heart disease and apparently had spent most of her 40s and 50s as a very unwell woman, continuously plagued with one health problem after another. Given this information, probably no one is surprised that she died. After all, the woman was a "walking time bomb." The funny thing is, everyone who loved her was shocked by her death. My great-grandmother bore the terrible fate of outliving almost all of her children, who were all obese; most of them died from complications related to Type 2 diabetes.

This is the book I wish my grandmother and her siblings had read. I want to give you the information my grandmother should have had, and might have used, *if it had been available to her.*

By 2004, one in four people over the age of 45 will be diagnosed with Type 2 diabetes. Currently, 1.5 million Canadians have been diagnosed with Type 2 diabetes; an estimated additional 750,000 Canadians have the disease but don't know it.

My grandmother was one of the original founders of the Winnipeg Art Gallery, and was particularly drawn to Aboriginal artwork. The irony is that she did not know how much she had in common with Aboriginal Canadians, whose rates of Type 2 diabetes have been soaring out of control since the 1940s. Today the rate of diabetes among Aboriginal Canadians is five times that of non-Natives—one of the highest rates of diabetes worldwide. In fact, the artists my grandmother loved the most probably suffered from the same disease she did. For this reason, I urge you to read Chapter 9.

Unless you live in a large Canadian city, you may not have immediate (or any!) access to the right health care professionals. Take heart—there are other ways to get the information you need to manage your disease. Every manufacturer of a diabetes product, be it a glucose meter, insulin pen or diabetes medication, has a 1-800 customer care line. These are excellent sources of information. As well, the Canadian Diabetes Association (CDA) should be the first call you make once you're diagnosed. CDA divisions and branches are listed in the resource section at the back of the book. I've also listed a range of Web sites you can visit for more information. And you can always visit me on-line, at www.sarahealth.com.

As I'll stress again and again in this book, Type 2 diabetes is a genetic disease, but by modifying your lifestyle and diet, you may be able to delay the onset of the disease.

If you have any of these signs or symptoms of Type 2 diabetes, this book can help:

▶ Weight gain (over a short time span)

▶ Blurred vision or any change in sight

▶ Drowsiness or extreme fatigue at times when you shouldn't be drowsy or tired

▶ Frequent infections that are slow to heal. (Women should be alert for recurring vaginal yeast infections.)

▶ Tingling or numbness in the hands and feet

▶ Gum disease

PART I

When Your Doctor Says "You Have Diabetes"

Chapter 1

WHAT IS TYPE 2 DIABETES?

● ● ● ● ● ● ● ● ● ● ●

You've just come home from your doctor's office. You can't remember anything he or she said other than those three horrible words: "You have diabetes." What does this mean? How will your life change? You've never been any good at diets, meal plans or exercising. And since you can't stand the sight of blood, how can you be expected to prick your finger every day to monitor your blood sugar? By 2004, one in four Canadians over the age of 45 will be diagnosed with Type 2 diabetes. Currently, 1.5 million Canadians have been diagnosed with Type 2 diabetes; an estimated additional 750,000 Canadians have the disease but don't know it. Whether you've just been diagnosed, or have been living with it for years, this is a difficult disease to understand.

NAMES, NAME CHANGES AND DEFINITIONS

Over the years, the names for different types of diabetes have changed, creating a lot of confusion for people who are newly diagnosed with Type 2 diabetes. Other names for this disease were used when our parents or grandparents were diagnosed, and a lot of people over 40 still remember them. When Canada's Dr. Frederick G. Banting first got the idea for developing a therapy for diabetes in 1921 (see Appendix 1), "diabetes," like the world war, wasn't yet numbered. It was long known, however, that there was a "milder" diabetes, and a more severe form, but diabetes wasn't officially labelled Type 1 and Type 2 until 1979.

When you see the word "diabetes" it refers to *diabetes mellitus*, which means, according to the Canadian Diabetes Association's *Diabetes Dictionary*, "a condition in which the body either cannot produce insulin or cannot effectively use the insulin it produces," causing in turn, high blood sugar (hyperglycemia). But the literal meaning of the word "diabetes" is from the Greek *siphon*. The word *mellitus* is Latin for "sweet." That doesn't mean much today, but it does make sense: In Ancient Greece, diabetes used to be diagnosed by "urine tasters" since the urine becomes sweet when blood sugar is dangerously high. The Greeks noticed that when people with sweet urine drank fluids, the fluids came out in the form of urine immediately—like a siphon. Hence the term "diabetes mellitus" was coined and has stuck to this day.

Confusing Type 2 with Type 1

Many people confuse Type 2 diabetes with Type 1 diabetes, a misunderstanding that interferes with getting accurate information about Type 2 diabetes, so here's what you need to understand: Type 2 diabetes can be managed, reversed or even prevented by modifying your lifestyle; managing Type 2 diabetes does not necessarily require insulin. Most diabetes experts agree that it is poor diet combined with a sedentary lifestyle that triggers the Type 2 gene for those of us who are genetically predisposed to it. In other words, a combination of environment and genes is at work with Type 2 diabetes.

Type 1 diabetes is *completely different*. It cannot be reversed or prevented through lifestyle modification. The working theory, believed by most diabetes experts, is that Type 1 diabetes is an *autoimmune* disease that just strikes without warning. Here, the immune system attacks the beta cells in the pancreas, effectively destroying them. The result is that no insulin is produced by the pancreas at all. Type 1 diabetes is usually diagnosed before age 30, often in childhood. For this reason, Type 1 diabetes was once known as *juvenile diabetes,* or *juvenile-onset diabetes.* Because of organizations such as the Juvenile Diabetes Foundation, we will still see "juvenile diabetes" widely used in the literature on diabetes, even though it is technically an outdated term. It is also misleading, since we are now diagnosing Type 2 diabetes in young children, especially in Aboriginal Canadians.

Because people with Type 1 diabetes depend on insulin injections to live, it was also once called *insulin-dependent diabetes mellitus* (IDDM). Only 10 percent of all people with diabetes have Type 1 diabetes.

The Many Names for Type 2 Diabetes

Ninety percent of all people with diabetes have Type 2 diabetes. Since Type 2 diabetes is a disease of resistance to, rather than an absence of, insulin, it often can be managed through diet and exercise, without insulin injections. For this reason, Type 2 diabetes was once called *non-insulin-dependent diabetes mellitus* (NIDDM). But since many people with Type 2 diabetes may require insulin down the road (see Chapter 5), NIDDM is an inaccurate and misleading name and is not used any more. In fact, about one-third of all people with Type 2 diabetes will eventually need to begin insulin therapy.

When people with Type 2 diabetes require insulin, they can mistakenly believe that their diabetes has "turned into" Type 1 diabetes. But this isn't so; in the same way that an apple cannot turn into a banana, Type 2 diabetes cannot turn into Type 1 diabetes. For reasons I will discuss later in this book, Type 2 diabetes can progress and become more severe over the years, requiring insulin therapy. That's why the terms "NIDDM" and "IDDM" were dropped; they are both inaccurate and misleading. Nonetheless, you may still see these terms widely used in diabetes literature currently circulating.

Since Type 2 diabetes doesn't usually develop until after age 45, before it was named NIDDM, it had even earlier names: *mature-onset diabetes* or *adult-onset diabetes. Mature-onset diabetes in the young* (MODY) referred to Type 2 diabetes in people under 30 years old. None of these terms is used any more.

"Type I and Type II" versus "Type 1 and "Type 2"

It's worth noting that since 1979, when the types of diabetes were numbered, most literature used Roman numerals (I and II) instead of the common usage Arabic numerals (1 and 2). As a result, many people remain confused over whether "Type I and Type II" diabetes were the same thing as "Type 1 and Type 2" diabetes. *Yes, Type I and Type II diabetes mean the same thing as Type 1 and 2 diabetes.* In the late 1990s, consensus in the diabetes medical community was reached over finally dropping the Roman numerals, and using only "1" and "2" in the literature to distinguish between the two types of diabetes.

WHAT HAPPENS IN TYPE 2 DIABETES?

If you have Type 2 diabetes, your pancreas is functioning. You are making plenty of insulin. In fact, you are probably making too much insulin, a condition called *hyperinsulinemia*. Insulin is a hormone made by your *beta cells*, the insulin-producing cells within the *islets of Langerhans*—small islands of cells afloat in your pancreas. The *pancreas* is a bird beak-shaped gland situated behind the stomach.

Insulin is a major player in our bodies. One of its most important functions is to regulate the blood sugar levels. It does this by "knocking" on your cells' door and announcing, "Sugar's here; come and get it!" Your cells then open the door to let sugar in from your bloodstream. That sugar is absolutely vital to your health and provides you with the energy you need to function.

Insulin Resistance

When the cell doesn't answer the door, this is called *insulin resistance:* The cell is resisting insulin. What happens if the cells don't answer the door? Two things. First, the sugar in your bloodstream will accumulate because it has nowhere to go. (It's the kind of situation that develops when your newspapers pile up outside your door when you're away.) Second, your pancreas will keep sending out more insulin to try to get your cells to open that door. This results in high blood sugar. The result is too much sugar and too much insulin. This is a bad combination of problems, which can lead to high blood pressure (a.k.a. hypertension) and high cholesterol, and a host of other complications (see Part 3).

It wasn't until the 1960s that researchers discovered that most people with Type 2 diabetes suffered from a *resistance* to insulin, not necessarily a *lack* of insulin. If insulin resistance goes on for too long, the pancreas can become over-worked and eventually may not make enough, or any, insulin. In effect, it's like a strike. This is why some people with Type 2 diabetes may require insulin injections one day. (I discuss this in more detail later on.)

When the body uses insulin properly, it not only lowers blood sugar but also assists in the distribution of fat and protein. Therefore, when your body doesn't use insulin properly, obesity can be the by-product. Insulin also increases the appetite, which can also lead to obesity. Some diabetes experts I've interviewed believe that insulin resistance may be what actually causes obesity, not the other way around.

High Blood Sugar

The high blood sugar that results from insulin resistance can lead to a number of other diseases, including cardiovascular disease (heart disease and stroke) and peripheral vascular disease (PVD), a condition in which the blood doesn't flow properly to other parts of your body. This can create a number of problems, discussed in Part 3. Many people who suffer a heart attack or stroke have Type 2 diabetes.

High blood sugar can also become aggravated by glycogen, a form of glucose that is stored in the liver and muscles, which is released when you need energy. Insulin enables your cells to store glucose as glycogen. But when your cells are resisting insulin, glycogen can be released in a confused response because it appears to the cells that there is no sugar in the blood.

When You Have Type 2 Diabetes but Require Insulin

Insulin resistance, characterized by the body's inability to use insulin, sometimes leads to a condition in which the pancreas stops making insulin altogether. The cells' resistance to insulin causes the pancreas to work harder, causing too much insulin in the system (a.k.a. hyperinsulinemia) until it just plumb tuckers out, as the saying goes. Your pancreas is making the insulin and knocking on the door, but the cells aren't answering. Your pancreas will eventually say, "Okay, fine! I'll shut down production, since you obviously aren't using what I'm making." But this isn't always the reason that you need insulin.

Often the problem is that your body becomes increasingly more resistant to the insulin your pancreas is producing. This is sometimes exacerbated by medications or by the progression of the disease over time. Controlling your blood sugar becomes harder and harder until, ultimately, you need to inject insulin.

You may also require insulin if you go for long periods with high blood sugar levels. In this case, the high blood sugar can put you at very high risk for other health complications, discussed in Part 3. It is not unusual to be diagnosed with Type 2 diabetes in a later stage and prescribed insulin.

CONDITIONS THAT CAN LEAD TO TYPE 2 DIABETES

There are a variety of risk factors for Type 2 diabetes, such as high cholesterol, or obesity, which I discuss in Chapter 10. The following conditions, however, are said to be definite precursors to Type 2 diabetes, meaning that if you have any of the following conditions, you are at very high risk of developing Type 2 diabetes.

Impaired Glucose Tolerance (IGT)

Prior to September 1998, many people with Type 2 diabetes were told they had *impaired glucose tolerance* (IGT), which was more widely known as "borderline diabetes." For the record, there is no such thing as borderline diabetes. But in light of new guidelines announced in 1998, many people once diagnosed with IGT will now be diagnosed with diabetes.

IGT was what many doctors referred to as the "grey zone" between normal blood sugar levels and "full-blown diabetes." Normal fasting blood sugar levels (what they are before you've eaten) are between 4 and 6 millimoles per litre (mmol/L). In the past, three fasting blood glucose levels between 5 mmol/L and 7.8 mmol/L meant that you had IGT. A fasting blood glucose level over 7.8 mmol/L or a random (any time of day) blood glucose level greater than 11.1 mmol/L meant that you had diabetes.

But that's all changed. Today, anyone with symptoms of diabetes, and with one fasting blood sugar level higher than 7.0 mmol/L, is considered to have diabetes and is officially diagnosed with Type 2 diabetes. People with no symptoms, who have a fasting blood sugar level greater than 7.0 mmol/L on two occasions, are also considered to have diabetes.

A new term, *impaired fasting glucose* (IFG), has also been introduced, which refers to blood glucose levels between 6.1 and 6.9 mmol/L. The term IGT is now used only when describing people who have a blood glucose level between 7. 8 and 11.1 *two hours after an oral glucose tolerance test.* Take a look at Table 1.1, "What Your Readings Mean," for more details.

It's also possible to have abnormally low blood glucose levels, which is called *hypoglycemia* (discussed in Chapter 14).

TABLE 1.1

What Your Readings Mean

Prior to September 1998, what constituted diabetes, impaired glucose tolerance (IGT) or normal blood sugar?

	Normal	IGT	Diabetes
Fasting	<7.8	<7.8	>7.8
Two hours after meals	<7.8	7.8–<11.1	≥11.1

Today, new guidelines stipulate the following:

	Normal	IFG	Diabetes
Fasting	<6.1 mmol/L	>6.1 mmol/L–<7.0 mmol/L	>7.0

Two hours after an oral glucose tolerance test

Normal	IGT	Diabetes
7.8 mmol/L >7.8 mmol/L–<11.1mmol/L		11.1 mmol/L

IFG = impaired fasting glucose

IGT = impaired glucose tolerance, referring to test results two hours after an oral glucose tolerance test

> = greater than / < = less than

Source: Canadian Medical Association Journal 1998; 159(8 Suppl): S12.

Syndrome X

Also known as the Metabolic Syndrome, the term "Syndrome X" was coined by Dr. Gerald Reaven, professor of medicine at Stanford University. It describes a group of people with high blood insulin levels and an elevated risk of heart disease. This is indistinguishable from IGT, but Dr. Reaven insists that people with Syndrome X do not generally develop full-blown Type 2 diabetes. The problem here is that the high insulin levels can still predispose you to risk factors for cardiovascular problems. Dr. Reaven's research showed that a high-carbohydrate diet could raise Syndrome X sufferers' insulin levels even more, as well as their risk of heart disease. People with Syndrome X tend to have higher "bad cholesterol" levels, as well as a reduced ability to break up blood clots. High blood pressure is also seen in people with Syndrome X. The myth about Syndrome X is that it causes obesity, which Reaven states is untrue.

Nonetheless, Syndrome X has now fuelled a whole industry of diet books, promoting low or no-carbohydrate diets (see Chapter 6). The best dietary advice if you have Syndrome X is to limit your carbohydrates to 45 percent of calories (Health Canada recommends 55 percent). On a 2,000-calorie diet, this would be roughly 225 g of carbohydrates per day. For more information on meal planning, see Chapter 6.

Gestational Diabetes Mellitus (GDM)

Gestational diabetes refers to diabetes that is first diagnosed during the 24th to 28th week of pregnancy. If you developed (or will develop) gestational diabetes during pregnancy, consider yourself put on alert. Approximately 20 percent of all women with gestational diabetes develop Type 2, presuming no other risk factors. If you are genetically predisposed to Type 2 diabetes, a history of gestational diabetes can raise your risk of eventually developing the disease. Gestational diabetes develops more often in women who were overweight prior to pregnancy, and women who are over 35; gestational diabetes increases with maternal age. If your mother had gestational diabetes, you are also more likely to develop it. For a more detailed discussion, see Chapter 11.

If you had diabetes prior to your pregnancy (Type 1 or Type 2), this is known in the medical literature as *pre-existing diabetes*, which is a completely different story and not at all the same thing as gestational diabetes.

Pancreatitis

Diabetes can be caused by a condition known as pancreatitis, which means inflammation of the pancreas. This occurs when the pancreas's digestive enzymes turn on you and attack your own pancreas. This can cause the gland to bleed, as well as serious tissue damage, infection and cysts. (Other organs, such as your heart, lungs and kidneys, could be affected in severe cases.) Pancreatitis is most often chronic, as opposed to acute (sudden), caused by years of alcohol abuse. In fact, 90 percent of all chronic pancreatitis affects men between 30 and 40 years of age. In rare cases, chronic pancreatitis is inherited, but experts are not sure why this is. People with chronic pancreatitis tend to have three main symptoms: pain, weight loss (due to poor food absorption and digestion), as well as diabetes (the type depends on how much damage was done to your islet or insulin-producing cells).

The treatment is to first stop drinking. Then you will need to be managed like any other diabetes patient: blood glucose monitoring, meal planning and possibly insulin injections.

Side-Effect Diabetes

This is a term I've coined to describe what's known as "secondary diabetes." This occurs when your diabetes is a *side effect* of a particular drug or surgical procedure.

A number of prescription medications, including steroids or Dilantin, can raise your blood sugar levels, which would affect the outcome of a blood sugar test, for example. Make sure you tell your doctor about all medications you're on prior to having your blood sugar checked.

If you've had your pancreas removed (a pancreatectomy), diabetes will definitely develop. It may also develop if you've experienced severe injury to your pancreas, liver disease or iron overload.

As you can see, this is a complicated disease to understand, and a disease that has gone through many name changes in recent years, making things even more confusing. By now, you should have a good understanding of what Type 2 diabetes is and how it is different from other types of diabetes you may have heard about. The next chapter is about who is most likely to develop Type 2 diabetes. The good news is that some lifestyle changes can reduce risk.

Chapter 2

WHO GETS TYPE 2 DIABETES?

● ● ● ● ● ● ● ● ● ●

Screening studies show that Type 2 diabetes is prevalent all over the world, particularly in countries that are becoming Westernized. Type 2 diabetes is increasing in the developed world at an annual rate of about 6 percent, while the number of people with Type 2 diabetes doubles every 15 years. Roughly 6 percent of all Caucasian adults have Type 2 diabetes, but the disease affects African-North Americans at a rate of 12 to 15 percent, Hispanics at a rate of 20 percent and Aboriginal-North Americans at a rate exceeding 30 percent. In some Aboriginal communities, up to 70 percent of adults have Type 2 diabetes. This is why I've devoted a separate chapter to this population.

Many people won't realize they have Type 2 diabetes until they develop a complication of Type 2 diabetes, such as eye problems, nerve problems, cardio-vascular disease or peripheral vascular disease—all discussed in Part 3. People with Type 2 diabetes are four times more likely to develop heart disease and five times more likely to suffer a stroke than people without Type 2 diabetes.

If you consume a diet higher in fat than carbohydrates, and low in fibre, you increase your risk for Type 2 diabetes if you are genetically predisposed to the disease. If you weigh at least 20 percent more than you should for your height and age (the definition of "obese"), are sedentary and are over the age of 45, you are considered at high risk for Type 2 diabetes. Your risk further increases if you

- are of Aboriginal descent (this is true for Aboriginal peoples all over the world, from Australia to North America; in Canada, First Nations people are at highest risk; in the United States, the Pima Indians are at highest risk)
- are of African or Hispanic descent

- have a family history of Type 2 diabetes
- are obese and female (73 percent of all women with diabetes are obese)
- are pregnant (one in 20 women will develop gestational diabetes by the third trimester; this number increases with age, while gestational diabetes can predispose you to Type 2 diabetes later in life)

Several cofactors contribute to your risk profile and can change your risk from higher to lower. The purpose of this chapter is to give you a clear idea of where you fit into this risk puzzle. That way, you'll be more aware of early warning signs of the disease, which will make it easier for you to get an accurate diagnosis. If you've already been diagnosed with Type 2 diabetes, this chapter will help you understand *why* you developed the disease, and what you can do today to eliminate some of the factors that may be aggravating your condition.

RISK FACTORS YOU CAN CHANGE

Type 2 diabetes more than meets the requirements of an epidemic. In 1985, the World Health Organization (WHO) estimated that roughly 30 million people globally had Type 2 diabetes. By 1993, that number jumped to 98.9 million people, and it's estimated that 250 million people worldwide will have Type 2 diabetes by 2020.

As mentioned earlier, one in four Canadians over the age of 45 will be diagnosed with diabetes by 2004. And, unless more people modify their risk factors, that number is likely to increase by the year 2020.

Thirty-two percent of people with at least three of the risk factors can *double* their risk of developing Type 2 diabetes, while 89 percent of people with the disease have at least one *modifiable* risk factor. That means you can lower your risk of developing diabetes by changing your lifestyle or diet.

Calculating your risk of getting a particular disease is a very tricky business. To simplify matters, I've divided this chapter into two sections: modifiable risk factors—risk factors you can change; and risk markers—risk factors you cannot change, such as your age or genes. It's also crucial to understand that risk estimates are only guesses that are not based on you personally, but on people *like* you, who share your physical characteristics or lifestyle patterns. It's like betting on a horse. You look at the age of the horse, its vigour and shape, its breeding, its training, and where the race is being run. Then you come up with odds. If you own the horse, you can't change your horse's colour or breeding, but you can change its training, its diet, its jockey and, ultimately, where it's being raced, when and how often. Chance, of course, plays a role in horse racing. You can't control acts of God. But you can decide whether you're going to tempt fate by racing your horse during a thunderstorm.

The following are modifiable risk factors. You can remove the risk if you make the change.

High Cholesterol

Cholesterol is a whitish, waxy fat made in vast quantities by the liver. It is also known as a lipid, the umbrella name for the many different fats found in the body. That's why liver or other organ meats are high in cholesterol! Cholesterol is needed to make hormones as well as cell membranes. Dietary cholesterol is found only in foods from animals and fish. The daily maximum amount of dietary cholesterol recommended by Health Canada is 300 mg. If you have high cholesterol, the excess cholesterol in your blood can lead to narrowed arteries, which in turn can lead to a heart attack. Saturated fat, discussed in detail in Chapter 7, is often a culprit when it comes to high cholesterol, but the highest levels of cholesterol are due to a genetic defect in the liver. Since people with diabetes are four times more likely to develop heart disease and five times more likely to suffer a stroke, lowering your cholesterol, especially if you're already at risk for Type 2 diabetes, is a good idea.

Insulin's role in "fat control"

Insulin not only keeps blood sugar in check, it also keeps the levels of "good" cholesterol (HDL—high-density lipoproteins), "bad" cholesterol (LDL—low-density lipoproteins) and triglycerides in check. When you're not making enough insulin or your body isn't using insulin efficiently, your LDL levels and your triglycerides rise, but more important, *your HDL levels fall,* which can lead to heart disease. When diabetes is in control, cholesterol levels will return to normal, which will cut your risk of heart disease and stroke as well.

Checking your cholesterol

In Canada, total blood cholesterol levels are measured in millimoles per litre. If you're over 30, cholesterol levels of less than 5.2 mmol/L is considered healthy. If your cholesterol levels are between 5.2 and 6.2 mmol/L, discuss with your doctor lifestyle changes that can lower cholesterol levels. If your levels are greater than 6.2 mmol/L, your doctor may recommend cholesterol-lowering drugs if your lifestyle changes were not successful.

For people 18 to 29 years of age, a cholesterol level less than 4.7 mmol/L is considered healthy, while a level ranging between 4.7 and 5.7 mmol/L is considered too high, warranting some lifestyle and dietary changes. In this age group, a reading greater than 5.7 may even warrant cholesterol-lowering drugs. High cholesterol is also called hypercholesterolemia. Another term used in conjunction with high cholesterol is hyperlipidemia, which refers to an elevation of lipids (fats) in the bloodstream; lipids include cholesterol and triglycerides (the most common form of fat from food sources in our bodies). For adults, a triglyceride level of less than 2.3 mmol/L is considered healthy.

Total blood cholesterol levels are guidelines only. You also have to look at the relative proportion of high-density lipoprotein (HDL) or "good cholesterol" to low-density lipoprotein (LDL) level or "bad cholesterol" in the blood. If you're over 30, an LDL reading of less than 3.4 mmol/L and an HDL reading of more than 0.9 mmol/L is considered healthy; if you're 18 to 29, an LDL reading of less than 3.0 mmol/L and an HDL reading of more than 0.9 is considered healthy.

Cholesterol-lowering drugs

For many, losing weight and modifying fat intake simply aren't enough to bring cholesterol levels down to optimal levels. You may be a candidate for one of the numerous cholesterol-lowering drugs. These medications, when combined with a low-fat, low-cholesterol diet, target the intestine, blocking food absorption, and/or the liver, where they interfere with the processing of cholesterol. These are strong drugs, however, and ought to be a last resort after really giving a low-fat, low-cholesterol diet a chance. You might be given a combination of cholesterol-lowering medications to try with a low-cholesterol diet. It's important to ask about all side effects accompanying your medication because they can include gastrointestinal problems, allergic reactions, blood disorders and depression. One study looking at male patients taking cholesterol-lowering drugs found an unusually high rate of suicide and accidental trauma. There have not been enough studies on women taking these drugs to know for certain how they interact with women's health conditions. At any rate, here's what's available as of this writing. Please note only the generic drug names are listed.

- **Niacin:** When taken properly, niacin is the best cholesterol treatment available. In 1986 the Coronary Drug Project (a National Institute of Health Study) found that prolonged use of niacin significantly reduced mortality rates among heart attack victims. It has since become one of the most popular cholesterol-lowering drugs on the market. Niacin, a water-soluble B vitamin, can lower LDL by 30 percent and triglyceride levels by as much as 55 percent. It also increases HDL by about 35 percent. Also known as nicotinic acid, niacin must be taken in large doses (1–3 mg/day) in order to be effective. Because the dosage is up to 76 times higher than the recommended daily allowance, side effects are common. Many patients experience itching, flushing and panic attacks. Switching to slow-release capsules, taking an aspirin 30 minutes before taking the medication, or taking it on a full stomach might help alleviate some of these symptoms. Niacin can aggravate both stomach ulcers and diabetes.

• **Statins:** Statins, such as lovastatin, hinder the liver's ability to produce cholesterol, keeping LDL levels to a minimum while increasing levels of HDL. When combined with the proper diet, statins can reduce your risk of death from heart disease by as much as 40 percent. However, certain statins have been known to cause liver damage, muscle pain and weakness. The official drug category for statins is 3-Hydroxy-3-Methylgluteryl-CoA Reductase Inhibitors. In Canada, altorvastatin, fluvastatin, lovastatin, prevastatin and simvastatin are available. Please note that cerivastatin was taken off the market in 2001.

• **Resins:** Technically called bile acid sequestrants, such as cholestyramine, these drugs help the body eliminate cholesterol through the gut. It is considered the safest of cholesterol-lowering drugs; it has also been around the longest. A National Institute of Health study in the early 1980s demonstrated that cholestyramine decreases heart attack deaths by lowering cholesterol levels. In fact, for each 1 percent drop in the cholesterol levels of participants, there was a 2 percent drop in death rates, which is pretty impressive when you consider that the average decline in blood cholesterol was 25 percent. Although cholestyramine reduces LDL or bad cholesterol, it can sometimes raise triglyceride levels. It can also trigger a host of side effects, the most unpleasant of which is *really bad* gas. Cholestyramine interferes with the effectiveness of digitalis, diuretics, warfarin, fat-soluble vitamins and beta-blockers. It can also lead to gallstones. Cholestyramine should be taken in the morning and at bedtime.

• **Fibrates (gemfibrozil, fenofibrate, clofibrate, bezafibrate):** These lower cholesterol and triglyceride levels in the blood. In a Finnish study, the rate of coronary artery disease among 4,000 men with high cholesterol dropped 34 percent.

- **Probucol:** Probucol can cut your LDL by as much as 15 percent, but it also lowers your HDL, or "good" cholesterol. Lately probucol has been generating new interest among doctors because it is also a powerful antioxidant. LDL creates arterial plaque through a change in its molecular makeup. This "change" is called oxidation, and an antioxidant like probucol can help to prevent it from happening.
- **Arginine:** Preliminary studies suggest that this amino acid may lower cholesterol levels and improve coronary blood flow by acting as an antioxidant and maintaining elasticity in blood vessel tissues. Arginine is currently available without a prescription.
- **Coenzyme Q10:** Japanese and European practitioners love this powerful antioxidant, but more studies are needed to prove its reputed effect on arterial plaque.

Hypertension (High Blood Pressure)

About 12 percent of Canadian adults suffer from hypertension, or high blood pressure. What is blood pressure? The blood flows from the heart into the arteries (blood vessels), pressing against the artery walls. The simplest way to explain this is to think about a liquid-soap dispenser. When you want soap, you need to pump it out by pressing down on the little dispenser pump, the "heart" of the dispenser. The liquid soap is the "blood" and the little tube, through which the soap flows, is the "artery." The pressure that's exerted on the wall of the tube is therefore the "blood pressure."

When the tube is hollow and clean, you needn't pump very hard to get the soap; it comes out easily. But when the tubing in your dispenser gets narrower as a result of old, hardened, gunky liquid soap blocking the tube, you have to pump much harder to get any soap, while the force the soap exerts against the tube is increased. Obviously, this is a simplistic explanation of a very complex problem, but essentially, the narrowing of the arteries forces your heart to work harder to pump the blood: high blood pressure. If this goes on too long, your heart muscle enlarges and becomes weaker, which can lead to a heart attack. Higher pressure can also weaken the walls of your blood vessels, which can cause a stroke.

The term "hypertension" refers to the tension or force exerted on your artery walls. (Hyper means "too much," as in "too much tension.") Blood pressure is measured in two readings: X over Y. The X is the systolic pressure, which is the pressure that occurs during the heart's contraction. The Y is the diastolic pressure, which is the pressure that occurs when the heart rests between contractions. In "liquid soap" terms, the systolic pressure occurs when you press the pump down; the diastolic pressure occurs when you release your hand from the pump and allow it to rise back to its "resting" position.

In the general population, target blood pressure readings are less than 130 over 85 (<130/85). Readings greater than 130/85 are considered by diabetes educators to be too high for people with diabetes, but in the general population, readings of 140/90 or higher are generally considered borderline, although for some people this is still considered a normal reading. For the general population, 140/90 is "lecture time," when your doctor will begin to counsel you about dietary and lifestyle habits. By 160/100, many people are prescribed a hypertensive drug, which is designed to lower blood pressure.

Let's examine some of the causes of hypertension. The same factors that put you at risk for Type 2 diabetes, such as obesity, can also put you at risk for hypertension. Hypertension is also exacerbated by tobacco and alcohol consumption and too much sodium or salt in the diet. (People of African descent tend to be more salt-sensitive.)

If high blood pressure runs in the family, you're considered at greater risk of developing hypertension. High blood pressure can also be caused by kidney disorders (which may be initially caused by diabetes) or pregnancy (known as pregnancy-induced hypertension). Medications are also common culprits. Estrogen-containing medications (such as oral contraceptives), non-steroidal anti-inflammatory drugs (NSAIDs)—such as ibuprofen, nasal decongestants, cold remedies, appetite suppressants, certain antidepressants and other drugs—can all increase blood pressure. Be sure to check with your pharmacist.

How to lower your blood pressure without drugs

- Change your diet and begin exercising (see discussion of obesity in Chapter 10).
- Limit alcohol consumption to no more than 60 mL (2 oz.) of liquor or 250 mL (8 oz.) of wine or 750 mL (24 oz.) of beer per day and even less for liver health.
- Limit your salt intake to about 7.5 mL (1 1/2 tsp.) per day by cutting out all foods high in sodium, such as canned soups, pickles, soy sauce and so on. Some canned soups contain 1,000 mg of sodium, for example. That's a lot!
- Increase your intake of calcium or dairy products and potassium (i.e., bananas). Some still-unproven studies suggest that people with hypertension are calcium- and potassium-deficient.
- Lower your stress levels. Studies show that by lowering your stress, your blood pressure decreases.

Blood pressure-lowering drugs

If you can't lower your blood pressure through lifestyle changes, you may be a candidate for some of the following blood-pressure–lowering drugs:

- **Diuretics:** Diuretics are the most commonly used blood pressure medication. Also known as water pills, diuretics work by flushing excess water and salt (often 1–2 kg/2–4 lb. worth!) out of your system. But diuretics may actually increase the risk of heart attack by leaching potassium salts needed by the heart, and the heart may respond to blocked nerve signals by trying harder and harder until it fails. Another common side effect of diuretic therapy is low potassium. Levels of potassium tend to drop when diuretics replace the low-fat diet you've worked so hard to maintain. If you make sure not to substitute one therapy for another, diuretics will not affect your potassium levels. Other side effects include increased blood sugar and cholesterol levels.
- **Beta-blockers:** Beta-blockers alter the way hormones like adrenaline control blood pressure. They slow the heart rate by decreasing the strength of its contractions. Beta-blockers are most often used by young people and/or people with coronary artery disease. Possible side effects include fatigue and an increase in blood sugar and cholesterol levels.
- **Centrally acting agents:** These drugs act through centres in the brain to slow the heart rate and relax the blood vessels. Possible side effects include stuffy nose, dry mouth and drowsiness.
- **Vasodilators:** Vasodilators dilate, or relax, the blood vessels, thereby reducing blood pressure.
- **Ace-inhibitors:** Ace-inhibitors lower blood pressure by preventing the formation of a hormone called angiotensin II, which causes the blood vessels to narrow. Ace-inhibitors are also used to treat heart failure. Possible side effects include a cough and swelling of the face and tongue.
- **Alpha-blocking agents:** Alpha-blocking agents block the effects of noradrenaline, a stress hormone, allowing the blood vessels to relax. Blood pressure decreases with treatment, as does cholesterol. You may also notice an increase in HDL, or "good" cholesterol. A possible side effect is blood pressure variation when standing versus reclining.
- **Calcium-channel blockers:** Calcium-channel blockers limit the amount of calcium entering the cells, allowing the muscles in the blood vessels to relax. Possible side effects include ankle swelling, flushing, constipation and indigestion.

Obesity

Many obese people say that they've "dieted themselves up" to their present weight. Obesity is the strongest risk factor for developing Type 2 diabetes. Basically, the longer you've been obese, the more you are at risk. I am not referring to people who need to lose weight for cosmetic reasons; I'm referring to people who weigh at least 20 percent more than their ideal weight for their age and height. If this describes you, don't panic. No one is asking you to lose *all* your weight, or any weight, at once. Instead of aiming to lose 5 kg (10 lb.), just aim for 2 (4 lb.). Even 2 kg (4 lb.) will allow your body to use insulin more effectively. For more on weight and Type 2 diabetes, see Chapter 2.

Sedentary Lifestyle

What's the definition of sedentary? *Not moving!* If you have a desk job or spend most of your time at a computer, in your car or watching television (even if it *is* PBS or CNN), you are a sedentary person. If you do roughly 20 minutes of exercise less than once a week, you're relatively sedentary. You need to incorporate some sort of movement into your daily schedule in order to be considered active. That movement can be anything: aerobic exercise, brisk walks around the block or walking your dog. If you lead a sedentary lifestyle and are obese, you are at significant risk of developing Type 2 diabetes in your 40s if you are genetically predisposed. If you are not obese, your risk is certainly lowered, but you are then predisposed to a number of other problems, particularly if you're female. Chapter 8 discusses exercise and Type 2 diabetes in detail.

Sleep Deprivation or Sleep Disorders

There are studies linking obesity, and hence Type 2 diabetes, to lack of sleep, snoring, loss of REM sleep and a range of other sleep disorders. When you don't sleep well or get enough sleep—particularly REM sleep (rapid eye movement, which occurs in deep sleep)—you will be irritable and drowsy during the day. That means you'll eat more and will likely crave fast-energy foods high in sugar or starch. By visiting a sleep-disorder clinic or, in some cases, by going to a time-management seminar, you should be able to get your ZZZs.

Smoking

Smoking and diabetes is a toxic combination. You already know that smoking leads to heart attacks. But what you might not know is that if you have Type 2 diabetes and do not smoke, you are *already* four times more likely to have a heart attack than a person without diabetes. If you smoke *and* have Type 2 diabetes, you have an even greater risk of having a heart attack than non-smokers without diabetes.

Smoking and obesity

Smoking and obesity often coexist. Women, in particular, begin to smoke in their teens as a way to lose weight. A 1997 study done by the Department of Psychology and Preventive Medicine at the University of Memphis in Tennessee shows that this approach doesn't work. Smoking teens are just as likely to become obese over time as non-smokers. Ironically, it was found that the more a person weighed, the more cigarettes he or she smoked. In the long run, smokers often wound up weighing more than non-smokers because they substituted food for nicotine when they quit or attempted to quit.

Smoking-cessation programs

Not everyone can quit smoking "cold turkey," although it's a strategy that many have used successfully. (Some "cold turkey" quitters report that keeping one package of cigarettes within reach reduces anxiety.) The symptoms of nicotine withdrawal begin within a few hours and peak at 24 to 48 hours after quitting. You may experience anxiety, irritability, hostility, restlessness, insomnia and anger. For these reasons, many smokers turn to smoking-cessation programs, which can include some of the following:

- **Herbal and homeopathic smoking-cessation aids:** There are many herbal and homeopathic smoking-cessation products available. Some use plant sources to reduce cravings; some work by using natural substances to help you "detox." For all the many natural smoking-cessation products available in Canada, contact Canada's leading natural pharmacy, Smith's Pharmacy at 1-800-361-6624 or visit www.smithspharmacy.com.
- **Behavioural counselling:** Behavioural counselling, either group or individual, can raise the rate of abstinence to 20 to 25 percent. This approach to smoking cessation aims to change the mental processes of smoking, reinforce the benefits of non-smoking and teach skills to help the smoker avoid the urge to smoke.
- **Nicotine gum:** Nicotine (Nicorette) gum is now available over the counter. It helps you quit smoking by reducing nicotine cravings and withdrawal symptoms. Nicotine gum helps you wean yourself from nicotine by allowing

you to gradually decrease the dosage until you stop using it altogether, a process that usually takes about 12 weeks. The only disadvantage with this method is that it caters to the oral and addictive aspects of smoking (i.e., rewarding the "urge" to smoke with a dose of nicotine).

- **Nicotine patch:** Transdermal nicotine or the "patch" (Habitrol, Nicoderm, Nicotrol) doubles abstinence rates. Most brands are now available over the counter. Each morning, a new patch is applied to a different area of dry, clean, hairless skin and left on for the day. Some patches are designed to be worn a full 24 hours. However, the constant supply of nicotine to the bloodstream sometimes causes very vivid or disturbing dreams. You can also expect to feel a mild itching, burning or tingling at the site of the patch when it is first applied. The nicotine patch works best when it is worn for at least seven to twelve weeks, with a gradual decrease in strength (i.e., nicotine). Many smokers find it effective because it allows them to tackle the psychological addiction to smoking before they are forced to deal with physical symptoms of withdrawal.

- **Nicotine inhaler:** The nicotine inhaler (Nicotrol Inhaler) delivers nicotine orally via inhalation from a plastic tube. Its success rate is about 28 percent, similar to that of nicotine gum. It's available by prescription only in the United States and has yet to make its debut in Canada. Like nicotine gum, the inhaler mimics smoking behaviour by responding to each craving or "urge" to smoke, a feature that has both advantages and disadvantages to the smoker who wants to get over the physical symptoms of withdrawal. The nicotine inhaler should be used for a period of 12 weeks.

- **Nicotine nasal spray:** Like nicotine gum and the nicotine patch, the nasal spray reduces craving and withdrawal symptoms, allowing smokers to cut back gradually. One squirt delivers about 1 mg of nicotine. In three clinical trials involving 730 patients, 31 to 35 percent were not smoking at six months. This compares to an average of 12 to 15 percent of smokers who were able to quit unaided. The nasal spray has a couple of advantages over the gum and the patch: Nicotine is rapidly absorbed across the nasal membranes, providing a kick that is more like the real thing, and the prompt onset of action, plus a flexible dosing schedule, benefits heavier smokers. Because the nicotine reaches your bloodstream so quickly, nasal sprays do have a greater potential for addiction than the slower-acting gum and patch. Nasal sprays are not yet available for use in Canada.

- **Alternative therapies:** Hypnosis, meditation and acupuncture have helped some smokers quit. In the case of hypnosis and meditation, sessions may be private or part of a group smoking-cessation program.

Smoking-cessation drugs

The drug bupropion (Zyban) is now available and is an option for people who have been unsuccessful using nicotine replacement. Formerly prescribed as an antidepressant, bupropion was "discovered" by accident: Researchers knew that quitting smokers were often depressed, so they began experimenting with the drug as a means to fight depression, not addiction, but found that it worked for both conditions. Bupropion reduces the withdrawal symptoms associated with smoking cessation and can be used in conjunction with nicotine-replacement therapy. Researchers suspect that bupropion works directly in the brain to disrupt the addictive power of nicotine by affecting the same chemical neurotransmitters (or "messengers") in the brain, such as dopamine, that nicotine does.

The pleasurable aspect of addictive drugs like nicotine and cocaine is triggered by the release of dopamine. Smoking floods the brain with dopamine. *The New England Journal of Medicine* published the results of a study of more than 600 smokers taking bupropion. At the end of treatment, 44 percent of those who took the highest dose of the drug (300 mg) were not smoking, compared to 19 percent of the group who took a placebo. By the end of one year, 23 percent of the 300 mg group and 12 percent of the placebo group were still smoke-free. Using Zyban *with* nicotine-replacement therapy seems to improve the quit rate a bit further. Four-week quit rates from the study were 23 percent for placebo; 36 percent for the patch; 49 percent for Zyban; and 58 percent for the combination of Zyban and the patch.

Vitamin Deficiency

Blood samples from people with diabetes show a tendency toward "oxidative stress," meaning that people with diabetes tend to be antioxidant-deficient. Antioxidants are vitamins found in coloured (i.e., non-green) fruits and vegetables, discussed in more detail in Chapter 7.

Many people make the mistake of cutting out nutrients along with the fat in their diets. Experts recommend that to meet all vitamin needs through food alone, you need 1,200 calories per day if you're female and 1,500 calories per day if you're male (unless you need more or fewer vitamins due to a medical condition). Studies reveal that when diets fall to 1,000 calories, these vitamins dropped to approximately 60 percent of their recommended levels. This is where vitamin supplements, meal-replacement drinks or health bars come in. They're designed to give you your daily requirement of vitamins and minerals. If you're on a low-fat diet, make sure that you're not cutting out all protein, calcium or carbohydrates. You do need some of these! (See Chapter 6.)

Studies also show that approximately 25 percent of North Americans skip breakfast, while an additional 38 percent skip lunch. Eating breakfast will help you to lower your fat intake because a small meal in the morning reduces that impulsive snacking in the late afternoon and actually improves your nutrient absorption.

Age can also interfere with vitamin intake. Research shows that seniors (over 65) tend to be deficient in vitamins A, C, D, protein and calcium. Yet these nutrients can boost the immune system and improve bone density, cardiovascular health and a thousand other things.

RISK FACTORS YOU CAN'T CHANGE

By *modifying* any of the modifiable risk factors above, you can help to offset your risk of developing Type 2 diabetes if you have any of the following risk markers. While you can't change your genetic makeup, medical history or age, you can significantly reduce the odds of these factors predisposing you to Type 2 diabetes.

Age

The risk of developing Type 2 diabetes increases with age. Perhaps at no other time in history have we seen so many people over age 45—the so-called baby boom generation. This may, in part, account for the increase we're seeing in Type 2 diabetes, as well as other age-related diseases. However, the lifestyle and dietary habits you practise before age 45 count—either against you or for you. So, by changing your diet and becoming more active before age 45, you may not necessarily be able to prevent your genetic fate, but you may certainly be able to delay it. And in the event that you develop Type 2 diabetes, a healthy diet and active lifestyle will go a long way in controlling the disease.

It's crucial to keep in mind that studies regarding diet, lifestyle and Type 2 diabetes are still unclear, although experts certainly agree that there is a strong relationship between genetic markers for diabetes and environmental factors, such as activity levels, weight and diet.

Menopause

When women reach menopause, estrogen loss can lead to some well-documented problems, such as osteoporosis (estrogen helps to maintain calcium levels) and heart disease (estrogen raises HDL levels, or "good" cholesterol, which protects premenopausal women from heart disease). Estrogen also helps to protect against insulin resistance. Even if you decide against hormone replacement therapy, diet and lifestyle changes can lower your risks of heart disease, osteoporosis and Type 2 diabetes substantially. See Chapter 12 for more details.

Genes

Most diabetes experts believe that Type 2 diabetes is a genetic disease, which means you have the "wiring" installed for Type 2 diabetes at birth. Fortunately, we do understand some of the outside factors that can trip the Type 2 switch. Body shapes, diet and activity levels are strong switch-trippers. On the other hand, if you don't have any Type 2 diabetes genes (in other words, you're not "wired" for this disease), these outside factors cannot, by themselves, cause you to develop Type 2 diabetes. For instance, there are plenty of obese and sedentary people walking around who do not have Type 2 diabetes, nor will they develop the disease in the future.

When underdeveloped populations become urbanized and adopt a Western lifestyle, there is an explosion in Type 2 diabetes. But the genes must be present in order to "allow" for the disease in the first place. This is more proof that there is a genetic-environmental combo platter at work when it comes to this disease. What aspect of Westernization triggers Type 2 diabetes in these regions? "Western" means many things, including a higher-fat diet, less physical activity, as well as access to medical care, which means populations are living longer.

And what role does earlier screening and better detection of Type 2 diabetes play in the global increase of the disease? As one doctor put it to me, "When you don't look for it, you don't find it." More and more evidence points to the fact that Type 2 diabetes has been around for a long time.

What are the odds?

Type 2 diabetes is caused by multiple factors. The odds of developing it have to do with some genes interacting with some environmental factors. Obesity, excess calories, deficient calorie expenditure and aging can all lead to a resistance to insulin. If you remove the environmental risks, however, you can probably modify the risk of Type 2 diabetes.

Your ethnic background

As discussed earlier, Aboriginal cultures develop Type 2 diabetes at far higher rates than other Canadians. On some reserves, Type 2 diabetes is present in 70 percent of the adult population. Approximately 15 percent of African-North American adults have Type 2 diabetes, while about 20 percent of all Hispanic-North Americans have Type 2 diabetes.

The "thrifty gene" is so named because it is believed to have evolved out of biological efficiency, or thriftiness. It is thought to be responsible for the higher rates of Type 2 diabetes in the Aboriginal and African-North American populations. This means that the more recently your culture has lived indigenously or nomadically (that is, living off the land you came from and eating seasonally), the more efficient your metabolism is. Unfortunately, it is also more sensitive to nutrient excess. If you're an Aboriginal North American, only about 100 years have passed since your ancestors lived indigenously. This is an exceedingly short amount of time to ask thousands of years of hunter-gatherer genes to adjust to a Western diet. If you're African-North American, your ancestors did not live here any longer than about 400 years; prior to that, they were living a tribal, nomadic lifestyle. Again, 400 years is *not* a long time.

As for Hispanic populations or other immigrant populations, many come from families who have spent generations in poverty. Their metabolisms adjusted to long periods of famine and are often overloaded by Western foods. The other problem is poverty in North America. Aboriginal, African and Hispanic populations tend to have much lower incomes and are therefore eating lower-quality food, which, when introduced to the "thrifty gene," can trigger Type 2 diabetes.

Type 2 diabetes seems to occur in South-East Asian populations at Western rates even when the diet is Eastern. East Indians, in particular, have very high rates of heart disease. In fact, India has the largest Type 2 population in the world. Urbanization is cited as a major factor.

Your risk of developing Type 2 diabetes depends on your mix of genes and your current and past lifestyle and diet. If you are part Aboriginal and part European, for example, you will probably need to be more conscientious about your diet than if you were part Asian and part European. Studying your family tree and family history of Type 2 diabetes is the best way to assess the "damage" and make the necessary changes in your own diet and lifestyle to repair it.

Other Medical Conditions

There are certain diseases such as Prader-Willi, Down's syndrome, Turner's syndrome, Cushing's disease or acromegaly (large face, long arms and hands) that can lead to diabetes in the long term. In this case, diabetes is a presenting feature of the disorder. Many diseases run together and this is another example of that.

SIGNS AND SYMPTOMS

These are the signs of Type 2 diabetes:

- Weight gain. When you're not using your insulin properly, you may suffer from excess insulin, which can increase your appetite. This is a classic Type 2 symptom.
- Blurred vision or any change in sight.
- Drowsiness or *extreme* fatigue at times when you shouldn't be drowsy or tired.
- Frequent infections that are slow to heal. (Women should be on alert for recurring vaginal yeast infections.)
- Tingling or numbness in the hands and feet.
- Gum disease. High blood sugar affects the blood vessels in your mouth, causing inflamed gums; the sugar content can get into your saliva, causing cavities in your teeth.

YOUR CHILD'S RISK OF TYPE 2

In recent years, there has been an alarming increase in Type 2 diabetes among children, teens and young adults. This is due to our environment: television, video, computers and more sedentary activities, combined with high-fat snacks, fast food and higher rates of obesity in children. Type 2 diabetes is highest among Aboriginal children. In the Sioux Lookout region, since 1994, the rate of Type 2 diabetes in children aged seven to fifteen more than doubled per 1,000 individuals.

As discussed earlier, Type 2 diabetes is believed by most diabetes experts to be a genetic disease. But, as mentioned, there are many outside factors that can "trip" the switch. The most influential factors are eating habits and lack of physical activity, which, thankfully, can be modified.

If one parent has developed Type 2 diabetes under age 30, your child has a 50 percent chance of developing it, too.

Breast-feed Your Baby

Breast-feed your baby. And do so for as long as possible. Lots and lots of studies say breast-fed children are healthier and have fewer diseases (including obesity-related diseases) than formula-fed babies. Breast milk is perfectly balanced to satiate your baby; the "foremilk" is more watery, while the "hindmilk" is creamier and fattier—the perfect meal for someone with no teeth. (And breast milk is more watery in hot climates for hydration, and creamier in cold climates for calories!)

A recent study concludes that nutrition is most important in infancy and adolescence. For example, the amount of salt in a newborn's diet could affect blood pressure later in life. The formula Similac contains 27 mg of sodium per 140 mL (5-oz.) serving, which is too high for a baby!

Feed Your Children a Varied Diet

Why is your toddler eating toys, mud and crayons? Because that toddler is communicating that he or she needs a *variety* of foods. And, fortunately, because we're not living in war or famine, we can give this to our children. Introduce a wide variety of "normal" foods (all colours of vegetables and fruits; whole grains, pastas and so on). Without a varied diet, a child will not consume the vitamins and minerals he or she needs. The lack of a varied diet could also lead to obesity in childhood, as the child loads up on carbohydrates, fat and junk foods.

Teach Your Children Good Eating Habits

You can't change your child's genes, but you can help to offset the genetic tendency toward Type 2 diabetes by teaching your child good habits early. Since you control much of your child's diet and environment, you can make sure that you lower these odds.

For example, in young children, try to limit what I call the Sugar Shows— television programming for children that is basically a vehicle to sell sugar cereals and junk food. Some foods aimed at children contain as much as 22 g of fat and 1,500 mg of sodium. (Add in the pudding cup and you can well imagine the damage!) And selling pies and cakes as "breakfast foods" to children raises some ethical questions as well.

Instead, play that Disney video again or limit programs to "safe channels." Some of the worst damage is done through children's shows run by commercial networks. You can also practise fast-food control by ordering some of the healthier foods for your kids (you know what they are) when they're begging for a burger or chicken fingers. Try to resist fat-in-a-box meals that boast enough grease to kill your whole family, *plus* a free chocolate layer cake when you buy two!

Everything your child eats today counts in adulthood. Research shows that even infant eating patterns can lead to obesity years later. One famous baboon study found that baboons overfed early in life became obese later on. This didn't happen with baboons who were fed a normal diet in infancy.

Stop Parenting with Food

Many bad habits begin with parents forcing children to finish food when they say they're full. We all start with biological mechanisms that tell us when we're hungry or full. But if we hear things like "Clean your plate" when we say, "But I'm full, Mom," and worse, "Good girl/boy" when we do cram that last bit of food in to "please," we *wreck* those biological signals designed to stop us from becoming obese. In essence, you're teaching your child not to follow natural instincts about food and eating. When your child is hungry, she or he will eat. If a food isn't palatable, unless your child is living in war or famine, don't force the food on your child. And *never* punish a child by withholding food or, worse, *rewarding* a child with dessert. By saying, "No chocolate until you finish your carrots," you're programming your child to feel *emotional* rewards when he or she eats that chocolate. In other words, both these parenting methods (which we learned from *our* parents) are recipes for eating disorders, chronic dieting or obesity down the road.

FINDING DIABETES EARLIER

Perhaps the most important change in the future of diabetes is revising the Clinical Practice Guidelines for Diabetes. This means that doctors will need to change the way they manage and treat diabetes. For example, the new guidelines may require that all health care providers do the following:

- Routinely screen for Type 2 diabetes in high-risk individuals (see Chapter 2). This means screening based on risk factors instead of symptoms.
- Provide prevention education to anyone at high risk for Type 2 diabetes. This means you'll be sent on a diabetes education course, even if you don't have the disease.
- Encourage people with Type 2 diabetes to self-monitor their blood sugar levels, if data proves this is useful.
- Not prescribe medication to people with Type 2 diabetes unless meal planning and lifestyle modification has been tried first and has not worked.

- Revisit who should use insulin and who can avoid it, and not prescribe insulin with pills.
- Prevent, at all costs, complications by making sure that Type 2 diabetes patients understand how to change their diet and lifestyle.
- Lobby to make more diabetes educators and special care centres available across Canada.
- Be alert to which medications can affect our insulin levels (see the box "Know Your Drugs" in Chapter 4).

Having Type 2 diabetes is a 24-hour, 7-day-a-week job. Despite this, 70 percent of people with Type 2 diabetes never receive any diabetes education whatsoever. Even when diabetes education is made available, educating people about diabetes will just get more challenging in the future, since increasingly many Canadians do not speak English as their first language or come from completely different cultures. Clearly diabetes is taking its toll on our health care system. Experts predict that as more people age and are diagnosed with Type 2 diabetes, less education will be available as doctors and diabetes educators become overburdened with patients.

The next chapter focuses on how to maximize your relationships with all your health care providers. Developing a good relationship with your doctor means *helping your doctor help you*! Actively managing your diabetes involves keeping health logs; choosing the right doctor to begin with; knowing the right questions to ask your doctors, educators and pharmacists; and avoiding duplication of efforts.

Chapter 3

YOUR DIABETES HEALTH CARE TEAM

• • • • • • • • • •

Diabetes is a major problem for the North American health care system. In the United States, for example, 14 percent of all health care dollars is spent on managing Type 2 diabetes. Canada reports similar statistics. As a result, there is really no such thing as one "diabetes doctor" who manages the disease completely. Your primary care physician often acts as overall supervisor of your condition, but ideally, this doctor should be working with a team of health care professionals, which includes the following:

- **A certified diabetes educator (CDE):** CDEs come from a variety of back-grounds. They can be dietitians, nurses, physicians or social workers; each of these professionals must write a CDE exam in Canada and practise within the scope of his or her own discipline and relevant legislation. CDEs are absolutely vital to managing diabetes. They will help you gain control of your disease by teaching you how to adjust your diet, incorporate physical activity into your routine, test your blood and record the results, as well as manage any medication or insulin that's been prescribed. CDEs can be found through the Canadian Diabetes Association, or you can be referred through your primary care doctor or endocrinologist (see page 44).
- **A dietitian:** In addition to a CDE, you should see a dietitian regularly during your first year with diabetes. If you learn to meal-plan accordingly, you may be able to control your diabetes without taking any medications.

- **An exercise/fitness instructor:** This is any professional who can tailor a fitness program that suits your lifestyle and level of ability. Check with your CDE, the Canadian Diabetes Association, the YMCA/YWCA or your local community centre for lists of fitness instructors. You do not need a referral to one; you can simply make an appointment independent of your doctor.
- **Community health representative (CHR):** This is someone from your community who works with you and your family, as well as with other health care professionals, to educate you about diabetes. CHRs are usually found in rural areas where access to doctors is poor. CHRs attend a four-day training session and complete a skills test, but skills training and experience vary widely, although CHRs are required to review and update their skills annually. CHRs are common in Aboriginal Canadian communities.
- **An endocrinologist and other specialists:** This is discussed further on page 44.
- **Pharmacist:** Since you may be expected to do home glucose tests, your pharmacist will recommend the right glucose meter for you and will become a valuable source of information on drug interactions and their effects on your blood sugar. Finding a diabetes care centre in your neighbourhood is an ideal place to purchase your diabetes products and consult with a pharmacist.

While clearly there is treatment for Type 2 diabetes, it is a complex disease that can only be managed through a multilayered approach. The goal of treatment is not just to relieve symptoms, but to prevent a range of other diseases in the future. Self-managing your disease while maintaining your quality of life can happen only if you're willing to learn and to change. That means asking questions and participating in your treatment.

There are various stops along this treatment highway. How many times you stop depends on how well you can control your blood sugar. Some of you may be able to control diabetes solely through diet and exercise (see Chapters 7 and 8). Some of you may need to combine diet and lifestyle modification with diabetes pills, while some of you may need to use insulin to control your disease.

This chapter will guide you through the maze of treatments and health care professionals you'll encounter. It will also feed you the right questions so you can get the right answers. Only then can you be expected to participate more fully in decisions that affect your diabetes and the rest of your life.

THE RIGHT PRIMARY CARE DOCTOR

A primary care doctor is the doctor you see all the time. For example, you would see this doctor for a cold, flu or an annual physical; this is the doctor who refers you to specialists.

In Canada, primary care doctors today are *general practitioners* (four years of medical school and one year of internship), *family practitioners* (four years of medical school, and a two-year residency in family medicine) or *internists* (four years of medical school, and a four-year residency in internal medicine). During medical training, rotations are done in a variety of specialties, such as psychiatry, endocrinology, obstetrics and gynecology, emergency medicine and so on. During a residency, the years are spent in a teaching hospital under the supervision of teaching faculty (assistant, associate or full professors of medicine) who teach one specialty. The number of years spent in a residency program after four years of medical school varies depending on the university and specialty. To qualify as a specialist, such as an endocrinologist, a doctor must do a residency in endocrinology. A fellowship year is required after that, and the doctor must be eligible to write exams for the Fellowship of the Royal College of Physicians of Canada. The letters "F.R.C.P." stand for Fellow Royal College of Physicians. ("F.R.C.S." stands for Fellow Royal College of Surgeons). In the United States, the "R" is replaced with "A" for American (College of Physicians/Surgeons).

Eighty percent of all people with Type 2 diabetes are cared for by their primary care doctors, but the quality of care may vary. What you'll find today is that most primary care doctors in Canada become very good at treating a few conditions. Some see a lot of patients with diabetes; others see more pregnant women; still others see more elderly patients requiring palliative care. It all depends on the magic phrase "patient population." *Where* is the doctor's practice located? *Who* are the people in that neighbourhood?

Therefore, a primary care physician may not be the best doctor to manage your diabetes if that doctor doesn't see many diabetes patients. Some doctors are also behind the times when it comes to diabetes and do not immediately recognize early warning signs or high-risk groups. Nor do all primary care doctors counsel their patients about newer approaches to therapy, namely, self-monitoring of blood glucose levels, which, though optional in Type 2 diabetes, may not be discussed as an option. (See Chapter 4.)

When you're diagnosed with diabetes, ask your doctor the following questions. It will help determine whether you should stay with your doctor or look for another one:

1. **What is your philosophy about blood sugar monitoring?** Any doctor who does not discuss the option of your purchasing a glucose meter and self-monitoring your blood sugar levels may not be up to date. The Canadian Diabetes Association recommends that people with Type 2 diabetes get into the habit of self-testing their blood sugar. A discussion about it with your doctor is warranted, even though self-testing remains optional pending more convincing data. A good family doctor should present the facts to date: "Here's what some people think; here's what I think; here are my recommendations." (Ultimately, the decision is yours.)

2. **How often will you be checking my glycosylated hemoglobin or glycohemoglobin levels?** If your doctor says, "Huh?" get out of there and find another doctor! This is a blood test (HbA_{1c}) that should be done every three to six months. (Note: In Quebec, family doctors report that this test is not uniformly available.)

3. **Will you be referring me to a specialist?** The answer should be "Yes!" If you've been diagnosed with diabetes, you need to see other health care professionals as soon as possible, such as an endocrinologist who specializes in diabetes, a certified diabetes educator, a dietitian and an ophthalmologist (or optometrist if the former isn't available). If your doctor says, "I can manage your condition without referring you elsewhere," get out of that office and go elsewhere.

4. **Where can I go for more information?** Any doctor who does not tell you to call the Canadian Diabetes Association as soon as you're diagnosed with diabetes is not worth seeing.

The Alarm Bells

If you hear the following words come out of your doctor's mouth, go elsewhere:

- You have borderline diabetes or "just a touch of sugar." (There's no such thing. There *is* such a thing as impaired glucose tolerance, discussed in Chapter 1.)
- You don't need to change your diet; I'll just give you a pill. (In general, no medication should be prescribed until you've been sent to a dietitian, who will work with you to modify your diet and lifestyle. In cases where medication is warranted immediately, you must still see a dietitian.)

- You don't need to see a specialist. (You *do* need to see a specialist.)
- You have a recurrent yeast infection. This is perfectly normal. (Chronic vaginal yeast infections are a classic sign of diabetes in postmenopausal women.)

WHAT ARE HEALTH CARE RIGHTS?

In a very general way, patients' rights in Western health care involve four basic umbrella principles. Since so many people with diabetes are mismanaged, this is important information for you to have. You can challenge your doctor on any of these principles and use the following information to launch a complaint to the Royal College of Physicians and Surgeons in your province if you feel your rights have been ignored. This section has been reviewed by experts at the University of Toronto's Joint Centre for Bioethics. For more information, you can also visit my Bioethics Page and links at www.sarahealth.com.

Respect for Persons

The phrase "respect for persons" refers to the concept that we must respect that each person has full human rights. That means you have a right to be fully informed about all things involving your care, your body or things being done to your body (if you're pregnant, you have the right to know about everything that affects the fetus you're carrying), and to make your own decisions about care based on accurate information. This is sometimes known as "patient autonomy." A health care provider has a duty to respect your personhood, wishes, bodily integrity and health care preferences. So information, counselling and informed consent (see further on) are all crucial aspects of care that support this principle. Here are some examples of when your health care provider is ignoring the concept of respect for persons:

- You are given no information about your condition, and your doctor refuses to answer or address your questions.
- You refuse a certain treatment or procedure after being fully informed of all the risks and benefits of that procedure, but your health care provider tries to force you or coerce you into having the procedure anyway, which does not respect your choice.
- You request a referral to a specialist and your doctor ignores your request.
- You do not speak English and your doctor refuses to speak to a translator you've appointed.

- Your doctor forces a feeding tube up the nose of your 92-year-old mother who suffers from severe dementia despite your express objections as her appointed decision-maker.
- Your confidentiality (see further on) is breached in some way.

What is "informed consent"?

Many of you have heard the term "informed consent," but may not truly understand what it means. To uphold the principle of respect for persons, you have the right to accurate and full information about your health so you can make an informed decision about your health care. This is known as informed consent. You cannot even know about refusing a procedure if you are not given information first. In order for informed consent to take place, three things have to happen:

- **Disclosure:** Have you been provided with relevant and comprehensive information by your health care provider? For example, a description of the treatment; its expected effects (e.g., duration of hospital stay, expected time required for recovery, restrictions on daily activities, scars); information about relevant alternative options and their expected benefits and relevant risks; and an explanation of the consequences of declining or delaying treatment. Have you been given an opportunity to ask questions, and has your health care provider been available to answer them?
- **Capacity and competency:** Do you understand information relevant to a treatment decision and appreciate the reasonably foreseeable consequences of a decision or lack of decision? Do you understand information and appreciate its implications? Do you understand what's being disclosed and can you decide on your treatment based on this information?
- **Voluntariness:** Are you being allowed to make your health care choice free of any undue influences? To answer the question, we need to take into consideration factors such as pain and manipulation (when information is being deliberately distorted or omitted).

Other barriers to informed consent include:
- language barriers
- wide gaps in knowledge (When you're not a doctor, how informed can you really be unless you go to medical school?)

• health care provider bias (when your health care provider makes assumptions about your intelligence or character and tailors the information to those assumptions)

What about confidentiality?

You may think your health care records or the information you disclose to your health care provider are confidential, but your medical records are, in fact, not confidential. These are the questions you must ask your health care provider if you're concerned about confidential information getting into the wrong hands:

1. **Who owns this information?** For example, if you test positive for a particular cancer gene or HIV, does your health care provider have a duty to report this information to anyone other than yourself? If you're placed on antidepressants, do you want this information to get out? Can you bar your physician from disclosing this information? And what about employers who demand that you have routine physicals?

2. **How will this information be used?** Can your health status information be used by employers or health insurers as tools of discrimination? In the 1970s, for example, African-North Americans who tested positive for sickle cell anemia were denied jobs by major airlines and were forced to pay higher insurance costs.

3. **How will your health status affect other family members?** If you test positive for a particular cancer gene, for example, do you have to disclose this information to your children? Ought you? Ought they be tested? And what are the consequences involved?

Beneficence and nonmalificence

This means that the health care provider must strive to maintain or promote the well-being of a patient and avoid harming that patient. This is known as "beneficence." At the same time, the health care provider must also strive not to inflict harm or evil on a patient. This is known as "nonmalificence." This means that a health care provider has a duty not to kill a patient, and a duty not to refrain from aiding a patient.

In order to promote the well-being of patients and avoid harming them, therapies, treatments or diagnostic tests that involve risks to your health need to be weighed against potential benefits. Here are some examples of when your health care provider is ignoring beneficence:

- Your doctor is recommending you try an experimental therapy that has not yet been proven to work better than a standard therapy and has unknown risks.
- You are given a drug or therapy and not provided with information on side effects or potential risks.
- You are in a drug study that involves some people taking a "dummy pill" (called a placebo) and some people taking a real pill. In this case, you may continue to suffer needlessly from an ailment if you are taking the dummy pill and are not offered a standard therapy that will help your ailment.
- Your health care provider breaches your confidentiality (see above).

Justice

This means that the health care provider or system has to ensure that all people have the same access to health care services (e.g., hospital beds, medicine, treatments, clinical trials, health care providers, preventive care, etc.) regardless of their ability to pay, gender, ethnicity or race, physical or mental ability, age or any other factors, such as behaviour or lifestyle.

In order to be fair, all people should have equal access to health care services and resources. Being just or fair means all lives and interests are of equal importance and must be given equal weight. As well, a health care provider has a duty to provide the same standard of care and options to all patients, regardless of income, education or race. Here are some examples of when the health care system—or your individual health care provider—is ignoring justice:

- When some people have more access to resources than other people due to privilege and wealth.
- When your health care provider places a greater value on some patients than on others.
- When poor people with diabetes have less access to good health care than affluent people with diabetes because they have fewer services in poorer areas.
- When an HIV-positive person is refused health care service by a health care provider who fears HIV.
- When certain groups of people die of curable diseases because they don't have the same access to screening for that disease than other groups of people.
- When vulnerable populations (the elderly, mentally ill, people in developing countries or certain ethnic groups) are selected for dangerous or risky medical experiments because they are perceived "expendable."

Problems with "Doing the Right Thing" for Patients

Ignoring one of the above principles can put you in jeopardy, which would make the health care provider negligent. But in many circumstances "the right thing" to do isn't always clear, and it isn't always possible to do the right thing:

- When people are unconscious, for example, it's impossible to inform them and ask them about their wishes. (In this case, someone close to the unconscious person may make decisions on his or her behalf.)
- When people are not competent to make their own decisions, it's difficult to inform them (here, again, someone close to the incompetent patient makes the decision).
- When the benefits of certain medications or therapies have to be weighed against certain risks, it's difficult to know what to do, and what's in the patient's best interests.
- When health care providers are faced with limited resources, such as funding for research, organs for transplant or even hospital beds, it's difficult to decide who should get the funds, the organ or the bed.
- When conducting drug studies, is it right to conduct a study where someone is taking a dummy pill (known as a placebo-controlled study)?

Whose life is worth saving? Whose life is worth risking? And who decides? These are all common, everyday questions and situations that health care providers face.

Legal Duties of Health Care Providers

Whether health care practitioners are considered to be trained in a conventional manner or unconventional manner, charging a fee for services ought to imply that there are standards of competence their patients or clients have a right to expect. Any health care professional who earns a salary is bound by tort law to uphold standards of care. Moreover, there is a duty of all health care practitioners of "due awareness," meaning that they have a duty to stay educated, informed and up to date on all aspects of legally enforceable duties of care to patients, their families, colleagues and staff members. Health care providers have a basic duty to diagnose, treat, manage or care for a health problem. They also have a duty to counsel you about potential harms you may be doing to yourself through medications you're taking, bad habits or other practices, or harms from outside forces beyond your control, such as environmental factors. And finally, when medical records need to be transferred or copied to a third party, health care providers have a duty to disclose potentially sensitive or stigmatizing information to that party, as well as to you.

Health care standards of practice in Canada have two legal checks: You can sue or you can complain to the professional regulatory authority, which monitors standards of practice to protect the public.

Patients' Rights Specific to Diabetes

Applying your rights as a patient to diabetes specifically, here are some things you should expect from your health care provider:

As much information about your diabetes as you want: Any doctor who is reluctant to give you literature, videos and a referral to a diabetes educator and dietitian is not giving you proper care.

Answers to your questions about diabetes: If there isn't time during an exam or checkup, make another appointment that serves as a question-and-answer period.

Regular assessments: When you have diabetes, you should be seen at least every three months for a checkup or at regular intervals. It's important to ask how much advance booking time you need to get an appointment.

Participation in treatment plans: You'll need to educate yourself about your diabetes before you can participate, but you have many options in treatment.

Decent emergency care and an opportunity to meet your doctor's substitute: Who looks after you when your doctor is on holidays or sick?

Privacy and confidentiality: Diabetes often taints relationships with employers, co-workers and insurance companies. Find out what your doctor's legal obligations are with respect to health records—and what are *yours?*

Information about fees and costs: What is covered by the province and what is not? How much of your medication and equipment is covered by your drug plan? Your doctor should be able to give you an estimate for your diabetes care products in case you are not covered. He or she should also be able to give you cheaper products if you cannot afford what is being prescribed. Pharmacists and the Canadian Diabetes Association are also helpful.

To be seen on time: If you're on time for an appointment, your doctor should be as well. Do you generally have to wait more than 30 minutes in the reception area before your doctor will see you? Although this sometimes can't be helped, the doctor should be aware that waiting creates anxiety—especially if appointments are timed close to meals, and you are taking insulin.

A change to another doctor: If you're unhappy with your current doctor, or simply need a change, you have every right to switch. Make sure you arrange for your records to be transferred. Some costs may be involved, however.

A second opinion, or a consultation with a specialist: No family doctor should deny you a referral to a specialist.

Your Doctor's Rights

Your doctor has the right to expect the following from you:

Honesty: If you're not being truthful about how often you're checking your blood sugar levels or about what you're eating, or if you are not being honest in recording your log to avoid a lecture, your doctor can't be blamed if your health deteriorates.

Courtesy and respect: Treat your doctor like a business associate. If you make an appointment, show up; if you need to cancel, give 24 hours' notice. If you have a problem, go through reasonable channels; dial the after-hours emergency number the doctor leaves with the answering service, or call your doctor's office during business hours.

Good reporting: Don't tell your doctor that you're not feeling well and expect a diagnosis. Tell your doctor what your *specific symptoms* are. Better yet, write them down before you visit your doctor.

Questions: If you don't ask a particular question, you can't blame your doctor for not answering it.

Follow-through: If you don't follow your doctor's advice, you can't blame the doctor if you experience side effects to medications or worsening symptoms. If you don't think your doctor's advice is reasonable, say so and discuss it. Maybe your doctor doesn't have a full understanding of your condition; maybe you don't have a full understanding of your doctor's suggestions.

Self-management: Don't call your doctor ten times a day with every little change in your blood sugar levels. You should be able to monitor your blood sugar levels and adjust your diet and medication regimen accordingly. Emergencies or illness are different situations, however, and your doctor should be notified since even a common virus will elevate your blood sugar level.

YOUR DIABETES SPECIALIST

A diabetes specialist is an endocrinologist who subspecializes in diabetes. Endocrinologists are hormone specialists. Some see more thyroid patients than diabetes patients. Some specialize in reproductive endocrinology (male and female hormones). Therefore, it's important that you wind up with someone who almost exclusively manages diabetes patients. The shortest route to a diabetes specialist is to ask your primary care doctor for a referral. If your primary care doctor refuses to refer you (this, by the way, is not unusual), call the Canadian Diabetes Association and ask them for a list of endocrinologists in your area.

If you live in an underserviced area (there are several of these in Canada!), ask people you know if they know someone with diabetes, and then call them! Who are *they* seeing? You may need to go outside your area to a larger city, but it's worth the trip to avoid being mismanaged.

Your primary care doctor can continue to manage the rest of your referrals to ophthalmologists (for diabetes eye disease), podiatrists for foot care, and so on. (See Chapter 20 for more details.)

Getting Along with Your Specialist

You may find your endocrinologist a little intimidating because he or she is more academic; he or she may use more technical terms to explain your disease and treatment. Endocrinologists often teach or run residency programs, are active in research, frequently lecture and regularly publish articles and books in their field. These doctors are usually harder to get in touch with; they're usually booked months in advance. That's why it's crucial to maximize the time you *do* have. The best way to do this is to tape-record the conversation at your appointment. That way, you can replay the information in the comfort of your own home. It's also important to take a list of questions with you. If there isn't time for all your questions to be answered, schedule a separate question-and-answer session. Finally, ask your specialist to draw you a picture of your condition. Visualizing your disease, and seeing how various medications may interact in your body, will help you understand what's going on, and what's being recommended.

A dozen good questions to ask

Of course, it's difficult to prepare questions in advance when you don't know what to ask, so here are few good questions to get you started:

1. How severe is my diabetes? (In other words, if you are experiencing other health problems as a result of your diabetes, the disease is likely more advanced.)

2. Does my hospital or treatment centre have a multidisciplinary diabetes education care team? (This means that a number of health care professionals—certified diabetes educators, clinical nurse specialists, dietitians, endocrinologists and other relevant specialists—discuss your case together and recommend treatment options.)

3. What treatment do you recommend, and why? (For example, if insulin therapy is being recommended over oral hypoglycemic agents, find out why. And find out how this particular treatment will reduce the odds of complications.)

4. How will my treatment help the risks and side effects associated with diabetes, and who will help me adjust my medications or insulin?

5. How long do you recommend this particular treatment? (Lifelong? On a wait-and-see basis?)

6. What if I forget to take a pill or insulin shot? What are the consequences?

7. What other health problems should I look out for? (You'll want to watch for symptoms of high or low blood sugar, as well as symptoms of long-term complications, such as eye problems or numbness in your feet.)

8. How can I contact you between visits?

9. Can I take other medications? Or how will my pills or insulin affect other medications I'm taking?

10. What about alcohol? How will alcohol consumption affect any pills or insulin I'm on? How do I compensate for it?

11. Will I be able to participate in new studies or clinical trials using new drugs or therapies?

12. Are there any holistic approaches I can turn to as a complement to diabetes pills or insulin therapy?

OTHER SPECIALISTS

Since diabetes can involve a variety of complications in the future, you may need to consult some or all of the following specialists:

Internist: This is a doctor who specializes in non-surgical treatment of a variety of medical problems, including diabetes.

Ophthalmologist: This is an eye specialist who will monitor your eyes and make sure that you're showing no symptoms of diabetes eye disease (see Chapter 17). If you are, this is the specialist who will treat your condition.

Cardiologist: This is a heart specialist. People with Type 2 diabetes are four times more likely to suffer from heart attacks. You may be sent here if you are experiencing symptoms of heart disease or angina.

Nephrologist: This is a kidney specialist. Since kidney disease is a common complication of diabetes, you may be sent here if you're showing symptoms of kidney disease (protein in your urine).

Gastroenterologist: This is a G.I. (gastrointestinal) specialist. Diabetes often results in a number of chronic gastrointestinal ailments. You may be sent here if you have symptoms of chronic heartburn, reflux and other gastric aches and pains.

Neurologist: This is a nerve specialist who will see you if you're experiencing nerve damage as a result of your diabetes.

Gerontologist: This is a doctor who specializes in diseases of the elderly. If you are over 65 and have a number of other health problems, this doctor will help you balance your various medications and conditions, in conjunction with your diabetes.

Obstetrician/Gynecologist: If you develop diabetes during pregnancy, you'll need to be under the care of an obstetrician for the remainder of your pregnancy. All women should see a gynecologist regularly for Pap smears, breast health and consultation regarding sexual health, contraception and hormone replacement therapy after menopause.

Urologist: This is a doctor who specializes in male reproductive problems. Impotence is often a complication with diabetes, and this is the doctor who will be able to determine the cause of your impotence.

Orthopedist: This is a foot doctor who can help you monitor foot health. If you're experiencing severe problems with your feet (see Chapter 20), your podiatrist will likely send you here.

When You Want a Second Opinion

Getting a second opinion means that you see two separate doctors about the same set of symptoms. If you answer yes to one of the questions below, you're probably justified in seeking a second opinion.

1. Is the diagnosis uncertain? If your doctor can't give you a straight answer about what's going on, you're justified in seeing someone else.
2. Is the diagnosis life-threatening? In this case, hearing the same news from someone else may help you cope better with your illness or come to terms with the diagnosis.

3. Is the treatment controversial, experimental or risky? You might not question the diagnosis but have problems with the recommended treatment. For example, if you're not comfortable with treatment approach A, perhaps another doctor can recommend treatment approach B.

4. Is the treatment not working? If your oral hypoglycemic agents can't seem to control your blood sugar levels, maybe it's time for insulin. In this case, getting a second opinion may help to clear up the problem.

5. Are risky tests or procedures being recommended? If you find a particular test or procedure frightening, a second opinion will either help confirm your suspicions, or confirm your original doctor's recommendations.

6. Do you want another approach? If you have poor control over your diabetes, your doctor may want you to begin taking insulin, while another doctor may prescribe dietary changes along with antidiabetic medication.

7. Is the doctor's competence in question? If you suspect that your doctor doesn't know what he or she is doing, go somewhere else to either reaffirm your faith in your doctor or confirm your original suspicions.

WHAT THE DOCTOR ORDERS

Throughout the year, your managing doctor (primary care physician or endocrinologist) should order a variety of blood tests to make sure that your blood sugar levels are as controlled as they can be, and that no complications from diabetes are setting in.

The Hemoglobin A_{1c} (HbA$_{1c}$) Test

The most important test is one that checks your glycolsylated hemoglobin levels, known as the hemoglobin A_{1c} test or the HbA$_{1c}$ test. Hemoglobin is a large molecule that carries oxygen to your bloodstream. When the glucose in your blood comes in contact with the hemoglobin molecule, it conveniently sticks to it. The more glucose stuck to your hemoglobin, the higher your blood sugar is. The HbA$_{1c}$ test actually measures the amount of glucose stuck to hemoglobin. And since each hemoglobin molecule stays in your blood about three to four months before it is replaced, this test can show you the average blood sugar level over the last three to four months. Therefore this test is recommended at least every six months. If you have cardiovascular problems, you will need to have the HbA$_{1c}$ test more often.

A similar test, known as a fructosamine test, can show the amount of glucose stuck to a molecule in your blood known as albumin. Albumin gets replaced every four to six weeks, however, so this test can therefore give you an average of blood sugar levels only over the last four to six weeks.

What's a good HbA$_{1c}$ result?

Just like your glucose monitor at home, the goal of the HbA$_{1c}$ test is to make sure that your blood sugar "average" is as close to normal as possible. Again, the closer to normal it is, the less likely you are to experience long-term diabetes complications.

This test result is slightly different from your glucose meter result. For example, an HbA$_{1c}$ level of 7.0 percent is equal to 144 mg/dl (8 mmol/L) on your blood glucose meter. A result of 9.5 percent is equivalent to 234 mg/dl (13 mmol/L) on your blood glucose meter. In a person without diabetes, an HbA$_{1c}$ ranges from 4 to 6 percent. The results are often expressed as percentages of "normal" such as <110 percent, 111 to 140 percent or >140 percent.

The new guidelines stipulate that values of 6 percent or less are good results and mean that your blood sugar is perfectly under control. Meanwhile, anything higher than 8.4 percent is alarming; this would be a poor result and means that your diabetes is not under control. Studies show that when your HbA$_{1c}$ result is 8.4 percent or higher, you have a greater chance of developing long-term complications. In fact, for every 1 percent drop in your HbA$_{1c}$ average (that is, 7.2 percent down from 8.2 percent), the risk of long-term complications falls by about 25 percent.

TABLE 3.1
What's a Good Glycosylated Hemoglobin Test (HbA$_{1c}$) Result?*

Non-Diabetic Range	Optimal	Suboptimal	Poor Control
4–6.0%	<7.0%	7.0–8.4%	>8.4%
<100%	<115%	116–140%	>140%

*Based on fasting blood glucose levels.

Source: Canadian Medical Association Journal 1998; 159(8 Suppl): S12.

Problems with the HbA$_{1c}$ test

If your child comes home with a report card showing a B average, it doesn't mean your child is getting a B in every course; it means that he or she could have received a D in one course and an A+ in another. Similarly, the HbA$_{1c}$ test is just an "average mark." You could have a decent result, even though your blood sugar levels may be dangerously low one day and dangerously high the next.

If you suffer from sickle cell disease or other blood disorders, the HbA_{1c} results will not be accurate either. In this case, you may wind up with either false high or low readings.

And at any time, if your home blood sugar tests (if you've opted for self-testing) over the past two or three months do not seem to match the results of the HbA_{1c} test, be sure to check the accuracy of your meter, and perhaps show your doctor or certified diabetes educator how you are using the meter in case your technique needs some refining.

Other Important Tests

It's important to have the following routine tests done at least once a year, and more often if you are at high risk for complications.

Blood pressure

As discussed in Chapter 2, high blood pressure can put you at greater risk for cardiovascular problems. Diabetes can also cause high blood pressure. That's why it's important to have your blood pressure checked every four to six months.

Cholesterol

As discussed in Chapter 2, high cholesterol is a problem for people with diabetes, while diabetes can also trigger high cholesterol. Your cholesterol is checked through a simple blood test that should be done once upon diagnosis, and once a year thereafter. See Table 3.2 for more details.

TABLE 3.2

Checking Your Cholesterol

The following are guidelines for people age 30 and over:

	Good	Poor
Total Cholesterol	below 5.2	above 6.2
LDL Cholesterol	below 3.4	above 3.4
HDL Cholesterol	above 0.9	below 0.9
Triglycerides	below 2.3	above 2.3

Source: Canadian Heart and Stroke Foundation, 2001.

Eye exam

Since diabetes can cause what's known as diabetes eye disease or diabetic retinopathy (damage to the back of your eye), annual eye exams are crucial. Your eye exam should also rule out cataracts and glaucoma.

When diabetic eye disease is caught early, laser treatment can be used to treat it and prevent blindness. If your exam uses the term *absent* on your chart, it means your retina is just fine. If you see the word *background*, it means that mild changes have occurred to your eye(s) and that you need more regular monitoring. If the terms *non-proliferative* or *proliferative* are used, it means that there is some damage to one or both eyes and you will require treatment and regular exams. See Chapter 17 for more details.

Foot exam

When you have diabetes, nerve damage and poor circulation can wreak havoc on your feet. Be sure to have a thorough foot exam each year to check for reduced sensation, feeling or circulation, and evidence of calluses or sores. See Chapter 20 for more details.

Glucose meter checkup

If you've opted to test your own blood sugar, it's important to compare your home glucose meter's test results to a laboratory blood glucose test. In fact, it's a good idea to do this every six months. All you do is bring your meter to the lab when you're having a blood glucose test done. After the lab technician takes your blood, do your own test within about five minutes and record the result. Your meter is working perfectly so long as your result is within 15 percent of the lab test (if your meter is testing whole blood, as opposed to plasma).

Kidney tests

One of the most common complications of diabetes is kidney disease, known in this case as *diabetic nephropathy* (diabetic kidney disease). This condition develops slowly over the course of many years, but there are usually few symptoms or warning signs. To make sure no damage to the kidneys has occurred, it's important to have your urine tested regularly to check the health of your kidneys. See Chapter 19 on kidney health in Part 3.

When you have diabetes, you are the most important part of your diabetes health care team. The next chapter will show you all the things you can do to maximize your health and stay in control of your diabetes. By helping yourself, you will help your health care providers do their job a little better: the job of taking care of you.

Chapter 4

DIABETES SELF-CARE

● ● ● ● ● ● ● ● ● ●

Diabetes self-care is all about eliminating your diabetes symptoms, and then remaining as symptom-free as possible. Meal planning (Chapter 6) combined with exercise (Chapter 8) is the best way to remain symptom-free. This will help you lose weight if you need to, as well as distribute an even amount of calories to your body throughout the day. By not putting any unusual strain on your body's metabolism, you will likely *not* experience any surprises when it comes to your blood sugar levels. Exercise makes insulin much more available to your cells, while your muscles use sugar as fuel.

If you can't seem to keep your blood sugar levels below 8 mmol/L, you are probably a candidate for diabetes medications, such as an oral hypoglycemic agent, discussed in Chapter 5.

TESTING YOUR OWN BLOOD SUGAR

In order to plan your meals and activities properly, you have to know what your blood sugar levels are throughout the day. One of the most important research projects ever undertaken was the Diabetes Control and Complications Trial (DCCT). This trial proved beyond a doubt that when people with Type 1 diabetes kept their blood sugar levels as normal as possible, as often as possible, they could dramatically reduce the odds of developing small blood-vessel diseases related to diabetes, such as kidney disease, eye problems and nerve disease, all discussed in Part 3.

In 1998, the results of a landmark British study, the United Kingdom Prospective Diabetes Study (UKPDS), showed that frequent blood sugar testing (meaning about three or four times a day) in people with Type 2 diabetes also helped reduce eye, kidney and nerve damage, as well as high blood pressure. (See Chapter 13 for more details.)

Glucose meters were first introduced in 1982. They allow people with diabetes to test their own blood sugar any time they want without having to rely on doctors. When your parents or grandparents struggled with diabetes in the past, there was no such thing as a glucose meter. They had to go to the doctor to get their blood sugar tested regularly. Amazingly enough, through interviews with individual diabetes patients and several doctors, my research shows that there are still people who rely on the doctor to test their blood sugar. If you are still going to your doctor for a blood sugar test, purchase a glucose meter before your next doctor's visit and ask your doctor to show you how it works. There is no good reason to continue to rely on a doctor to test your blood sugar.

How Frequently Should You Test?

A healthy pancreas measures its owner's blood sugar levels once a second or 3,600 times an hour. It produces exactly the right amount of insulin for that second. In light of this, testing your blood sugar frequently makes sense, which has been confirmed by two major studies, mentioned above.

There is no official position in Canada regarding how frequently you should test your blood sugar. As a result, two management philosophies have emerged regarding frequent self-testing of blood sugar and Type 2 diabetes. Most physicians feel that the more involved you become in managing your blood sugar, the better off you'll be in the long run, and therefore, they support frequent self-testing of blood sugar in their Type 2 patients. The Canadian Diabetes Association also recommends that people with Type 2 diabetes frequently self-test their blood sugar. In fact, in a newly diagnosed person with Type 2 diabetes, frequent daily testing will show *individual patterns* of glucose rises and dips. This information may help your health care team tailor your meal plans, exercise routines and medication regimens. And if you do have to take insulin in the future, you will need to get into the habit of testing your own blood sugar anyway.

Not all physicians agree with this policy, however. Some physicians have told me that for some of their patients with Type 2 diabetes, the struggle to make necessary diet and activity changes is hard enough, and the frequent blood sugar testing can complicate that goal. In other words, for some people, it's too much to handle; the blood sugar testing interferes with more crucial goals, such as losing weight.

You have to be able to find a plan that works for you and put together realistic goals with your diabetes health care team. Regardless of your doctor's approach to frequent self-testing of blood sugar, there are a host of easy-to-use home blood sugar monitors that give you more choice in diabetes self-care than ever before, so you should take advantage of them. Your doctor, pharmacist or diabetes educator can recommend the right glucose meter for you. When you get your glucose monitor, experts suggest you compare your results to one regular laboratory test to make sure you've purchased a reliable and accurate machine.

Use the information in the boxed text below as a general guideline for testing times, and take it to your health care provider to help design a reasonable plan that works for you. Testing schedules are usually tailored for each individual.

WHEN TO TEST YOUR BLOOD SUGAR

In the days when diabetes patients went to their doctors' offices for blood sugar testing, they were usually tested first thing in the morning before eating (called a fasting blood sugar level) or immediately after eating (known as a postprandial or postmeal blood sugar level). It was believed that if either the fasting or postprandial levels were normal, the patient was stable. This is now known to be *completely false*. In fact, your blood sugar levels can bounce around all day long. Because your blood sugar is constantly changing, a blood sugar test in a doctor's office is pretty useless because it measures what your blood sugar is only for that nanosecond. In other words, what your blood sugar is at 2:15 p.m. is not what it might be at 3:05 p.m.

It makes the most sense to test yourself before each meal, so you know what your levels are before you eat anything, as well as about two hours after meals. Immediately after eating, blood sugar is normally high, so this is not the ideal time to test anybody. In a person without diabetes, blood sugar levels will drop about two hours after eating, in response to the natural insulin the body makes. Similarly, test yourself two hours after eating to make sure that you are able to "mimic" a normal blood sugar pattern, too. Ideally, this translates into at least four blood tests daily:

When you wake up
After breakfast/before lunch (i.e., two hours after breakfast)
After lunch/before dinner (i.e., two hours after lunch)
After dinner/or at bedtime (i.e., two hours after dinner)

The most revealing information about your blood sugar control is in the answers to the following questions:

1. What is your blood sugar level as soon as you wake up? (In people with Type 2 diabetes, it is often at its highest point in the morning.)

2. What is your blood sugar level two hours after a meal? (It should be much lower two hours after eating than one hour after eating.)

3. What is your blood sugar level when you feel ill? (You need to avoid dipping too low or high since your routine is changing.)

Variations on the theme

▶ Test yourself four times a day (times indicated above) two to three times a week, and then test yourself two times a day (before breakfast and before bedtime) for the remainder of the week.

▶ Test yourself twice a day three to four days a week in a rotating pattern (before breakfast and dinner one day; before lunch and bedtime the next).

▶ Test yourself once a day every day, but rotate your pattern (day 1 before breakfast; day 2 after dinner; day 3 before bedtime, and so on).

▶ Test yourself four times a day (times indicated above) two days a month.

A Brief History of Blood Sugar Tests

At one time, the only way you could test your blood sugar level yourself was by testing your urine for sugar; if the result showed that sugar was in your urine, you had already reached your renal threshold (kidney limit). Renal thresholds vary between about 6 and 11 mmol/L, but the limitations of urine testing were that it could only test for *really* high blood sugar levels and the results were delayed, meaning that you could be getting readings on urine that had been in the bladder for hours versus "fresh" urine (urine that has been in the bladder for less than an hour). Urine testing is also useless for checking low blood sugar. Far more accurate home blood sugar testing became available with the development of glucose meters in 1982, but the first meters were very expensive—about $600. Thankfully, meters today are quite affordable.

The first models measured glucose levels in whole blood, while laboratories were still measuring glucose levels in blood plasma. The difference is technical and not important to you personally. What you need to know, however, is that the readings vary. This meant that doctors needed to add about 12 percent to the glucose meter's recordings in order to get an accurate picture. This standard has changed. Today, all glucose meters measure glucose levels in plasma. If you're using an older glucose meter, don't panic when your next glucose meter suddenly gives you readings that are 12 percent higher than your last meter. It doesn't mean that you are losing control of your diabetes; rather, your meter is measuring glucose levels in your plasma instead of whole blood. Some diabetes literature recommends that you ask the pharmacist if the meter is a whole blood test or a plasma test, but most diabetes educators will tell you that this question is pretty redundant these days as all glucose meters are now plasma tests.

Choosing and Using Your Glucose Meter

As in the computer industry, glucose meter manufacturers tend to come out with technological upgrades every year. In fact, newer models allow you to download the time, date and blood sugar values for as many as 250 tests right onto your personal computer or personal organizer device. The information can help you gauge whether your diet and exercise routine is working, or whether you need to adjust your medications or insulin. If you've never purchased a glucose meter, keep in mind that the lowest-tech glucose meters all provide the following:

- a battery-powered, pocket-sized device
- an LED or LCD screen (that is, a calculator-like screen)

- accurate results in seconds
- at least a one-year warranty
- the opportunity to upgrade
- a 1-800 customer service hotline
- mailings and giveaways every so often
- a few free lancets with your purchase; you may have to separately purchase a lancing device, a dispenser for your lancets; eventually, you'll run out of lancets and have to buy those, too

The directions for using a glucose meter vary according to manufacturer. Be sure to read the directions carefully and ask your pharmacist for guidance if there's something you don't understand. It's a good idea to record your results in a logbook. *For example, a normal reading before meals ranges from 4–7 mmol/L; a normal reading after meals ranges from 5–10 mmol/L.*

Factors That Can Taint Your Test Results

Keep in mind that the following outside factors may interfere with your meter's performance.

Other medications you're taking: Studies show that some meters can be inaccurate if you're taking acetaminophen, salicylate, ascorbic acid, dopamine or levodopa. As a rule, if you're taking any medications, check with your doctor, pharmacist and glucose meter manufacturer (call their 1-800 number) about whether your medications can affect the meter's accuracy.

Humidity: The worst place to keep your meter and strips is in the bathroom, where humidity can ruin your strips unless they're individually wrapped in foil. Keep your strips in a sealed container away from extreme temperatures. Don't store your meter and strips, for example, in a hot glove compartment; don't keep them in the freezer either.

Bright light: Ever tried to use a calculator or portable computer in bright sunlight? It's not possible because the light interferes with the screen. Some meters are photometric, which means they are affected by bright light. If you plan to test in sunlight, get a biosenser meter that is unaffected by bright light (there are several).

Touching the test strip: Many glucose meters come with test strips that cannot be touched with your fingers or a second drop of blood. If you're all thumbs, purchase a meter that is unaffected by touch and/or allows a second drop of blood.

Wet hands: Before you test, thoroughly dry your hands. Water can dilute your blood sample.

Motion: It's always best to test yourself when you're standing still. Testing on planes, trains, automobiles, buses and subways may affect your results, depending on the brand of glucose meter.

Dirt, lint and blood: Particles of dirt, lint and old blood can sometimes affect the accuracy of a meter, depending on the brand. Make sure you clean the meter regularly (follow the manufacturer's cleaning directions) to remove buildup. If your meter requires battery changes, make sure you change them! There are meters on the market that do not require cleaning and are unaffected by dirt, but they may cost a little more.

Glycosylated Hemoglobin

The most detailed blood sugar test cannot be done at home yet. This is a blood test that checks for glycosylated hemoglobin (glucose attached to the protein in your red blood cells), known as *glycohemoglobin* or HbA_{1c} levels. This test can tell you how well your blood sugar has been controlled over a period of two to three months by showing what percentage of it is too high. It's recommended that you get an HbA_{1c} test every three months. This test is discussed in more detail in Chapter 5.

OTHER WAYS TO SELF-CARE

Diabetes self-care is also about managing your overall health, which has an impact on your diabetes.

Losing Excess Weight

Statistics suggest that about 80 percent of the people reading this book weigh 20 percent more than their ideal weight, the technical definition of "obese." If you begin a meal-planning program—which means eating the right combination and amount of food—with a diabetes educator and dietitian, as well as incorporate exercise into your routine, you'll lose weight. Weight loss can greatly improve your body's ability to use insulin. There is no need to start a crash diet or panic about your weight, however. Meal planning *is* managing your diabetes. Weight loss will become a fringe benefit. As you lose weight, your blood sugar levels will drop, which may affect any diabetes medication you're on. For example, if you're taking pills that stimulate your body to make insulin and if you don't adjust your dosage to your weight loss, you may experience hypoglycemia (low blood sugar, discussed in Chapter 14). Weight loss will also decrease the odds of developing complications from diabetes, such as heart disease.

Watching Highs and Lows

Once you begin meal planning and exercising, your body will operate more efficiently, which could mean that your blood sugar levels might be too low, especially if you're taking an oral hypoglycemic agent. A blood sugar level less than 3.5 mmol/L is too low. Immediately ingesting sugar in the form of juice, candy or a sweet soft drink will raise your sugar to normal levels again. In addition, if you're taking insulin, it will be some time before you get "good" at it, and you may also suffer from a "low." For this reason, I devote all of Chapter 14 to hypoglycemia, which will explain what happens during a low, what to do when it occurs and how to avoid it in the future.

Management errors can cause high blood sugar (hyperglycemia) as well, which will cause all the classic diabetes symptoms discussed in Chapter 2. Early signs of high blood sugar are extreme thirst, dry and flushed skin, mood swings or unusual fatigue, but many people notice no symptoms at all.

Common reasons for a change in blood sugar levels revolve around the following:

- overeating, or eating more than usual
- eating less than is in your usual meal plan
- a change in exercise routine
- missing a medication dose or an insulin shot (if you're taking insulin)
- an out-of-the-ordinary event (illness, stress, upset, excitement)
- a sudden mood change (extreme fright, anger or sadness)
- pregnancy

In response to unusual strains or stress, your body taps into its stored glucose supplies for extra energy. This will raise your blood sugar level as more glucose than usual is released into your system. Whether you're fighting off a flu or fighting with your mother, digesting all that food you ate at that all-you-can-eat buffet or running away from a black bear, your body will try to give you the extra boost of energy you need to get through your immediate stress.

A word about ketones

When blood sugar levels are excessively high, the body tries to get energy from other things: fat and muscle. Ketones (a.k.a. ketoic acid) are the by-product when the body breaks down fat or muscle. The body tries to get rid of them through the kidneys by flushing them into the urine. High ketones along with high blood glucose cause *diabetic ketoacidosis* (DKA), which results in an emergency. Signs of DKA include frequent urination (polyuria), excessive thirst (polydipsia), excessive hunger (polyphagia) and a fruity smell to the breath.

It's rare for people with Type 2 diabetes to form ketones because most of them are still producing insulin, which tends to inhibit ketone formation, but this isn't always the case. Just be aware of the signs of DKA, and if you're concerned about your risk for DKA, discuss it with your doctor.

Adjusting Your Routine When You're Sick

If you have Type 2 diabetes, it's important to call your doctor whenever you're sick with even just a cold or flu. Fighting off even the common viruses will elevate your blood sugar levels and will require some juggling of your regular routine until you get the hang of it yourself.

Until you can get in to see your doctor, stay on your meal plan. If that's not possible, drink about a half a cup of calorie-free fluid (could be water or calorie-free diet soda), alternating with half a cup of calorie-containing fluid (such as juice or broth) every hour you are awake. Over-the-counter medications may alter your blood sugar levels unless they are sugar-free. You should also test your blood sugar every four hours when you're ill to accommodate higher blood sugar levels, especially if there is vomiting or diarrhea. If you're taking any medication, stick to your usual plan and take it as prescribed at the usual times. You may need to go on insulin temporarily if your blood sugar levels remain high. This would not be the case with a cold, but may be necessary if you have a flu.

When you're not ill, but you have an unusually high blood sugar reading (over 11 mmol/L), it's time to see your doctor, too.

YOUR DIABETES HEALTH DIARY

One of the best ways to care for yourself is to keep a health diary, in which you record any unusual symptoms, and the times and dates those symptoms occur. Without your diary or health record, your doctors could be working in the dark and may not be able to design the right therapy program for you.

What Your Health Diary Should Record

The most important information your health diary will contain is the pattern of your blood sugar's peaks and valleys. Dates and times of these peaks and valleys may be important clues to establish the pattern. Your meal plan, exercise routine and medication regimen should be tailored to anticipate these peaks and valleys. You may need to incorporate a snack to prevent a low, or go for a 20-minute walk after dinner to prevent a high. Since there are a variety of factors that can affect your blood sugar levels, your diary should also record

- any medication you're taking
- unusually high or low readings that fall outside your pattern
- stressful life events or situations
- illness
- out-of-the-ordinary events (no matter how insignificant)
- changes in your health insurance or status
- severe insulin reactions (if you're taking insulin)
- general medical history (surgeries, tests you've had done, allergies, past drug reactions)

KNOW YOUR DRUGS

If you take any of the following prescription drugs, make sure you let your doctor know which ones can raise or lower blood sugar levels. (Some doctors aren't aware of all of these drugs.)

Drugs That Can Raise Blood Sugar Levels

Certain diuretics

Minoxidil

Corticosteroids

Cyclosporine

Diphenylhydantoin (e.g., Dilantin, used for seizures)

High-dose estrogen-containing oral contraceptives

Nicotinic acid and niacin (used to lower cholesterol)

Phenothiazines

Thyroid hormone

Beta-blockers

Calcium-channel blockers

Drugs That Lower Blood Sugar

Salicylates and acetaminophen

Ethanol in any form of alcohol

Angiotensin converting enzyme inhibitors (used for high blood pressure)

Alpha-blockers

Fibric acid derivatives (used to treat certain fat disorders)

One of the most important tools to self-care is understanding your medications. There's a lot to know, so the next chapter should be your next stop, whether you're taking oral hypoglycemic agents or insulin.

Chapter 5

DIABETES MEDICATIONS

● ● ● ● ● ● ● ● ● ● ●

Less than 10 percent of people with Type 2 diabetes are able to make the necessary lifestyle changes to keep their diabetes under control. First, the older we get, the harder it is for us to change our eating habits. Second, many of us are not able to incorporate enough exercise or physical activity into our routines.

Today there are pills to help you manage your diabetes if the lifestyle changes you've made aren't doing the trick. Going on diabetes medication is in no way a cure-all; taking a pill will help you stay as healthy as possible in the event that you cannot or will not make the necessary lifestyle changes.

There are several kinds of medications that may be prescribed for you. It's crucial to note, however, that these medications can only be prescribed for people who still produce insulin. They have no effect on people with Type 1 diabetes or insulin-dependent diabetes.

WHEN YOUR DOCTOR TELLS YOU TO TAKE A PILL

When diet and lifestyle changes make no impact on your blood sugar levels, you may be prescribed pills. Before you fill your prescription for oral diabetes medications, you should know that between 40 and 50 percent of all people with Type 2 diabetes require insulin therapy after ten years. Continuing insulin resistance may cause you to stop responding to oral medications. Furthermore, these pills are meant to complement your meal plan, exercise routine and glucose monitoring; they are not a substitute.

Bear in mind, too, that physicians who prescribe the medications discussed in this section without also working with you to modify your diet and lifestyle are not managing your diabetes properly. These medications should be prescribed only after you've been unsuccessful in managing your Type 2 diabetes through lifestyle modification and frequent blood sugar testing.

If you cannot get down to a healthy body weight, you are probably a good candidate for antidiabetic medication. And anyone with Type 2 diabetes who cannot control his/her blood sugar levels *despite* lifestyle changes is also a good candidate.

Oral Hypoglycemic Agents (OHAs)

OHAs account for about 75 percent of all prescriptions for people with Type 2 diabetes. This medication can make your insulin-producing cells more sensitive to glucose and stimulate them to secrete more insulin, which will lower your blood sugar. If your average blood-glucose levels are greater than 8 mmol/L, you will likely be prescribed an OHA. About 15 percent of people on OHAs will not respond to them, while an additional 3 to 5 percent of people on OHAs will stop responding to them.

Sulfonylureas and biguanides are common oral hypoglycemic agents (OHAs). Sulfonylureas are pills that help your pancreas release more insulin. There are many brands of sulfonylureas, which are listed here by their generic trade names, including gliclazide, glyburide and tolbutamide. Another oral hypoglycemic agent, repaglinide, technically classified as a "nonsulfonylureas," also lowers blood glucose levels by stimulating the release of insulin from the pancreas, but is considered a "short-acting" drug, which means it takes less time to take effect. Sulfonylureas or repaglinide would generally be the initial oral agent of choice for people who are *not* obese and/or have high blood sugar levels (or suffer from symptoms of high blood sugar). Any drug that stimulates your pancreas to release insulin is also called an "insulin secretogogue."

Biguanides (Metformin) are pills that help your insulin work better. This medication primarily stops your liver from producing glucose, thus helping to lower your blood sugar levels and increase glucose uptake by your muscle tissue. These pills also help your tissues respond better to your insulin. Ultimately, biguanides can lower premeal and postmeal blood sugar levels in 75 to 80 percent of people with Type 2 diabetes. This medication also seems to lower the "bad" cholesterol levels. These pills do not increase insulin levels and will not directly cause low blood sugar. A biguanide is appropriate for people who *are* obese and have milder levels of high blood sugar. That's because biguanides do not result in weight gain, which is typically associated with sulfonylurea and insulin therapy. Note: In some diabetes literature, the terms "antidiabetic agents" or "antidiabetic pills" are used; these terms refer to OHAs. The Canadian Diabetes Association does not use this terminology in its literature, although many doctors, other Canadian sources, such as the CPS (Compendium of Pharmaceuticals and Specialties), and most American sources use this terminology at times.

Initially, 75 percent of people with Type 2 diabetes will respond well to sulfonylureas, while biguanides will lower blood sugar in 80 percent of people with Type 2 diabetes. But about 15 percent of all people treated with OHAs fail to respond to them at all, while 3 to 5 percent of all people on OHAs will stop responding to them each year, so don't get too comfortable on these pills.

Dosages for sulfonylureas

There is no fixed dosage for sulfonylureas. It all depends on your brand. If you are taking a dosage higher than the recommended initial dose, indicated in Table 5.1 below, you should divide your dose into two equal parts. Your pills should be taken before or with meals, and your doctor should start you on the lowest, effective dose. If your blood sugar levels are high when you start your pills, it's a good idea to have a short trial period of six to eight weeks to make sure your drug is working.

TABLE 5.1

Most Commonly Prescribed Sulfonylureas

	Daily/mg	Initial	Per Day
**Gliclazide	40–320	160	1–2
**Glyburide	2.5–20	5	1–2
*Tolbutamide	500–3,000	1,000	1–3

*First generation—not prescribed very much. Older first-generation sulfonylureas, such as aceto-hexamide and chloropropamide, are no longer listed in the CPS and have been discontinued.
**Second generation—more commonly prescribed

Source: Compendium of Pharmaceuticals and Specialties, 2000.

Dosage for repaglinide

There is no fixed dosage for repaglinide. Dosing is based on your overall health and your blood sugar pattern (e.g., your rises and dips). Since this is a shorter-acting OHA, if you were previously on a longer-acting OHA, such as chloro-propramide (now discontinued), you must be monitored closely.

Dosages for biguanides (Metformin)

There is only one biguanide available in Canada; it goes by the generic trade name Metformin. In this case, the usual dose is 500 mg three or four times a day or 850 mg two or three times a day. Your dose is not to exceed 2.5 g a day. If you're elderly, a lower dose will probably be prescribed.

When OHAs Should Not Be Used

If you've had Type 2 diabetes for longer than ten years, this is not the time to start OHAs. And, of course, nobody with Type 1 or insulin-dependent diabetes (IDDM) should ever take OHAs; they will not work. OHAs should never be taken under the following conditions either:

- alcoholism
- pregnancy
- kidney or liver failure (Metformin only)

Side effects

Sixty percent of people taking OHAs continue to have high blood sugar levels two hours after meals. These pills can also cause increased appetite and weight gain. However, the main side effect with first-generation OHAs is hypoglycemia (low blood sugar), which occurs in one in five people treated with OHAs. If you're over age 60, hypoglycemia may occur more often, which is why it's dangerous for anyone over age 70 to take certain OHAs.

About one-third of all people taking OHAs will experience gastrointestinal side effects (no appetite, nausea, abdominal discomfort and, with Metformin, diarrhea). Adjusting dosages and taking your pills with your meals or afterward often clears up these symptoms.

Alpha-glucosidase Inhibitors

Introduced in 1996, these pills delay the breakdown of sugar in your meal. Acarbose was the first oral diabetes medication to be introduced since the introduction of sulfonylureas and biguanides in the 1950s. Acarbose goes by the brand name Prandase in Canada and is very similar in structure to the sugars found in foods. Acarbose reduces high blood sugar levels after you eat. Glucose, the main sugar in blood, is a *simple sugar* that is made from starch and sucrose (table sugar). Starch and sucrose are turned into glucose by enzymes in the lining of the small intestine called alpha-glucosidase. Acarbose stalls this process by forcing the starch and sugar you eat to "take a number" before they're converted into glucose. This slows down the absorption of glucose into the cells, preventing a rise in blood glucose after a meal. But in order to work, acarbose must be taken with the first bite of each main meal. You'll also need to test your blood sugar two hours after eating to see how well you're responding to the medication. Research is underway to determine if acarbose can be used worldwide as a preventive for people with impaired glucose tolerance (IGT).

Acarbose is prescribed for people who cannot seem to get their after-meal (that is, postmeal or postprandial) blood sugar levels down to acceptable levels. A major benefit of acarbose is that it may reduce the risk of hypoglycemic episodes during the night, particularly in insulin users. Investigators are studying whether acarbose may be used one day as a substitute for that "morning insulin." The usual rules apply here: Acarbose should complement your meal plan and exercise routine; it is not a substitute or way out, and does not, by itself, cause hypoglycemia.

Who should take acarbose?
- Anyone who cannot control his/her blood sugar through diet and lifestyle modification alone.
- Anyone who is on OHAs but is still experiencing high blood sugar levels after meals.
- Anyone who cannot take OHAs and for whom diet and lifestyle modifications have failed.
- Anyone not doing well on an OHA, but who wants to avoid starting insulin treatment.

Who should not take acarbose?
Anyone with the following conditions should not be taking this drug:

- inflammation or ulceration of the bowel (that is, inflammatory bowel disease, ulcerative colitis or Crohn's disease)
- any kind of bowel obstruction
- any gastrointestinal disease
- kidney or liver disorders

- hernias
- pregnancy or lactation
- Type 1 diabetes

Dosage

The usual starting dosage for acarbose is 25 mg (half of a 50 mg tablet), with the first bite of each main meal. After four to eight weeks, your dosage may be increased to 50 mg, three times a day. Or you may start by taking one 50 mg tablet once daily with supper. If that's not working, you'll move up to two 50 mg tablets twice daily with your main meals or three 50 mg three times daily with main meals. The maximum dosage of acarbose shouldn't go beyond 100 mg three times a day.

For best results, it's crucial that you take acarbose with *the first bite* of each main meal. In fact, if you swallow your pill even five to ten minutes before a meal, acarbose will pass through your digestive system and have no effect. It's also important that you take acarbose with a carbohydrate; the medication doesn't work if there are no carbohydrates in your meal. You shouldn't take acarbose between meals, either, because it won't work. Nor should acarbose be used as a weight-loss drug.

Side effects

The good news is that acarbose doesn't cause hypoglycemia. However, since you may be taking this drug along with an OHA, you may still experience hypoglycemia, as acarbose doesn't prevent it, either. (See the section "Recognizing the Symptoms" in Chapter 14 for warning signs and treatment for hypoglycemia.)

The only side effects that acarbose causes are gastrointestinal: gas, abdominal cramps, softer stools or diarrhea. But acarbose combined with Metformin can produce unacceptable gastrointestinal symptoms. You'll notice these side effects after you've consumed foods that contain lots of sugar. Avoid taking antacids; they won't be effective in this case. Adjusting the dosage and making sure you're taking acarbose correctly will usually take care of the side effects.

Thiazoladinediones (Avandia or Actos)

Thiazoladinediones are pills that make your cells more sensitive to insulin, thereby improving insulin resistance. And when this happens, more glucose gets into your tissues, and less glucose hangs around in your blood. The result is that you'll have lower fasting blood glucose levels, without the need to increase insulin levels. Both rosiglitazone (Avandia) and pioglitazone (Actos) work by stimulating muscle tissue to "drink in" glucose. They also decrease glucose production from the liver and make fat tissue more receptive to glucose. These drugs are reserved for people with Type 2 diabetes who must take insulin to reduce their blood sugar levels.

When the first generation of this drug, troglitazone (Rezulin), was released in 1997, there was great hope that it would be a wonder drug for people with Type 2 diabetes. Unfortunately, several incidents of severe liver damage were associated with Rezulin. In March 1999, the U.S. Food and Drug Administration's Endrocrine and Metabolic Drugs Advisory Committee recommended that only a select group of people with Type 2 diabetes be prescribed Rezulin. But since then, two newer drugs, Avandia and Actos, have been released, which have less risk of severe liver damage. In light of this, Rezulin was withdrawn from the market in March 2000 by its makers, Warner-Lambert Company.

In early studies done with the troglitazone, only 1.9 percent of people in the trial developed mild liver problems. But as soon as the drug was more widely prescribed, the U.S. Food and Drug Administration received reports of several cases of severe liver disease that led to death or the need for a liver transplant. For example, in one case, a 55-year-old woman using insulin and a daily dose of 400 mg of troglitazone for about three months developed liver failure. Avandia, released in Canada in April 2000, and Actos, released in Canada in June 2000, are very similar in chemical structure to troglitazone but seem to have a much lower risk of liver damage than troglitazone. Nevertheless, it's very important to *ask your doctor* about the risks of either drug if they are prescribed. If you've ever had hepatitis (A, B or C), you should not take this drug. A number of other factors in your history may prevent you from being on the drug, which you must discuss with your doctor.

The average starting dose for Avandia is 4 mg per day, but dosages range between 2 and 8 mg. The starting dose for Actos is either 15 mg or 30 mg per day, with a maximum dosage of 45 mg per day.

Other side effects

Trials with troglitazone showed that people with cardiovascular problems or who were immune-suppressed for any reason should not be on it. Therefore, please discuss the risks of Avandia or Actos if you have cardiovascular problems or are immune-suppressed, since the chemical structure of these drugs is similar to troglitazone.

Questions to Ask About Oral Diabetes Medications

Before you fill your prescription, it's important to ask your doctor or pharmacist the following:

1. What does this drug contain? If you are allergic to particular ingredients, such as dyes, it's important to find out the drug's ingredients before you take it.
2. Are there any medications I shouldn't combine with this drug? Be sure to ask about interactions with cholesterol or hypertension medications, as well as any antidepressants or antipsychotics.
3. If this drug doesn't work well, am I a candidate for combination therapy? This means that your drug could be combined with another drug. Common combo platters include a sulfonylurea and biguanide; acarbose and an OHA; a thiazoladinedione and a biguanide. Either the first drug you started is raised to its maximum dosage before the second drug is started at its lowest dosage, or both drugs are started at their lowest dosages and then raised gradually.
4. If this drug doesn't work well, would insulin ever be prescribed along with this pill? It remains controversial whether combining insulin with a pill has any benefits. Nevertheless, some studies have shown that there is some benefit.
5. How will you measure the effectiveness of my drug? You should be testing your blood sugar with a glucose monitor, particularly two hours after eating, to make sure that the lowest effective dose can be prescribed. Your doctor should also be doing a glycosylated hemoglobin or HbA_{1c} test two or three times per year (see above).
6. How should I store my drugs? All pills should be kept in a dry place at a temperature between 15°C and 25°C (59°F and 77°F). Keep these drugs away from children, don't give them out as "samples" to your sister-in-law (or anyone else!) and don't use tablets beyond their expiry date.
7. What symptoms should I watch out for while on these drugs? You'll definitely want to watch for signs of high or low blood sugar.

Natural Alternatives

If you don't like the idea of taking pills to control your diabetes, you can try to incorporate more natural methods to see if you can avoid taking medication.

You'll have to discuss this approach with your doctor, of course, but here are some options:

- *Guar gum.* This is a high source of fibre (which is a polysaccharide—see Glossary) made from the seeds of the Indian cluster bean. When you mix guar with water, it turns into a gummy gel, which slows down your digestive system and is similar in effect to acarbose (see above). Guar has often been used as a natural substance to treat high blood sugar as well as high cholesterol. Guar can cause gas, some stomach ache, nausea and diarrhea. (These are also side effects of acarbose.) The problem with guar is that there are no scientific studies, to date, concluding that it improves blood sugar control. Nevertheless, most experts agree that it can certainly provide some marginal benefits.
- Delay glucose absorption by eating more fibre, avoiding table sugar (sucrose) and eating smaller meals more often to space out your calories. Meal planning is discussed in detail in Chapter 6.

WHEN YOUR DOCTOR PRESCRIBES INSULIN

Let me dispel a common fear about insulin: Since insulin is not a blood product, you don't have to worry about being infected with a blood-borne virus such as HIV or hepatitis.

Many doctors often delay insulin therapy for as long as possible by giving you maximum doses of the pills discussed above. This isn't considered good diabetes management. If you need insulin, you should take insulin. The goal is to get your disease under control. Therefore, anyone with Type 2 diabetes with the following conditions is a candidate for insulin:

- high blood sugar levels, despite maximum doses of oral hypoglycemic agents
- fasting glucose levels consistently over 9 mmol/L
- illness or stress (insulin may be needed until you recover)
- major surgery
- complications of diabetes (see Part 3)
- pregnancy (insulin may be temporary)

If going on insulin will affect your job security, you should discuss this issue with your doctor so that appropriate notes or letters can be drafted to whomever it may concern. You should also keep in mind that if insulin therapy does not bring your diabetes under control within six months of treatment, it may be necessary to return to your oral drug therapy after all.

Most people think insulin needs to be prescribed by a doctor. Doctors will prescribe insulin, but you can walk into any pharmacy, identify yourself as a person with diabetes, and get at least one dosage of insulin over the counter anywhere in Canada. This policy is designed for emergencies, since people can damage or lose insulin while travelling, and so on. Insulin is not a patentable drug, which is one reason it remains an over-the-counter product. It is also not the sort of product that people would want unless they had diabetes. By supplying it over the counter, it remains a life-giving product that is not withheld from those in need; that doesn't mean it's given out free, but it is given out *hassle-free*, without the need to reach your doctor for permission.

The Right Insulin

The goal of a good insulin program is to try to mimic what your pancreas would do if it were working properly. Blood sugar rises in a sort of "wave" pattern. The big waves come in after a big meal; the small waves come in after a small meal or snack. The insulin program needs to be matched to your own particular wave pattern. So what you eat—and when—has a lot to do with the right insulin program. Therefore, the right insulin for someone who eats three square meals a day may not be appropriate for someone who tends to "graze" all day. And the right insulin for an active 47-year-old man in a stressful job may not be the right insulin for a 67-year-old woman who does not work and whose heart condition prevents her from exercising regularly.

You and your health care team will also need to decide how much control you need over your blood sugar. Insulin "recipes" depend on whether you need tight control (4–6 mmol/L), medium control (4–10 mmol/L) and even loose control (11–13 mmol/L). Loose control is certainly not encouraged, but on rare occasions, when a person is perhaps quite elderly and suffering from a number of other health problems, it is still "done." To determine the appropriate insulin recipe for you, your health care team should look at who you are as a person— what you eat, where you work (do you work shifts?), your willingness to change your eating habits and other lifestyle factors.

There are many kinds of insulins available. Every manufacturer has a different brand name of insulin and a separate letter code for the insulin action. To make things as easy to understand as possible, I've provided a table on page 79 with a translation of all these codes. Once you and your diabetes health care team choose the right insulin for you, you will need to have a minicourse on how to use and inject insulin. This is usually done by a certified diabetes educator (CDE).

Insulin Brands

As you can see, insulin is highly individualized. It's simply not possible for me to tell you in this book which insulin you need to be on any more than I can tell you what, exactly, you need to eat each day. This is why a diabetes health care team, discussed in Chapter 3, is so crucial. Your meal plans, medications and insulin (when needed) are tailored to suit *you*. And that has everything to do with who you are, not which brand of insulin is popular. The following is a description of what's available as of this writing.

Human insulin

All human insulin is biosynthetic, which means that the biochemically created "product" normally made by the human pancreas has been recreated in a test tube through DNA technology.

Today, most manufacturers produce only these insulins, which are considered the purest form of insulin available. Human insulins come in four different actions: immediate-acting, short-acting (clear fluid), intermediate-acting (cloudy fluid) and long-acting (cloudy fluid). Short-acting means that it stays in your body for the shortest duration of time; long-acting means that it stays in your body for the longest duration of time. (See Table 5.2, "Getting to Know Your Insulin," for details.)

Insulin lispro

The newest insulin is known as insulin lispro, an insulin analogue ("copycat"). This is a synthetic insulin that does not have an animal or human source. With traditional human insulins, you need to be extremely good at calculating when you're going to eat, how much you're going to eat and how much insulin to inject. Basically, you need to be in excellent control of your diabetes. The problem with traditional, longer-acting insulin is that you can wind up with too much of it in your system, which can cause insulin shock or hypoglycemia (low blood sugar, see Chapter 14). Insulin lispro is an immediate-acting insulin, which means that you inject it about 15 minutes before you eat (while you're cooking dinner or when ordering food in a restaurant). Therefore some experts consider it an easier insulin to work with.

Premixed insulin

Premixed insulin means that both the short-acting insulin and the intermediate-acting insulin are mixed together. These are extremely popular insulins for people with Type 2 diabetes for reasons explained in Table 5.2, "Getting to Know Your Insulin." They work well for people who have a very set routine and don't want to take more than one or two insulin injections daily.

Premixed insulins are labelled as 10/90 (10 percent short-acting; 90 percent intermediate-acting), 20/80, 30/70, 40/60 and 50/50. Premixed insulin is always cloudy. It's also possible to mix together short-acting with long-acting, or long-acting with intermediate-acting.

A word about beef/pork insulin

Eli Lilly still makes pure pork insulin. For information about obtaining it, visit www.diabetes.ca/about_diabetes/animal_insulin.html. The Canadian Diabetes Association frequently tells people that animal insulin is no longer available, but this refers to beef/pork insulin. Animal insulin is never recommended to people newly diagnosed with diabetes, but some people with Type 1 diabetes, who developed a rhythm with their animal insulin years ago and are reluctant to switch to human insulin or an insulin analogue, can still obtain pork insulin as of this writing.

Learning to Use Insulin

Insulin must be injected. It cannot be taken orally because your own stomach acids digest the insulin before it has a chance to work. Your doctor or a registered nurse (frequently a CDE is a registered nurse, too) will teach you how to inject yourself painlessly. Don't inject insulin by yourself without a training session. One convenient way to use insulin is with an insulin pen, but not all insulin can be used with the pen. If you use the pen, your insulin (if human or biosynthetic) will come in a cartridge. If you are not using a pen, your insulin will come in a bottle and you will need a needle and syringe. Always know the answers to these questions before you inject your insulin:

1. How long does it take before the insulin starts to work? (Known as the *onset of action*.)
2. When is this insulin working the hardest? (Known as the *peak*.)
3. How long will my insulin continue to work? (Known as the *duration of action*.)

How many injections will I need?

This really depends on what kind of insulin you're taking and why you're taking it. A sample routine may be to take an injection in the morning, a second injection before supper and a third before bed. What you want to prevent is low blood sugar while you're sleeping. You may need to adjust your insulin if there is a change in your food or exercise routine (which could happen if you're sick). Your insulin schedule is usually carefully matched to your meal times and exercise periods.

Where to inject it

The good news is that you do not have to inject insulin into a vein. As long as it makes it under your skin (but *not* in your muscle) you're fine. This is called a subcutaneous injection. Thighs and tummies are popular injection sites. These areas are also large enough that you can vary your injection site. (You should space your injections 2–3 cm/about an inch apart.) Usually you establish a rotating pattern. Other injection sites are the upper outer area of the arms, the upper outer surfaces of the buttocks and lower back areas. Insulin injected in the abdomen is absorbed more quickly than insulin injected in the thigh. In addition, strenuous exercise will speed up the rate of absorption of insulin if the insulin is injected into the limb you've just "worked out." Other factors that can affect insulin's action is the depth of injection, your dose, the temperature (it should be room temperature or body temperature) and what animal your insulin came from (human or pig). A hardening of skin due to overuse will affect the rate of absorption. Your doctor or CDE will show you how to actually inject your insulin (angles, pinching folds of skin and so on). There are lots of tricks of the trade to optimize comfort. With the fine needle points available today, injection doesn't have to be an uncomfortable ordeal. The needle length also affects the absorption rate; the longer the needle, the deeper it goes, and the faster it's absorbed. With shorter needle lengths, patient advocates with diabetes recommend leaving the needle in for about five seconds to increase the rate of absorption.

Side Effects

The main side effect of insulin therapy is low blood sugar, which means that you must eat or drink glucose to combat symptoms. This side effect is also known as insulin shock. Low blood sugar or hypoglycemia is discussed in Chapter 14.

A rare side effect is *lipodystrophy* (a change in the fatty tissue under the skin) or *hypertrophy* (an enlarged area on your skin). Rotating your injection sites will prevent these problems. A sunken area on your skin surface may also occur, but usually only when using animal insulin. Rashes can sometimes occur at injection sites, too. Less than 5 percent of all insulin users notice these problems.

Questions to Ask About Insulin

The answers to the following questions will depend on your insulin brand. Pharmacists and doctors should know the answers to all these questions, but if they don't, call the customer care 1-800 number provided by your insulin manufacturer.

- How do I store this insulin?
- What are the characteristics of this insulin (that is, onset of action, peak and duration of action)?
- When should I eat after injecting this insulin?
- When should I exercise after injecting this insulin?
- How long are opened insulin bottles or cartridges safe at room temperature?
- What about the effect of sunlight or extreme temperatures on this insulin?
- Should this insulin be shaken or rolled?
- What should I do if the insulin sticks to the inside of the vial or cartridge?
- Should this insulin be clear or cloudy? And what should I do if the appearance looks "off" or has changed?
- What happens if I accidentally inject out-of-date insulin?
- What other medications can interfere with this particular brand?
- Who should I see about switching insulin brands?
- If I've switched from animal to human insulin, what dose should I be on?

Your Insulin Gear

If you've graduated to insulin therapy, here's what you'll need to buy:

- a really good glucose monitor that is made for people who test frequently
- lancets and a lancing device for testing your blood sugar
- insulin pens and cartridges (this is far easier) or traditional needles and syringes (a diabetes educator will need to walk you through the types of products available)
- the right insulin brand for you

Travelling with Insulin

When travelling, you'll need to make sure you pack enough insulin for your trip, as well as identification (a doctor's note) that clearly states you have diabetes, so you don't get harassed over carrying needles, syringes and vials. In fact, many experts suggest that for a trip, you switch to an insulin pen, if you can. (Again, not all insulins work with the pen.) In some cases, even lancets and a glucose meter may be suspect without identification. Experts recommend the following supplies for travel:

- a backup supply of insulin *on you*, as well as extra cartridges, needles, syringes and testing supplies; vials break, baggage gets lost, and planes, trains or buses get delayed
- a doctor's written prescription for your insulin and a doctor's note explaining why you're carrying your equipment
- a Medic Alert tag or card stating that you have diabetes
- a day's supply of food (especially if you're flying)
- an extra sugar source, such as dextrose tablets
- a list of hospitals in your travel-destination areas

It's also important never to part with your insulin; always carry it with you in carry-on baggage. Dividing your supplies between two bags is best in case vials break. If you're flying, drink lots of liquids prior to boarding, as well as one glass of non-alcoholic liquid for every hour of flight. If you've ordered a special meal, keep in mind that these meals have a nasty habit of never making it to the plane; frequently there are not enough regular meals to cover for the mistake. So it's best to stick with the regular meal and pick at it, while bringing your own supply of food to fill in the gaps. You should also stroll up and down the cabin as much as possible to avoid high blood sugar. (This bit of exercise will use up some sugar.) If you're travelling to a different time zone, consult your doctor or diabetes educator about adjusting insulin injections to the new time zone.

TABLE 5.2

Getting to Know Your Insulin

Short-acting Insulin (This is the "hare." It gets there fast but tires easily.)

Starts working in 30 minutes
   (Insulin Lispro or Insulin Aspart: 15–30 minutes)
Peaks in 2–4 hours
   (Insulin Lispro or Insulin Aspart: 30 minutes–2.5 hours)
Duration of action: 6–8 hours
   (Insulin Lispro or Insulin Aspart: 3–4 hours)
When to eat: Within 30 minutes of injecting
   (Insulin Lispro or Insulin Aspart: Within 10 minutes of injecting)
Peak effect
   (maximum action): 1 1/2–5 hours
Exits body in 8 hours
Appearance: Clear. Don't use if cloudy, slightly coloured or if solid chunks
   are visible.

Intermediate-acting Insulin (This is the "tortoise." It gets there at a slower pace, but it lasts longer.)

Starts working in 1–2 hours
Peaks in 4–12 hours (usually around 8 or less)
Duration of action: 24 hours (or less)
When to eat: Within 2 hours
Exits body in 24 hours
Appearance: Cloudy. Do not use if the white material remains at the
   bottom of the bottle after mixing, leaving a clear liquid above; or if
   clumps are floating in the insulin after mixing; or if it has a "frosted"
   appearance.

Long-acting Insulin (This is the "two-legged turtle." It's really slow, and it hangs around for a long time.)

Starts working in 8 hours

Peaks in 18 hours

Duration of action: 36 hours

When to eat: Within 8 hours

Exits body in 36 hours or more

Appearance: Cloudy. Do not use if the white material remains at the bottom of the bottle after mixing, leaving a clear liquid above; or if clumps are floating in the insulin after mixing; or if it has a "frosted" appearance.

Source: "Getting to Know Your Insulin," copyright 1997, 1999, 2001, M. Sara Rosenthal. *For information about brand names, premixed insulins and specific products, consult your doctor, pharmacist, diabetes educator or insulin manufacturer.*

TABLE 5.3

Breaking the Codes

Insulin Lispro: This is an immediate-acting insulin under the brand name Humalog, which starts to work in 15–30 minutes. It is a biosynthetic insulin made from two amino acids, LYS and PRO. It's ideal for people with Type 1 diabetes.

Insulin Aspart: This is an immediate-acting insulin under the brand name NovoRapid, manufactured by Novo Nordisk Canada Inc., which became available in 2001. Like Insulin Lispro, it is ideal for people with Type 1 diabetes. In the United States, Insulin Aspart goes by the brand name Novolog®.

R: This stands for "regular" biosynthetic human insulin. Regular means that it is short-acting insulin.

"ge" Toronto: "ge" is the name Connaught-Novo gives to all of its biosynthetic insulin. It stands for "genetically engineered." Toronto is the brand name of this company's regular insulin, like "Kraft" or "President's Choice."

N or NPH: NPH is simply the initials of the man who invented this type of insulin, which is an intermediate-acting insulin that is said to have an "abrupt" peak. ("ge"-NPH stands for genetically engineered NPH.)

L or Lente: This is also an intermediate-acting insulin that is very similar to NPH except it has a more "lumbering" peak. ("ge"-Lente stands for genetically engineered Lente.)

Novolin ultra "ge": Connaught-Novo's long-acting insulin, which starts acting in 4 hours, peaks within 8–24 hours and exits within 28 hours. Again, "ge" stands for genetically engineered.

Ultra Lente "ge": The same as above except it peaks in 10–30 hours and exits in 36 hours.

Semi Lente-NPH: This is a very long-acting insulin that is rarely used. Most diabetes educators haven't seen someone on this stuff for years!

Beef/Pork: This was animal insulin made from cows or pigs. It's no longer available. Pure pork is still available through Eli Lilly.

Humulin 10/90: This is a premixed insulin, meaning that it is 10% regular and 90% NPH. Also available in 20/80, 30/70, 40/60 and 50/50. (Note: Many people with Type 2 diabetes do well on 30/70.)

Novolin 10/90 "ge": Exactly the same as above, except "ge," which stands for genetically engineered, is the label Connaught-Novo gives to its biosynthetic insulin.

Source: "Breaking the Code," copyright 1997, 1999, 2001, M. Sara Rosenthal.

Chapter 6

HOW SWEET: COUNTING SUGAR, PLANNING MEALS

● ● ● ● ● ● ● ● ● ● ●

The diabetes meal plan is not just for people with diabetes; it's healthy eating that everyone in North America could be following. So when you begin to plan your meals, your entire family will benefit. The results will be that through food, you'll be able to gain control of your condition, while the rest of your family may be able to prevent or delay it.

Only carbohydrates influence blood sugar levels, while cholesterol-containing foods increase blood *fat* levels—cholesterol and triglycerides. What lowers the sugar in your bloodstream are exercise and medications you may be taking, such as oral hypoglycemic pills or insulin. Ideally, by balancing your food with activity, most of you will be able to control your diabetes. How do you know if you're balancing well? And how do you know what to eat so you can create all this balance? That's what this chapter is all about.

A FEW GOOD FOODS

Before the discovery of insulin in 1921, people with diabetes went on the Allen Diet, a very low-calorie diet that required low quantities of carbohydrates, followed by exercise.

Dr. Frederick Madison Allen, a leading diabetologist who spent four years working with diabetic patients at the Rockefeller Institute in New York City, published a 600-plus–page paper in 1919 called "Total Dietary Regulation in the Treatment of Diabetes." Allen's work showed that diabetes was largely a problem of carbohydrate metabolism. He introduced a radical approach to diabetes, the traces of which are apparent in current meal planning. It was known as the starvation treatment, which consisted of fasting followed by a gradual building up of diet. Allen's treatment also included exercise, which is now a vital aspect of diabetes treatment. The idea of emaciated patients fasting and exercising was controversial, but at the time it was the best treatment available without insulin. Although in some cases, Allen's patients did die of starvation, Allen ultimately prolonged the lives of many through his system of dietary regulation. Allen's diets were found to be more tolerable than any of the fad diabetes diets that were popular in Allen's day. Doctors were doing everything from feeding patients with diabetes as much sugar as possible to compensate for the sugar lost in the blood, to putting them on low-carbohydrate diets, which were so unappetizing that most patients wouldn't stick to them. Oatmeal diets, milk diets, rice diets and potato diets were also popular. The most logical diet, however, was the low-carbohydrate diet, which included recipes such as "thrice-boiled vegetables." Although this diet was effective in eliminating sugar from the urine (which produced the same effects as food rationing), it didn't seem to work with patients who had insulin-dependent or Type 1 diabetes.

Allen and his predecessors understood something central to diabetes meal planning: *Carbohydrates were key*. And they are. Allen recognized the ability of carbohydrates to convert into glucose. The timing of this glucose conversion will affect how quickly and how high the blood glucose level rises after eating. But what's changed drastically since the Allen Diet is that variety, quantity and timing of meals are crucial, too.

What to Eat

To live, you need three basic types of foods: carbohydrates, protein and fat. Carbohydrates are the main source of fuel for muscles. Protein is the "cell food" that helps cells grow and repair themselves. Fat is a crucial nutrient that can be burned as an alternative fuel in times of hunger or famine. Simple sugars that do not contain any fat will convert quickly into energy or be stored as fat.

Your body will change carbohydrates into glucose for energy. If you eat more carbohydrates than you can burn, your body will turn the extra into fat. The protein your body makes comes from the protein you eat. As for fats, they are not broken down into glucose and are usually stored as fat. The problem with fatty foods is that they have double the calories per gram compared with carbohydrates and protein, so you wind up gaining weight. Too much saturated fat, as discussed in Chapter 7, can increase your risk of developing cardiovascular problems. What we also know is that the rate at which glucose is absorbed by your body from starch and sugars is affected by other parts of your meal, such as the protein, fibre and fat. If you're eating only carbohydrates and no protein or fat, for example, your blood sugar will go up faster.

The Bad News About Low-Fat Diets

All that said, if you think the key to weight loss is avoiding fat, think again. There is new thinking about what many perceive to be the dangers of low-fat dieting. Not only do they *not* work according to many critics, but they promote insulin resistance. A low-fat diet is a diet in which most of your calories come from carbohydrates rather than protein or fat. Carbohydrates convert into glucose quickly in the body, so you eat, feel full and then feel very hungry again. In order to feel satisfied and satiated, we must have some fat in our diets. But in addition to this, fat in our diets triggers fat-burning compounds in our bodies. Years of conditioning us to no fat has made most people fatter and has dramatically increased our risk of developing Type 2 diabetes because of the amount of insulin we require to "clean up" the carbohydrates that convert so quickly into sugar. And as you know from earlier discussions in this book, higher insulin levels increase your appetite. The best advice now is to limit carbohydrates in each meal to about 40 percent, and be sure to have about 30 percent protein and 30 percent of "helpful" fat. Canadian nutrition guidelines stipulate that your daily intake of protein (animal products) shouldn't exceed 20 percent (British guidelines stipulate 15 percent). The American Diabetes Association guidelines state that a healthy diet should consist mainly of complex carbohydrates (roughly 50 percent) with about 30 percent of your energy from fat—and less than 10 percent from saturated fats. Chapter 7 discusses fat in more detail, but the 40/30/30 breakdown reflects newer thinking.

Variety, Variety, Variety

Variety is the key to a good meal plan. If your meal contains mostly carbohydrates (50 to 55 percent), some protein (15 to 20 percent), not much fat (less than 30 percent) and limited sugar, you're eating well. See Table 6.4, "How Your Food Breaks Down," for some examples of simple and complex carbohydrates, proteins and fat. (I think you know what sugar is, but there are examples provided there, too.) The outside aisles of a supermarket contain the food items you need to eat. It's the middle aisles that have all the extras we don't need.

The Glycemic Index

The glycemic index (GI) shows the rise in blood sugar from various carbohydrates. Therefore, planning your diet using the GI can help you control your blood sugar by using more foods with a low GI and fewer foods with a high GI. Encouraging people with IGT or Type 2 diabetes to use the GI is now recommended by the Canadian Diabetes Association in its latest position statement regarding new guidelines for nutritional management of Type 2 diabetes.

TABLE 6.1

The Glycemic Index at a Glance

This glycemic index, developed at the University of Toronto, measures the rate at which various foods convert to glucose, which is assigned a value of 100. Higher numbers indicate a more rapid absorption of glucose. This is not an exhaustive list and should be used as a sample only. This is not an index of food energy values or calories; some low GI foods are high in fat, while some high GI foods are low in fat. Keep in mind, too, that these values differ depending on what else you're eating with that food and how the food is prepared.

Sugars

Glucose = 100	Honey = 87
Table sugar = 59	Fructose = 20

Snacks

Mars bar = 68	Potato chips = 51
Sponge cake = 46	Fish sticks = 38
Tomato soup = 38	Sausages = 28
Peanuts = 13	

Cereals

Corn Flakes = 80	Shredded wheat = 67
Muesli = 66	All Bran = 51
Oatmeal = 49	

Breads

Whole wheat = 72	White = 69
Buckwheat = 51	

Fruits

Raisins = 64

Orange juice = 46

Apple = 39

Banana = 62

Orange = 40

Dairy Products

Ice cream = 36

Milk = 34

Yogurt = 36

Skim milk = 32

Root Vegetables

Parsnips = 97

Instant mashed potatoes = 80

Beets = 64

Sweet potato = 48

Carrots = 92

New boiled potato = 70

Yam = 51

Pasta and Rice

White rice = 72

Spaghetti (white) = 50

Brown rice = 66

Spaghetti (whole wheat) = 42

Legumes

Frozen peas = 51

Chickpeas = 36

Butter beans = 36

Green beans = 31

Lentils = 29

Baked beans = 40

Lima beans = 36

Black-eyed peas = 33

Kidney beans = 29

Dried soybeans =15

Source: Adapted from David Drum and Terry Zierenberg, R.N., CDE, *The Type 2 Diabetes Sourcebook.* (Los Angeles: Lowell House, 1998), p. 130. Used with Permission.

How Much to Eat

Meal plans recommended by registered dietitians are tailored to your individual goals and medication regimen. Men and women will usually require different quantities of food. The goal is to keep the supply of glucose consistent by spacing out your meals, snacks and activity levels accordingly. If you lose weight, your body will use insulin more effectively, but not all people with Type 2 diabetes need to lose weight. If you're on insulin, meals will have to be timed to match your insulin's peak. A dietitian can be helpful by prescribing an individualized meal plan that addresses your specific needs (weight control, shiftwork, travel, etc.).

Anatomy of a Carbohydrate

Carbohydrates are like people; they can be simple or complex. Simple carbohydrates are found in any food that has natural sugar (honey, fruits, juices, vegetables, milk) and anything that contains table sugar or sucrose.

Complex carbohydrates are more sophisticated foods that are made up of larger molecules, such as grain foods, starches and foods high in fibre. The fibre foods, both soluble and insoluble (an important distinction), such as cereals, oatmeal, or legumes, are discussed in Chapter 7.

All About Sugar

Sugars are found naturally in many foods you eat. Sucrose and glucose (table sugar), fructose (fruits and vegetables), lactose (milk products) and maltose (flours and cereals) are all naturally occurring sugars. What you have to watch out for is *added sugar*; these are sugars that manufacturers add to foods during processing or packaging. Foods containing fruit juice concentrates, invert sugar, regular corn syrup, honey or molasses, hydrolyzed lactose syrup or high-fructose corn syrup (made out of highly concentrated fructose through the hydrolysis of starch) all have added sugars. Many people don't realize, however, that pure, *unsweetened* fruit juice is still a potent source of sugar, even when it contains no added sugar. Extra lactose, dextrose and maltose are also contained in many of your foods. In other words, the products may have naturally occurring sugars anyway, and then *more* sugar is thrown in to enhance consistency, taste and so on. With the exception of lactose, which breaks down into glucose and galactose, all of these added sugars break down into fructose and glucose during digestion. To the body, no one sugar is more nutritional than the other; everything is broken down into either single sugars (called monosaccharides) or double sugars (called disaccharides), which are carried to cells through the bloodstream. See Table 6.2, "Sugar on the Table," for the complete sugar breakdown. The best way to know how much sugar is in a product is to look at the nutritional label for carbohydrates.

However, *how fast* that sugar is ultimately broken down and enters the bloodstream greatly depends on the amount of fibre in your food, how much protein you've eaten and how much fat accompanies the sugar in your meal. Theoretically, while the Canadian Diabetes Association guidelines allow you to substitute relative quantities of table sugar for starch, fruit or milk in your meal plan (e.g., one bread slice equals 15 mL/3 tsp. of sugar; one orange equals 10 mL/2 tsp. of sugar), substituting may be a tricky balancing act you'll need to discuss with your dietitian.

As far as your body is concerned, all sugars are nutritionally equal. Honey and table sugar, for instance, are nutritionally comparable. Ultimately, all the sugars from the foods you eat wind up as glucose; your body doesn't know whether the sugar started out as maltose from whole grain breads or lactose from milk products. Glucose then travels through your bloodstream to provide energy. If you have enough energy already, the glucose is stored as fat for later use. Different forms of sugars and starches (in equal "doses") affect blood sugar differently because of the time involved in conversion to glucose. Different forms of carbohydrates are converted at different rates, so it's important to discuss sugar conversion with your dietitian.

Why is sugar added?

Sugar is added to food because it can change consistencies of foods and, in some instances, act as a preservative, as in jams and jellies. Sugars can increase the boiling point or reduce the freezing point in foods; sugars can add bulk and density, and make baked goods do wonderful things, including helping yeast to ferment. Sugar can also add moisture to dry foods, making them "crisp," or balance acidic tastes found in foods like tomato sauce or salad dressing. Invert sugar is used to prevent sucrose from crystallizing in candy, while corn syrup is used for the same purpose.

Since the 1950s, a popular natural sugar in North America has been fructose, which has replaced sucrose in many food products in the form of high-fructose syrup (HFS), made from corn. HFS was developed in response to high sucrose prices and is very cheap to make. In other parts of the world, the equivalent of high-fructose syrup is made from whatever starches are local, such as rice, tapioca, wheat or cassava. According to the International Food Information Council in Washington, D.C., the average North American consumes about 37 g of fructose daily.

GOING SHOPPING

Food shopping can be daunting because most foods are not purely carbohydrate, protein, fat or sugar, but often a mixture of two or three. That's where the Canadian Diabetes Association Food Choice Values and Symbols come in.

Instead of forcing you to eyeball the ingredients of your foods, the categories and symbols in "The Food Choice Values System" section on the following page are designed to do this for you. If you can count, you can plan a meal that has everything you need. A good meal plan will ensure that you are getting enough nutrients to meet your body's needs, and that your food is spread out over the course of the day. For example, if your meal plan allots for three meals with one or two snacks, meals should be spaced four to six hours apart so your body isn't overwhelmed. A meal plan should also help you to eat consistently rather than bingeing one day and starving the next.

A good meal plan will also ensure that you're getting the vitamins and minerals you need without taking supplements, such as iron, calcium, folic acid, vitamins A, B_1, B_2, B_3, C, D and E. By consuming a variety of foods from each of the four food groups (in Canada's Food Guide) at every meal, you'll be meeting your vitamin and mineral requirements.

GOLDEN RULES OF DIABETES MEAL PLANS

▶ Eat three meals a day at fairly regular times (spaced four to six hours apart).

▶ Ask your dietitian to help you plan your meals and snacks.

▶ Try to eat a variety of foods each day from all food groups.

▶ Learn how to gauge serving sizes, volume of bowls and glasses, and so on.

▶ Ask your dietitian or diabetes educator about how to adjust your diet if you're travelling. (This depends on whether you're on medication, where you're going, what foods will be available, and so on.)

▶ Draw up a sick days plan with your dietitian (see Chapter 4, "Adjusting Your Routine When You're Sick). This special plan will depend on what your regular meal plan includes.

▶ Ask about any meal supplements, such as breakfast bars, sports bars or meal-replacement drinks. How will these figure into your meal plan?

▶ Choose lower fat foods more often. (See Chapter 7.)

The Food Choice Values System

The first thing you need to learn before you shop for food is the Food Choice Values and Symbols System, developed by the Canadian Diabetes Association, which will tell you how various foods can be incorporated into your meal plan. The CDA has created seven symbols (colour- and shape-coded) to represent various food groups. (Many of these food categories are a combination of carbohydrates, protein or fat).

 Starch Choice (breads, grains, cereals, pasta, corn, rice, potato)
1 Starch Choice contains 15 g carbohydrate (CHO) and 2 g protein.

 Fruits and Vegetables Choice (all fruits and sweet vegetables, such as squash, carrots or peas)
1 Fruits and Vegetables Choice contains 10 g CHO and 1 g protein.

 Milk Choice (all milk and yogurt products; cheese not included)
1 skim milk choice contains 6 g CHO, 4 g protein and 0 g fat.
1 1% milk choice contains 6 g CHO, 4 g protein and 1 g fat.
1 2% milk choice contains 6 g CHO, 4 g protein and 2 g fat.
1 homogenized milk choice contains 6 g CHO, 4 g protein and 4 g fat.

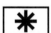 Sugars Choice (sweet)
1 Sugar Choice contains 10 g CHO.

 Protein Choice (all lean meats, poultry, fish, eggs and cheeses)
1 Protein Choice contains 7 g protein and 3 g fat.

 Fats and Oils Choice (anything high in fat, including butter, fatty meats, any oils and so on)
1 Fats and Oils Choice contains 5 g fat.

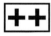 Extras (all low-calorie foods such as leafy greens, herbs and spices, artificially sweetened and/or zero-calorie foods, all cruciferous veggies such as broccoli and a few others)
All Extras have no more than 2.5 g CHO and 60 kilojoules (14 calories) energy.

*Canadian Diabetes Association Food Choice Values and Symbols, Copyright 1999. Used by permission of the Canadian Diabetes Association.

Your dietitian or diabetes educator will work with you to create an individual meal plan using food choices within the above food groups. One person, for example, may need eight starch choices daily while another person may need six. I cannot tell you in this book how many choices you can have; I can only explain how the foods are categorized.

A wide assortment of packaged goods have the CDA symbol on their labels to provide information for people with diabetes; this is not a legal requirement, however. Food manufacturers ask the Canadian Diabetes Association to assign the appropriate CDA Food Choice Symbols. Consumers often assume that CDA symbols mean that the product is better or more nutritious than products that do not carry those symbols. This assumption is false. CDA symbols on food packages are equivalent to the Braille symbols on elevator buttons; they're a courtesy to people with diabetes to assist in meal planning—that's all.

The Outside Aisles

What you need to live is usually found on the outside aisles of any supermarket or grocery store. Outside aisles stock the foods you can buy at outdoor markets: fruits, vegetables, meat, eggs, fish, breads and dairy products. Natural fibre (both soluble and insoluble), discussed in Chapter 7, is also found in the outside aisles. (See the categories and symbols in Table 6.4, "How Your Food Breaks Down," for a list of foods high in fibre.)

But remember: Foods you buy in the outside aisles can also be high in fat unless you select wisely, as discussed in Chapter 7.

The Inside Aisles

These are not only the aisles of temptation; they may also have complicated food labels. In Canada, ingredients on labels are listed according to weight, with the "most" listed first. If sugar is the first ingredient, you know the product contains mostly sugar. The lower sugar is on the list, the less sugar in the product. The nutrition information on the label should also list the total amount of carbohydrates in a *serving* of the food. That amount includes both natural and added sugars, as well as fibre, which is not digested by the body.

Planning to pick up some cough syrup for that cold of yours when you hit the pharmacy section? How about vitamin pills? Check the sugar content first. Your pharmacist will recommend a sugar-free remedy.

Whenever a product says it is "calorie-reduced" or "carbohydrate-reduced" it means there are 50 percent fewer calories or carbohydrates compared to the original product. But something that was originally 7,000 calories isn't much better at 3,500!

"Cholesterol-free" or "low cholesterol" means that the product doesn't have any, or much, animal fat (hence, cholesterol). This doesn't mean "low fat." Pure vegetable oil doesn't come from animals, but it is pure fat!

A label that screams "Low Fat" means that the product has less than 3 g of fat per serving. In potato-chip country, one serving means about six potato chips. (I don't know anybody who ever ate one serving of potato chips!) So if you eat the whole bag of "low-fat" chips, you're still eating a lot of fat. Be sure to check serving sizes.

"Light" (or Lite) product labels mean that there is 25 to 50 percent less of some ingredient in that product. It could be fat, cholesterol, salt, or sugar, or less food colouring, and therefore the designation is frequently misleading.

"Sugar-free"

Careful! Sugar-free in the language of labels simply means "sucrose-free." That doesn't mean the product is *carbohydrate-free*, as in dextrose-free, lactose-free, glucose-free or fructose-free. Check the labels for all ingredients ending in "ose" to find out the sugar content; you're not just looking for sucrose. Watch out for "no added sugar," "without added sugar" or "no sugar added." This simply means "We didn't put the sugar in, God did." Again, reading the number of carbohydrates on the nutrition information label is the most accurate way to find out the amount of sugar in the product. Nutrition claims in big, bold statements can be misleading.

Born in the U.S.A.

Labels on food produced in the United States that say "sugar-free" contain less than 0.5 g of sugars per serving, while a "reduced-sugar" food contains at least 25 percent less sugar per serving than the regular product. If the label also states that the product is not a reduced- or low-calorie food, or if it is not for weight control, it's got enough sugar in there to make you think twice.

Serving sizes in the United States are also listed differently. Foods that are similar are given the same *type* of serving size defined by the U.S. Food and Drug Administration (FDA). That means that five cereals that all weigh X g per cup will share the same serving sizes.

Calories (how much energy) and calories from fat (how much fat) are also listed per serving of food in the United States. Total carbohydrate, dietary fibre, sugars, other carbohydrates (which means starches), total fat, saturated fat, cholesterol, sodium, potassium, and vitamin and minerals are given in Percent Daily values, based on the 2,000-calorie diet recommended by the U.S. government. (In Canada, Recommended Nutrient Intake [RNI] is used for vitamins and minerals.)

TABLE 6.2
Sugar on the Table

What's in a sugar?

Fructose: a monosaccharide or single sugar. It combines with glucose to form sucrose and is one and a half times sweeter than sucrose.

Glucose: a monosaccharide or single sugar. It combines with fructose to form sucrose. It can also combine with glucose to form maltose, and with galactose to form lactose. It is slightly less sweet than sucrose.

High-fructose corn syrup (HFCS): a liquid mixture of about equal parts glucose and fructose from cornstarch. It has the same sweetness as sucrose.

Sucrose: a disaccharide or double sugar made of equal parts of glucose and fructose. Known as table or white sugar, sucrose is found naturally in sugar cane and sugar beets.

SWEETENERS

We gravitate toward sweet flavours because we start out with the slightly sweet taste of breast milk. A product can be sweet without containing a drop of sugar, thanks to the invention of artificial sugars and sweeteners. Artificial sweeteners will not affect your blood sugar levels because they do not contain sugar; they may contain a few calories, however. It depends on whether that sweetener is classified as nutritive or non-nutritive.

Nutritive sweeteners have calories or contain natural sugar. White or brown table sugar, molasses, honey and syrup are all considered nutritive sweeteners. *Sugar alcohols* (see below) are also nutritive sweeteners because they are made from fruits or produced commercially from dextrose. Sorbitol, mannitol, xylitol and maltitol are all sugar alcohols. Sugar alcohols contain only 4 calories per gram, like ordinary sugar, and will affect your blood sugar levels like ordinary sugar. How much sugar alcohols affect your blood sugar levels all depends on how much is consumed, and the degree of absorption from your digestive tract.

Non-nutritive sweeteners are sugar substitutes or artificial sweeteners; they do not have any calories and will not affect your blood sugar levels. Examples of non-nutritive sweeteners are saccharin, cyclamate, aspartame, sucralose and acesulflame potassium.

TABLE 6.3
Acceptable Daily Intake for Sweeteners

Sweetener	Intake based on mg/kg body weight
Aspartame	40
Ace-K	15
Cyclamate	11
Saccharin	5
Sucralose	9*

*Note: Outside Canada, this figure reads 15.

Source: Canadian Diabetes Association, "Guidelines for the Nutritional Management of Diabetes Mellitus in the New Millennium. A Position Statement." Reprinted from *Canadian Journal of Diabetes Care* 23 (3): 56–69.

The Sweetener Wars

The oldest non-nutritive sweetener is saccharin, which is what you get when you purchase Sweet'n Low or Hermesetas. In Canada, saccharin can be used as a tabletop sweetener only in either tablet or powder form. Saccharin is 300 times sweeter than sucrose (table sugar), but has a metallic aftertaste. At one point in the 1970s, saccharin was also thought to cause cancer, but this link was never proven.

In the 1980s, aspartame was invented; it is sold as NutraSweet. It was considered a nutritive sweetener because it was derived from natural sources (two amino acids, aspartic acid and phenylalanine), which means that aspartame is digested and metabolized the same way as any other protein foods. Every gram of aspartame has 4 calories, but since aspartame is 200 times sweeter than sugar, you don't need very much of it to achieve the desired sweetness. In at least 90 countries, aspartame is found in more than 150 product categories, including breakfast cereals, beverages, desserts, candy and gum, syrups, salad dressings, and various snack foods. Here's where it gets confusing: aspartame is also available as a tabletop sweetener under the brand names Equal and, most recently, PROSWEET. An interesting point about aspartame is that it's not recommended for baking or any other recipe where heat is required. The two amino acids in it separate with heat and the product loses its sweetness. That's not to say it's harmful if heated, but your recipe won't turn out.

For the moment, aspartame is considered safe for everybody, including people with diabetes, pregnant women and children. The only people who are cautioned against consuming it are those with a rare hereditary disease known as phenylke-tonuria (PKU) because aspartame contains phenylalanine, which people with PKU cannot tolerate.

Another common tabletop sweetener is sucralose, sold as Splenda. Splenda is a white crystalline powder actually made from sugar itself. It's 600 times sweeter than table sugar, but is not broken down in your digestive system, so it has no calories at all. Splenda can also be used in hot or cold foods and is found in hot and cold beverages, frozen foods, baked goods and other packaged foods.

In the United States, you can still purchase cyclamate, a non-nutritive sweetener sold under the brand name Sucaryl or Sugar Twin. Cyclamate is also the sweetener used in many weight-control products and is 30 times sweeter than table sugar, with no aftertaste. Cyclamate is fine for hot or cold foods. In Canada, however, you can find cyclamate only as Sugar Twin or as a sugar substitute in medication.

The Newest Sweeteners

The newest addition to the sweetener industry is acesuflame potassium (Ace-K), approved by Health Canada in the late 1990s. About 200 times sweeter than table sugar, Ace-K is sold as Sunett and is found in beverages, fruit spreads, baked goods, dessert bases, tabletop sweeteners, hard candies, chewing gum and breath fresheners. While no specific studies on Ace-K and diabetes have been done, the only people who are cautioned against ingesting Ace-K are those on a potassium-restricted diet or people who are allergic to sulpha drugs.

Researchers at the University of Maryland have discovered another sweetener that can be specifically designed for people with diabetes. This sweetener would be based on D-tagatose, a hexose sugar found naturally in yogurt, cheese or sterilized milk. The beauty of this ingredient is that D-tagatose has no effect on insulin levels or blood sugar levels in people both with and without diabetes. Experts believe that D-tagatose is similar to acarbose (see Chapter 5) in that it delays the absorption of carbohydrates.

D-tagatose looks identical to fructose and has about 92 percent of the sweetness of sucrose, except only 25 percent of it will be metabolized. Currently,

D-tagatose is being developed as a bulk sweetener. As of this writing, it is a few years away from being marketed and sold as a brand-name sweetener.

Stevia

Stevia is a natural, non-fattening sweetener that is 30 to 100 times sweeter than sugar, without any of the aftertaste that is common in many sugar substitutes. It is a herb that has been used in Paraguay and Brazil as a natural sweetener for centuries. It is declared safe to use in Japan and is commonly found in soy sauce, chewing gum and mouthwash. Stevia also is high in chromium (a mineral that helps to regulate blood sugar); is a high source of manganese, potassium, selenium, silicon, sodium and vitamin A; and contains iron, niacin, phosphorus, riboflavin, thiamine, vitamin C and zinc.

There has been an explosion of interest in stevia because it is a natural alternative to sugar that contains many nutrients to boot. Stevia is not approved as a sweetener by the U.S. FDA; instead it is legal only as a "dietary supplement." It also remains unapproved as a "food additive" in the United States. Stevia is available in Canada as a herbal product but is not officially approved as a sweetener or food additive by Health Canada, Agrafood Canada or the Canadian Diabetes Association. Please consult with your diabetes educator about the safety of stevia in your meal planning.

Sugar alcohols

Not to be confused with alcoholic beverages, sugar alcohols are nutritive sweeteners, like regular sugar. They are found naturally in fruits or are manufactured from carbohydrates. Sorbitol, mannitol, xylitol, maltitol, maltitol syrup, lactitol, isomalt and hydrogenated starch hydrolysates are all sugar alcohols. In your body, these types of sugars are absorbed lower down in the digestive tract and will cause gastrointestinal symptoms if you use too much. Because sugar alcohols are absorbed more slowly, they were once touted as ideal for people with diabetes, but since they are a carbohydrate, they still increase your blood sugar, just like regular sugar. Now that artificial sweeteners are on the market in abundance, the only real advantage of sugar alcohols is that they don't cause cavities. The bacteria in your mouth don't like sugar alcohols as much as real sugar.

According to the FDA, even foods that contain sugar alcohols can be labelled "sugar-free." Sugar alcohol products can also be labelled "Does not promote tooth decay," which is often confused with "low-calorie."

AT THE LIQUOR STORE

The one thing missing from the CDA food choices is alcohol. As a food choice, alcohol is as fattening as a Fats & Oils choice (see Table 6.4, "How Your Food Breaks Down"), delivering about 7 calories per gram or 150 calories per drink. Many people with diabetes think they have to avoid alcohol completely because it converts into glucose. This is not so. Alcohol *alone* doesn't increase blood sugar since alcohol cannot be turned into glucose. It's the sugar *in* that alcoholic beverage that can affect your blood sugar level. The problem with alcohol is that it's so darned fattening, something people with Type 2 diabetes may need to watch for. That said, alcohol has been proven to raise your "good" cholesterol (HDL). This fact was discovered in the late 1980s when researchers probed why France, with all its rich food, had such low rates of heart disease. It was the wine; red wine, in particular, was shown to decrease the risk of cardiovascular disease. But any alcohol will do this, so it's okay to drink this stuff, so long as *you plan for it* with your dietitian, discuss it with your doctor and *count it* as an actual food choice.

It's crucial to note that alcohol can cause hypoglycemia (low blood sugar) if you're on oral hypoglycemic agents or insulin. Please discuss the effects of alcohol and hypoglycemia with your health care team.

Fine Wine

Dry wines that are listed as (0), meaning no added sugar (in Ontario and British Columbia), or "dry" are fine to ingest if you are diabetic. Wine is the result of natural sugar in fruits or fruit juices fermenting. Fermentation is a process in which natural sugar is converted into alcohol. A glass of dry red or white wine has calories (discussed below) but no sugar. And unless extra sugar is added to the wine, there's no way that alcohol will change back into sugar, even in your digestive tract. The same thing goes for cognac, brandy and dry sherry that contain no sugar.

On the other hand, a sweet wine listed as (3) in Ontario or British Columbia means that it contains 3 g of sugar per 100 mL or 3.5-oz. portion. Dessert wines or ice wines are really sweet; they contain about 15 percent sugar or 10 g of sugar for a 60 mL (2-oz.) serving. Sweet liqueurs are 35 percent sugar.

A glass of dry wine with your meal adds about 100 calories, or the equivalent calories of fat or oil. Half soda water and half wine (a spritzer) contains half the calories. When you cook with wine, the alcohol evaporates, leaving only the flavour. If your wine has no sugar, it counts as two Fats & Oils choices. If it has sugar, it counts as a Sugars choice plus two Fat & Oils choices (see Table 6.4, "How Your Food Breaks Down").

At the Pub

If you're a beer drinker, you're basically having some corn, barley and a couple of teaspoons of malt sugar (maltose) when you have a bottle of beer. The corn and barley ferment into mostly alcohol and some maltose. Calorie-wise, that's about 150 calories per bottle plus 15 mL (3 tsp.) of malt sugar. Beer can be defined as one Sugar plus Fats & Oils choice.

A light beer has fewer calories but contains at least 100 calories per bottle. De-alcoholized beer still has sugar and counts as two Fruits & Vegetables choices.

The Hard Stuff

The stiffer the drink, the fatter it gets. Hard liquors such as scotch, rye, gin and rum are made out of cereal grains—the grains ferment into alcohol; vodka, the Russian staple, is made out of potatoes. Hard liquor averages about 40 percent alcohol, but has no sugar. Nevertheless, you're looking at about 100 calories per small shot glass, so long as you don't add fruit juice, tomato or clamato juice, or sugary soft drinks. As bizarre as it sounds, a Bloody Mary or Bloody Caesar is actually a Fruits & Vegetables choice: potatoes and tomatoes!

The Glycogen Factor

If you recall from Chapter 1, glycogen is the stored sugar your liver keeps handy for emergencies. If your blood sugar needs a boost, the liver will tap into its glycogen stores and convert it into glucose. Alcohol in the liver *blocks* this conversion process. So, if you've been exercising and then go out with friends for a few drinks, unless you've eaten something after your exercise, you may need that glycogen. If you drink to the point of feeling tipsy, that glycogen can be cut off by the alcohol, causing hypoglycemia. What complicates matters even more is that your hypoglycemia symptoms can mimic drunkenness. This glycogen problem can affect people with either Type 1 or Type 2 diabetes because it can result when either insulin or oral hypoglycemic agents are used. (See Chapter 14 for details on hypoglycemia, and below for the alcohol and diabetes rules.)

Don't Drink and Starve

If you're going to drink, *eat*! Always have food with your alcohol. Food delays absorption of alcohol into the bloodstream, providing you with carbohydrates and therefore preventing hypoglycemia.

Diabetes experts also recommend the following:

- Avoid alcohol when your blood sugar is high.
- Remember that two drinks a day is fine for someone with a healthy liver, but less is recommended for liver health.
- Choose dry wines or alcoholic beverages with no sugar. (Or rum and diet cola rather than rum and cola.)
- Remember that juice has sugar, even tomato and clamato juice.
- Never substitute alcohol for food if you're taking insulin or pills.
- Don't be afraid to ask your dietitian about how to count your favourite wine or cocktail as a food choice. Again, as long as it's planned for, it's fine.
- Talk to your doctor about how to safely balance alcohol and insulin, and alcohol and oral hypoglycemic agents.

TABLE 6.4

How Your Food Breaks Down

Complex Carbohydrates (digests more slowly)	Defined by CDA
fruits*	Fruits & Vegetables
vegetables* (corn, potatoes, etc.)	Fruits & Vegetables or Starch or Extras
grains (breads, pastas and cereals)	Starch
legumes (dried beans, peas and lentils)	Starch

*Note: The following vegetables and herbs are Extra: artichokes, asparagus, mushrooms, bean sprouts, okra, onions, parsley, peppers, radish, celery, rapini, cucumber, shallots, eggplant, endive, tomato, kohlrabi, zucchini.

Simple Carbohydrates (digests quickly)	Defined by CDA
*fruits/fruit juices	Fruits & Vegetables or Extra
sugars (sucrose, fructose, etc.)	Sugars or Starch
honey	Sugars or Starch
corn syrup	Sugars or Starch
sorghum	Sugars or Starch
date sugar	Sugars or Starch
molasses	Sugars or Starch
lactose	Milk

*Note: Lemon and lime juice are Extra. So are artificial sweeteners, clear coffee and tea.

Proteins (digests slowly)	**Defined by CDA**
*lean meats	Protein
*fatty meats	Fats & Oils + Protein
poultry	Protein
fish	Protein
eggs	Protein
low-fat cheese	Protein
high-fat cheese	Fats & Oils + Protein
legumes	Starch
grains	Starch

*Note: Bouillon, broth and consommé are Extra. So are garlic, mustard, vinegar, herbs and spices, Worcestershire sauce, uncreamed horseradish and soy sauce.

Fats (digests slowly)	**Defined by CDA**
high-fat dairy products (butter and cream)	Fats & Oils
oils	Fats & Oils
(canola, corn, olive, safflower, sunflower)	
lard	Fats & Oils
avocados	Fats & Oils
olives	Fats & Oils
nuts	Fats & Oils
fatty meats	Fats & Oils

Fibre (doesn't digest; goes through you)	**Defined by CDA**
whole-grain breads	Starch
cereals (e.g., oatmeal)	Starch
all fruits	Fruits & Vegetables
legumes (beans and lentils)	Starch + Protein
leafy greens	Extras
cruciferous vegetables	Extras

Source: "How Your Food Breaks Down" copyright 1997, 1999, 2001, M. Sara Rosenthal.

TABLE 6.5

Commonly Used U.S. and Canadian Nutrient Claim Comparisons

Claim	U.S.	Canada
"Low Calorie"	40 calories or less per serving	50 percent less energy than a regular product and 15 calories or fewer per serving
"Low Fat"	3 g of fat or less per serving	3 g of fat or less per serving
"Low Cholesterol"	20 mg of cholesterol or less per serving (in addition to saturated fat and total fat restrictions)	20 mg of cholesterol or less per serving (in addition to the saturated fat restrictions only)

TABLE 6.6

Comparing the U.S. and Canadian Food Group Systems

American Diabetes Association	Canadian Diabetes Association
Exchange System	Choice System
1 Starch	1 Starch
1 Fruit	1 1/2 Fruits & Vegetables
1 Vegetable	1 1/2 Fruits & Vegetables
1 Milk	2 Milk
(No equal food group)	Sugars
1 Lean Meat	1 Protein
1 Fat	1 Fats & Oils
Free Foods	Extras

Chapter 7

LOW FAT AND HEALTHY EATING

• • • • • • • • • •

Meal planning will necessarily get you thinking about low fat and healthy eating. And with all the information we are bombarded with daily on low-fat products and diets, it can get pretty confusing. This chapter tells you what you need to know about fat. Reducing your intake of certain fats, and increasing your intake of others, can dramatically reduce the risk of cardiovascular disease, one of the chief complications of Type 2 diabetes. Studies show that reducing dietary fat may also prevent various cancers, such as colorectal and estrogen-dependent cancers such as breast cancer.

When you begin to conscientiously eat a balanced diet and reduce your fat intake, you'll notice that you're much more aware of the "organic matter" that goes into your mouth, be it animal, vegetable or mineral. Almost without exception, people who adopt a lower-fat diet will begin to incorporate less of the animal and more of the vegetable into their diets. This, by itself, makes a significant contribution to the environment (see "The Costs of High-Fat Eating" below). And once you begin to eat more fruits and vegetables, you may want to know whether they are organically grown or laden with pesticides. Therefore, this chapter includes information on organic produce. (And don't forget, many of those animals we eat are grazing on pesticides, which remain in their fat, which then winds up in ours!)

Yet despite all the information you may read here, you may be unable to change your eating habits. That's because you may not fully understand *why* you're eating. I recommend you review Chapter 10 for some insights into our eating behaviours.

THE SKINNY ON FAT

Fat is technically known as *fatty acids*, which are crucial nutrients for our cells. We cannot live without fatty acids, or fat. Fat is therefore a good thing—in moderation. But like all good things, most of us want too much of it. Excess dietary fat is by far the most damaging element in the Western diet. A gram of fat contains twice the calories as the same amount of protein or carbohydrate. Decreasing the fat in your diet and replacing it with more grain products, vegetables and fruits is the best way to lower your risk of cardiovascular problems and many other diseases. Fat in the diet comes from meats, dairy products and vegetable oils. Other sources of fat include coconuts (60 percent fat), peanuts (78 percent fat) and avocados (82 percent fat). There are different kinds of fatty acids in these sources of fats: saturated, unsaturated and trans-fatty acids (a.k.a. transfat), which is like a saturated fat in disguise. Some fats are harmful while others are considered beneficial to your health.

Understanding fat is a complicated business. This section explains everything you need to know about fat, and a few things you probably don't *want* to know but should.

Saturated Fat

Saturated fat is solid at room temperature and stimulates cholesterol production in your body. In fact, the way the fat looks prior to ingesting it is the way it will look when it lines your arteries. Foods high in saturated fat include processed meats, fatty meats, lard, butter, margarine, solid vegetable shortening, chocolate and tropical oils (coconut oil is more than 90 percent saturated). Saturated fat should be consumed only in very low amounts.

Unsaturated Fat

Unsaturated fat is partially solid or liquid at room temperature. This group of fats includes monounsaturated fats, polyunsaturated fats and omega-3 oils (a.k.a. fish oil), which protect you against heart disease (see below). Sources of unsaturated fats include vegetable oils (canola, safflower, sunflower, corn) and seeds and nuts. To make it easy to remember, unsaturated fats, with the exception of tropical oils, such as coconut, come from plants. The more liquid the fat, the more polyunsaturated it is, which, in fact, *lowers* your cholesterol levels. However, if you have familial hyperlipidemia (high cholesterol), which often occurs alongside diabetes, unsaturated fat may not make a difference in your cholesterol levels.

What Is a Triglyceride?

Each fat molecule is a link chain made up of glycerol, carbon atoms and hydrogen atoms. The more hydrogen atoms that are on that chain, the more saturated or solid the fat. If you looked at each fat molecule carefully, you'd find three different kinds of fatty acids on it: saturated (solid), monounsaturated (less solid, with the exception of olive and peanut oils) and polyunsaturated (liquid) fatty acids, or three fatty acids plus glycerol, chemically known as triglycerides (see Chapter 2).

The liver breaks down fat molecules by secreting bile, which is stored in the gallbladder (the gallbladder's sole function). The liver also makes cholesterol (see Chapter 2). Too much saturated fat may cause your liver to overproduce cholesterol, while the triglycerides in your bloodstream will rise, perpetuating the problem. Too much cholesterol can clog your blood vessels, get into the bile and crystallize, causing gallstones and gallbladder disease.

Fish Fat (Omega-3 Oils)

The fats naturally present in fish that swim in cold waters, known as omega-3 fatty acids (crucial for brain tissue), or fish oils, are all polyunsaturated. They lower your cholesterol levels and protect against heart disease. These fish have a layer of fat to keep them warm in cold water. Mackerel, albacore tuna, salmon, sardines and lake trout are all rich in omega-3 fatty acids. In fact, whale meat and seal meat are enormous sources of omega-3 fatty acids, which were once the staples of the Inuit diet. Overhunting and federal moratoriums on whale and seal hunting have dried up this once-vital source of Inuit food, which clearly offered real protection against heart disease.

Artificial Fats

An assortment of artificial fats has been introduced into our diet, courtesy of food producers who are trying to give us the taste of fat without all the calories or harmful effects of saturated fats. Unfortunately, artificial fats offer their own bag of horrors.

Trans-fatty acids (a.k.a. hydrogenated oils)

These are harmful fats that not only raise the level of "bad" cholesterol (LDL) in your bloodstream, but lower the amount of "good" cholesterol (HDL) that's already there. Trans-fatty acids are what you get when you make a liquid oil, such as corn oil, into a more solid or spreadable substance, such as margarine. Trans-fatty acids, you might say, are the "road to hell, paved with good intentions." Someone, way back when, thought that if you could take the "good fat"—unsaturated fat—and solidify it so it could double as butter or lard, you could eat the same things without missing the spreadable fat. That sounds like a great idea. Unfortunately, to make an unsaturated liquid fat more solid, you have to add hydrogen to its molecules. This is known as *hydrogenation*, the process that converts liquid fat to semisolid fat. That ever-popular chocolate bar ingredient, hydrogenated palm oil, is a classic example of a trans-fatty acid. Hydrogenation also prolongs the shelf life of a fat, such as polyunsaturated fats, which can oxidize when exposed to air, causing rancid odours or flavours. Deep-frying oils used in the restaurant trade are generally hydrogenated.

Trans-fatty acid is sold as a polyunsaturated or monounsaturated fat with a line of copy such as "Made from polyunsaturated vegetable oil." In your body, it is treated as a saturated fat. This is why trans-fatty acids are a saturated fat in disguise. The advertiser may, in fact, say that the product contains "no saturated fat" or is "healthier" than the comparable animal or tropical oil product with saturated fat. So be careful: READ YOUR LABELS. The magic word you're looking for is "hydrogenated." If the product lists a variety of unsaturated fats (monounsaturated X oil, polyunsaturated Y oil, and so on), keep reading. If the word "hydrogenated" appears, count that product as a saturated fat; your body will!

Margarine versus butter

There's an old tongue twister: "Betty Botter bought some butter that made the batter bitter; so Betty Botter bought more butter that made the batter better." Are we making our batters bitter or better with margarine? It depends.

Since the news of trans-fatty acids broke in the late 1980s, margarine manufacturers began to offer some less "bitter" margarines; some contain no hydrogenated oils, while others have much smaller amounts of them. Margarines with less than 60 to 80 percent oil (9 to 11 g of fat) will contain 1.0 to 3.0 g of trans-fatty acids per serving, compared to butter, which is 53 percent saturated fat. You might say it's a choice between a bad fat and a *worse* fat.

It's also possible for a liquid vegetable oil to retain a high concentration of unsaturated fat when it's been partially hydrogenated. In this case, your body will metabolize this as some saturated fat and some unsaturated fat.

Fake fat

We have artificial sweeteners; why not artificial fat? This question has led to the creation of an emerging yet highly suspicious ingredient: *fat substitutes*, designed to replace real fat and hence reduce the calories from real fat without compromising the taste. This is done by creating a fake fat that the body cannot absorb.

One of the first fat substitutes was Simplesse, an all-natural fat substitute made from milk and egg-white protein, which was developed by the NutraSweet Company. Simplesse apparently adds 1 to 2 calories per gram instead of the usual 9 calories per gram from fat. Other fat substitutes simply take protein and carbohydrates and modify them in some way to simulate the textures of fat (creamy, smooth, etc.). All of these fat substitutes help to create low-fat products, discussed in Chapter 6.

The calorie-free fat substitute being promoted is called olestra, developed by Procter & Gamble. It's currently being test-marketed in the United States in a variety of savoury snacks such as potato chips and crackers. Olestra is a potentially dangerous ingredient that most experts feel can do more harm than good. Canada has not yet approved it.

Olestra is made from a combination of vegetable oils and sugar. Therefore, it tastes just like the real thing, but the biochemical structure is a molecule too big for your liver to break down, so olestra just gets passed into the large intestine and is excreted. Olestra is more than an "empty" molecule, however. It causes diarrhea and cramps and may deplete your body of vital nutrients, including vitamins A, D, E and K, necessary for blood to clot. If the FDA approves olestra for use as a cooking-oil substitute, you'll see it in every imaginable high-fat product. The danger is that instead of encouraging people to choose nutritious foods, such as fruits, grains and vegetables, over high-fat foods, products like these encourage a high *fake*-fat diet that's still too low in fibre and other essential nutrients. And the no-fat icing on the cake is that these people could potentially wind up with a vitamin deficiency to boot. Products like olestra should make you nervous.

TABLE 7.1

New Millennium Recommendations for Fat

Type of Fat	How Much to Eat
Total fat	No more than 30% of daily energy requirements
Saturated and polyunsaturated fat	No more than 10% of daily energy requirements
Monounsaturated fat	As much as possible
Fish fat	A serving at least once a week
Trans-fatty acids	Limit as much as possible

Source: Canadian Diabetes Association, "Guidelines for the Nutritional Management of Diabetes Mellitus in the New Millennium. A Position Statement." Reprinted from *Canadian Journal of Diabetes Care* 23 (3): 56–69.

THE INCREDIBLE BULK

For every action, there is an equal and opposite reaction. When you decrease your fat intake, you should increase your bulk intake, or fibre. Complex carbohydrates are foods that are high in fibre. Fibre is the part of a plant your body can't digest; it comes in the form of both water-soluble fibre (which dissolves in water) and water-insoluble fibre (which does not dissolve in water but instead absorbs water).

Soluble versus Insoluble Fibre

Soluble and insoluble fibre do differ, but they are equally good things. Soluble fibre—somehow—lowers the "bad" cholesterol, or LDL, in your body. Experts aren't entirely sure how soluble fibre works its magic, but one popular theory is that it gets mixed into the bile the liver secretes and forms a type of gel that traps the building blocks of cholesterol, thus lowering your LDL levels. It's akin to a spider web trapping smaller insects. Sources of soluble fibre include oats or oat bran, legumes (dried beans and peas), some seeds, carrots, oranges, bananas and other fruits. Soybeans are also high sources of soluble fibre. Studies show that people with very high cholesterol have the most to gain by eating soybeans. Soybean is also a *phytoestrogen* (plant estrogen) that is believed to lower the risks of estrogen-related cancers (for example, breast cancer), as well as lower the incidence of estrogen-loss symptoms associated with menopause.

Insoluble fibre doesn't affect your cholesterol levels at all, but it regulates your bowel movements. How does it do this? As the insoluble fibre moves through your digestive tract, it absorbs water like a sponge and helps to convert your waste into a solid form faster, making the stools larger, softer and easier to pass. Without insoluble fibre, your solid waste just gets pushed down to the colon or lower intestine as always, where it is stored and dried out until you're ready to have a bowel movement. High-starch foods are associated with drier stools. This is exacerbated when you "ignore the urge," as the colon will dehydrate the waste even more until it becomes harder and difficult to pass, a condition known as constipation. Insoluble fibre will help to regulate your bowel movements by speeding things along. It is also linked to lower rates of colorectal cancer. Good sources of insoluble fibre are wheat bran and whole grains, skins from various fruits and vegetables, seeds, leafy greens and cruciferous vegetables (cauliflower, broccoli or Brussels sprouts).

Fibre and Diabetes

Soluble fibre helps delay glucose from being absorbed into your bloodstream, which not only improves blood sugar control but helps to control postmeal peaks in blood sugar. This stimulates the pancreas to produce more insulin. Fibre in the form of all colours of vegetables will also ensure that you're getting the right mix of nutrients. Experts suggest that you have different colours of vegetables daily—for example, carrots, beets and spinach. An easy way to remember what nutrients are in which vegetable is to remember that all green vegetables are for cellular repair; the darker the green, the more nutrients the vegetable contains. All red, orange and purplish vegetables contain antioxidants (vitamins A, C and E), which boost the immune system and fight off toxins. Studies suggest that vitamin C, for example, is crucial for people with Type 2 diabetes because it helps to prevent complications, as well as rid the body of sorbitol, which can increase blood sugar. Another study suggests that vitamin E helps to prevent heart disease in people with Type 2 diabetes by lowering levels of "bad" cholesterol, but this isn't yet conclusive. Other minerals, such as zinc and copper, are essential for wound healing. The recommendation is to eat all colours of vegetables in ample amounts to get your vitamins, minerals and dietary fibre. It makes sense when you understand diabetes as a disease of starvation. In starvation, there are naturally lower levels of nutrients in your body that can be replenished only through excellent sources of food.

Breaking Bread

For thousands of years, cooked whole grains were the dietary staple for all cultures—rice and millet in the Orient; wheat, oats and rye in Europe; buckwheat in Russia; sorghum in Africa; barley in the Middle East; and corn in pre-European North America.

Whole-grain breads are good sources of insoluble fibre (flax bread is particularly good because flaxseeds are a source of soluble fibre, too). The problem is understanding what is truly "whole grain." For example, there is an assumption that because bread is dark or brown, it's more nutritious; this isn't so. In fact, many brown breads are simply enriched white breads dyed with molasses. ("Enriched" means that nutrients lost during processing have been replaced.) High-fibre pita breads and bagels are available, but you have to search for them. A good rule is to simply look for the words "whole wheat," which means that the wheat is, indeed, whole.

What's in a grain?

Most of us will turn to grains and cereals to boost our fibre intake, which experts recommend should be at 25–35 g per day. Use Table 7.2 to help you gauge whether you're getting enough. The following list measures the amount of insoluble fibre. If you're a little under par, an easy way to boost your fibre intake is to simply add pure wheat bran to your foods, which is available in health food stores or supermarkets. Forty-five millilitres (3 tbsp.) of wheat bran is equal to 4.4 g of fibre. Sprinkle 15–30 mL (1–2 tbsp.) onto cereals, rice, pasta or meat dishes. You can also sprinkle it into orange juice or low-fat yogurt. It has virtually no calories, but it's important to drink a glass of water with your wheat bran, as well a glass of water after you've finished your wheat bran-enriched meal.

TABLE 7.2

What's in a Grain?

Cereals	Grams of Fibre
(Based on 125 mL/1/2 cup unless otherwise specified)	
Fiber First	15.0
Fiber One	12.8
All Bran	10.0
Oatmeal (250 mL/1 cup)	5.0
Raisin Bran (190 mL/3/4 cup)	4.6
Bran Flakes (250 mL/1 cup)	4.4
Shreddies (160 mL/2/3 cup)	2.7
Cheerios (250 mL/1 cup)	2.2
Corn Flakes (375 mL/1 1/2 cup)	0.8
Special K (375 mL/1 1/2 cup)	0.4
Rice Krispies (375 mL/1 1/2 cup)	0.3

Breads	Grams of Fibre
(based on 1 slice)	
Rye	2.0
Pumpernickel	2.0
12-grain	1.7
100% whole wheat	1.3
Raisin	1.0
Cracked-wheat	1.0
White	0

Keep in mind that some of the newer high-fibre breads on the market today have up to 7 g of fibre per slice. This chart is based on what is normally found in typical grocery stores.

Fruits and Veggies

Another easy way of boosting fibre content is to know how much fibre your fruits and vegetables pack per serving. All fruits, beans (a.k.a. legumes) and vegetables listed here show measurements for insoluble fibre, which is not only good for colon health, but for your heart. Some of these numbers may surprise you!

TABLE 7.3

What's in a Fruit or Veggie?

Fruit	Grams of Fibre
Raspberries (190 mL/3/4 cup)	6.4
Strawberries (250 mL/1 cup)	4.0
Blackberries (125 mL/1/2 cup)	3.9
Orange (1)	3.0
Apple (1)	2.0
Pear (1/2 medium)	2.0
Grapefruit (1/2 cup)	1.1
Kiwi (1)	1.0

Beans	Grams of Fibre
(Based on 125 mL/1/2 cup unless otherwise specified)	
Green beans (250 mL/1 cup)	4.0
White beans	3.6
Kidney beans	3.3
Pinto beans	3.3
Lima beans	3.2

Vegetables	Grams of Fibre
(Based on 125 mL/1/2 cup unless otherwise specified)	
Baked potato with skin (1 large)	4.0
Acorn squash	3.8

Peas	3.0
Creamed, canned corn	2.7
Brussels sprouts	2.3
Asparagus (190 mL/3/4 cup)	2.3
Corn kernels	2.1
Zucchini	1.4
Carrots (cooked)	1.2
Broccoli	1.1

FOOD PILLS

Countries where high-fibre and plant-rich diets are the norm have far lower rates of cancer, heart disease and diabetes. This fact has led to research into specific foods or food ingredients that you can now buy in pill or capsule form: Garlic capsules, broccoli pills and hundreds of other food supplements have sprung onto the health food market. Should you be taking supplements or simply eating a healthy diet? The answer is boring and not one you want to hear: Eat a variety of good foods that are high in fibre and low in fat! The problem with taking a "plant pill" instead of eating the plant is that by taking the pill, you're missing out on other benefits, such as fibre, taste or the biochemical reaction that results from a known ingredient in the plant and the dozens of unknown ingredients.

Phytochemicals

Phytochemicals, or "plant chemicals" (*phyto* is Greek for "plant"), are the natural ingredients found in plant foods such as tomatoes, oats, soya, oranges and broccoli. As researchers strive for some magic wellness ingredient, they're finding all kinds of disease-fighting chemicals inside common fruits and vegetables. While phytochemicals, such as *isoflavones* (found in soybeans), *allylic sulphides* (found in garlic, onions and chives), *isothiocyanates* (found in cruciferous vegetables like Brussels sprouts, cabbage and cauliflower), *saponins* (spinach, potatoes, tomatoes and oats), *lignin* and *alphalinolenic acid* (flaxseeds), sound exotic, you can easily get them by simply eating a variety of fruits, grains and vegetables.

Another hot phytochemical right now is *betaglucan* (found in legumes, oats and other grains). Betaglucan is believed to help prevent diabetes by delaying gastric emptying and by slowing down glucose absorption in the small intestine, so if you have diabetes, it can help to regulate your blood sugar.

In fact, biologically engineered foods, which alter the natural genetic codes in vegetables (see below), may interfere with these natural phytochemicals.

Functional Foods

Functional foods are foods that have significant levels of biologically active disease-preventing or health-promoting properties. Tomatoes, oatmeal, soy and garlic are all examples of functional foods because they contain phytochemicals. Functional foods are therefore different from nutraceuticals (from the words *nutrition* and *pharmaceutical*), which are manufactured health foods, such as dietary fibre drinks or Zbars.

In the next few years, you may even see tomato sauces or canned goods with a "functional food" label touting, for example, that the food "may prevent prostate cancer" because it contains lycopene (a phytochemical in tomatoes, red peppers and red grapefruit).

CHANGING YOUR DIET (AND HELPING THE ENVIRONMENT, TOO!)

It's difficult enough to stick to a meal plan without having to worry about pesticides, toxins and "saving the world" all at the same time. Now that you may be making dramatic changes to your lifestyle and diet, it's important to have a more complete picture of what you're eating so you can be as healthy as you can.

Animal Farm

When you eat meat, you're eating a lot of other things you may not want. Sulphonamides and penicillin, first used to a limited extent in the 1930s and 1940s, were routinely added to feed by the late 1950s, when farmers began raising animals in concentrated areas to meet increased demands. (Tight quarters triggered the spread of disease, necessitating antibiotics.) Today, antibacterial drugs, antiparasitic drugs and hormones are in widespread use in meat-producing farms. Anabolic hormones or steroids are used to increase growth and muscle in cattle (so we can have our thick, juicy steaks). A few years ago, the European Community banned the raising or importing of any animal that was given hormones. The United States and Canada continue to use growth hormones.

When you see statements such as "low incidence" or "acceptable levels" of drug residue in animals, it means that the said meat or milk has drugs in it. It's like saying "acceptable levels of toxins," when, in fact, *no level* of toxin should be acceptable! The U.S. Food and Drug Administration has defined "no residue" as a level of drug that presents no more than one in a million risk of cancer over a lifetime; that's not the same thing as "no level of drug."

Bovine somatotropin (BST)

It gets worse. Bovine somatotropin, or BST, is a hormone that causes cows to overproduce milk. And when that happens the cows can become engorged and develop a bacterial infection called mastitis, necessitating the use of even more antibiotics. Although the FDA has concluded that milk and meat from BST-treated cows are safe for human consumption, Canada has not yet approved it. We don't know whether BST can affect human lactation hormones, nor do we know what effect "mastitis milk" or the antibiotics used to treat mastitis may have on us. Clear labelling guidelines of BST milk products must also be introduced before it is sprung onto unsuspecting milk consumers.

Mad cows

An almost biblical lesson in eating foods that are not indigenous can be seen with the revolting tale of mad cow disease, or *bovine spongiform encephalopathy* (BSE). BSE is an infectious disease that causes degenerative changes in the brains of cattle and degenerative brain disease in humans who ingest "mad cow" brains. This is not old news, but ongoing news. BSE is passed on to the cow through other animal brains, commonly sheep with a sheep disease known as *scrapies* (although humans cannot get this disease by eating sheep with scrapies).

The only way a cow can contract this disease is to eat the brain of an infected animal, which wouldn't happen in nature because cows are vegetarian. In the interest of cost-effective farming, the agriculture industry began using animal parts (slaughterhouse waste, dead pets and road kill) in cattle feed. This brain disease was passed on to "Cow Number 1" when it unwittingly ate a piece of another animal brain, probably from a sheep that was a carrier of the infection. Cow Number 1 gets slaughtered and becomes a hamburger. Its leftover brain parts get mixed into another sack of cattle feed and Cow Number 2 eats infected Cow Number 1's brain parts and *also* becomes infected. The cycle continues as the cows eat one another's brains—something that Mother Nature never meant to happen. Ultimately, when a human being eats the hamburger made with ground beef, which may have some remnants of mad cow brains and spinal cords (through the slaughtering and meat-recovery process), he or she will contract mad cow disease as well.

What's truly frightening is that BSE has a five-year incubation period. So even if you became a vegetarian today, the hamburger you ate three years ago could still have infected you. And in that time period, BSE can spread to other animals in many other countries that use slaughtered-cattle products in their feed. Mad cows have been identified throughout the developed world. By eating organically raised beef (this is where cows are raised grazing—what Mother Nature intended), you can prevent BSE.

Vegging Out

By simply becoming more vegetarian, you can actually change the world, lessening the demand for meat. Cleaning up the environment starts at your own kitchen table, in your own house, not in the House of Parliament.

It's estimated that at least 7 to 10 percent of North Americans practise some form of vegetarianism. Semivegetarians eat poultry, fish, eggs and dairy foods; pesco-vegetarians eat fish, eggs and dairy foods; lacto-ovo-vegetarians eat eggs and dairy foods. Stricter forms of vegetarianism include ovo-vegetarians, who do not eat dairy but will consume eggs; lacto-vegetarians will not eat eggs but will have dairy; and vegans, who will not eat any sort of animal-derived foods.

When you compare the health of vegetarians to that of the general population, vegetarians have lower rates of heart disease, colon cancer, colitis (inflammation of the colon), hypertension, Type 2 diabetes and obesity. Keep in mind that becoming more vegetarian isn't a licence to overdo it on high-fat, meatless food either. You should still choose lower-fat dairy products if you are still eating dairy. See "Milk Tips" for details.

Indigenous Eating

Earlier I discussed how the loss of ecology and environment has led to an epidemic of diabetes in Aboriginal Canadians. There are many reasons to support an indigenous diet. Eastern health practitioners (from Asia and India) maintain that the right diet is based on where you live. Canadians need no further proof than to look at the traditional Aboriginal diet. In hotter climates, such as India and other tropical regions, lighter diets based on grains and vegetables, and even certain spices, are more conducive to good health.

Eating seasonally

Eating foods that are seasonal to our own habitat ensures that we are getting the most bang from our produce. Food begins to lose its natural phytochemicals (or healthful properties) when it travels long distances in refrigeration units. Since most of us don't have the luxury of living on a farm, we may feel that we haven't much choice in controlling the produce that is in our local grocery stores, but does it seem "natural" for Winnipeg to eat tropical fruits in January, or for Tokyo to turn into a steak-and-potatoes society? What are the consequences of this?

For one thing, there may be some health-related reasons that we plant in the spring, harvest and preserve in the fall and make soups in the winter. Eastern nutritionist Mushio Kushi advises against foods that are not in harmony with the seasons. In cold weather, for example, food that is cooked longer—soups and stews—is considered better than salads and tropical fruits; in summer, lighter fare is healthier than heavy meats and starches.

Epidemiologists observe that as we send our meat and dairy to vegetarian-based societies, we notice that the incidence of Western diseases, such as Type 2 diabetes, rises. Yet as we meat-eaters adopt a more vegetarian diet, which need not mean tropical but rather *indigenous* fruits and vegetables and a wide variety of nuts that we can grow right here in Canada, we see a decrease in disease.

Discovering Canadian Roots

According to many horticulturists and organic growers, the future of farming is learning how to grow *native plants* from seed, which is called *sustainable farming*. This isn't anything new, but rather centuries old! Sustainable farming creates a sustainable vegetation system or "web" that keeps rebuilding upon itself for decades to come. Planting in this way helps to renew and protect soil, allowing the diverse range of organisms—some even pests—to coexist within the food chain. You see, when the food chain is left intact, parasites are taken care of by their natural predators, or natural repellents. Organic farmers therefore practise what's known as *companion planting*, which is simply ethical "biological pest management." In other words, if Vegetable A is always pestered by Beetle X, you simply plant Vegetable B next to it, which together with Vegetable A produces an odour that turns off Beetle X so that it doesn't go near either plant. Or you can plant Herb A next to Vegetable A, which is a more tempting treat for Beetle X. Vegetable A grows beautifully, Herb B gets devoured and then you simply hand-pick Herb B and throw it out at the end of the season. Companion planting is used to confuse insects, repel them or trap them. Companion planting is also used to make crops healthier. Vegetable A, for example, will grow better when it's beside Herb A for reasons not completely understood.

Why Not Just Use Pesticides?

Pesticides cause mutations in wildlife and humans, and have definitively and scientifically been shown to cause cancer. Because of this mutation and the destruction of wildlife, the food chain is dying off, which has led to disastrous consequences for planetary health. The entire pesticide story is, however, another big book. For the purposes of this chapter, all you need to understand is that by eating more indigenous and seasonable foods, you are supporting an enormous network of organic growers and farmers, who, in the next century, will be leading the way for sustaining and maintaining life on earth. We simply cannot continue to eat as we once did. It makes us fat; it makes us sick; and it can trigger Type 2 diabetes if you are genetically predisposed. Not only that, it wastes billions of acres of arable farmland that could be used to feed people nutritious foods, and it wastes billions of dollars of natural resources we can't afford to lose.

But I Don't Want to Be a Farmer!

You don't have to be a farmer to eat organic produce. Hundreds of organic farmers, united under the Canadian Organic Growers Association, will be happy to sell you their organic produce, from vegetables and beef to clothing (made with cotton that was grown without pesticides). By buying organic spinach instead of spinach that was sprayed with endosulphan (a pesticide), you are supporting organic farming, eating well and saving the world, all at the same time. To find out where your organic farmers are, contact the Organic Trade Association (serving both Canada and the United States) at www.ota.com.

As for your supermarket's produce, many supermarkets are getting into the organic act. In fact, a chain of U.S. supermarkets, called Bread and Circus, sells only organic produce. To get your local supermarkets to disclose where your produce was grown, how it was raised or where it swam, demand labelling that provides this information. You can exert your consumer power (and you do have power!) by contacting the head office of your supermarket and asking to speak to the head of Consumer Relations, Public Relations or Marketing. You can also exert pressure by calling manufacturers' 800/888 numbers that appear on your food labels, starting a newsgroup or banning products to help change standards. You have a right to a label that reads: This produce sprayed with pesticide A. By visiting www.cfia-acia.agr.ca, you can find out

- what your meat product source has eaten, and whether it was injected with anything
- what waters your fish swam in
- what your grown produce was sprayed with

In Your Own Backyard

While yes, you do have a beautiful flower garden, which may be the envy of all your neighbours, if you're using pesticides you're part of the problem, not the solution, as they said in the 1960s. Contact the Canadian Organic Growers Association for literature on organic insecticides and fungicides for lawns and gardens, as well as for companion planting tips for the backyard (such as planting garlic beside roses).

HOW TO GET MORE FRUITS AND VEGETABLES

Fruits and vegetables must be planned for in a diabetes meal plan.

▶ Go for one or two fruits at breakfast, one fruit and two vegetables at lunch and dinner, and a fruit or vegetable snack between meals.

▶ Consume many differently coloured fruits and vegetables. For colour variety, select at least three differently coloured fruit and vegetables daily.

▶ Put fruit and sliced veggies in an easy-to-use, easy-to-reach place (sliced vegetables in the fridge; fruit out on the table).

▶ Keep frozen and canned fruit and vegetables on hand to add to soups, salads or rice dishes.

Source: Adapted from June V. Engel, Ph.D., "Beyond Vitamins: Phytochemicals to Help Fight Disease," *Health News,* June 1996, Volume 14, No. 3.

MILK TIPS

▶ In North America, we consume a lot of milk. Know what you're getting:

▶ Whole milk is made up of 48 percent calories from fat.

▶ Two percent milk gets 37 percent of its calories from fat.

▶ One percent milk gets 26 percent of its calories from fat.

▶ Skim milk is completely fat-free.

▶ Cheese gets 50 percent of its calories from fat, unless it's skim milk cheese.

▶ Butter gets 95 percent of its calories from fat.

▶ Yogurt gets 15 percent of its calories from fat.

The Costs of High-Fat Eating

Our entire agricultural economy is designed to support livestock and animal products, which we consume in huge quantities. This is making us too fat, requires a large amount of resources to support its production and is ruining our environment. The land on which animals are raised for food production

- uses 85 percent of all cropland and 55 percent of all agricultural land in the United States
- destroys forest land and range land, through erosion and depletion
- uses 80 percent of all piped water in the United States
- uses pesticides, which pollute two-thirds of U.S. waters and more than half of U.S. lakes and streams
- destroys wildlife, through conversion and preemption of forest and range land habitats and through poisoning and trapping of predators
- takes up 14 percent of the U.S. energy budget, greater than twice the energy supplied by all our nuclear power stations
- uses large amounts of scarce raw materials, such as aluminum, copper, iron, steel, tin, zinc, potassium, rubber, wood and petroleum products, used for processing, storing and packaging
- uses 90 percent of our grains and legumes, and half of our fish catch to feed livestock

- affects our incomes: meats cost five to six times as much as foods with equivalent amounts of vegetable protein; the average U.S. household spends roughly $7,500 annually on meat
- uses 50 percent of the world's tropical forests to expand land for cattle production; the average hamburger is made from meat imported from Central or South America and represents the loss of 5 square metres (55 square feet) of rain forest
- depletes the ozone layer: the rain forests are the "lungs of the planet," which absorb excess carbon dioxide and clear methane, a greenhouse gas; cattle, however, produce methane, while the clearing of rain forests interferes with the ecosystem
- destroys arable land: cloud seeding, which upsets natural atmospheric weather patterns and weather cycles, results in rapid loss of arable land and the spread of desert regions across Africa, Central Asia and parts of Latin America

Source: Mischio Kushi. *The Cancer Prevention Guide.* New York: St. Martin's Press, 1993.

Chapter 8

THE ROLE OF ACTIVE LIVING

● ● ● ● ● ● ● ● ● ●

The purpose of this chapter is to explain how exercise affects your body when you have diabetes. It is not intended as a workout program, however. Anybody reading this chapter needs to design a *doable* exercise program that is appealing and convenient; for most people, that will mean combining some kind of simple stretching routine with some aerobic activity. As one expert aptly put it on her video, the program you *can* do is the one you *will* do.

Most people who have been sedentary most of their lives are intimidated by health-and-fitness clubs. Walking into a room with complex machines, filled with young, fit, supple bodies, is not exactly an inviting atmosphere for somebody who doesn't understand how to program a StairMaster. And the "language" of exercise is intimidating, too. Not only do you need an anatomy lesson to understand which movements stretch which group of muscles, but you need to take a crash course in cardiology to understand exactly how long you have to hyperventilate and have your pulse at X beats per minute, with the sweat pouring off you, before you burn any fat. The concept of "gaining muscle" over existing fat is also a hard one to grasp. (My stupid question is always: "How come, if I've been doing my program for six months, I weigh *more* than when I started?")

Aerobics classes are another problem; many people (like me) are uncomfortable with their lack of finesse in public. And many aerobics classes assume that you've had formal training with the National Ballet of Canada; after all, you need the grace of a dancer to perform half the moves! So let me stress something before you continue with this chapter: You're wearing all the equipment you will ever need to exercise. If you can breathe, stretch and walk, you can become a lean, mean exercise machine without paying a membership fee.

WHAT DOES EXERCISE *REALLY* MEAN?

The *Oxford English Dictionary* defines exercise as "the exertion of muscles, limbs, etc., especially for health's sake; bodily, mental or spiritual training." In the Western world, we have placed an emphasis on "bodily training" when we talk about exercise, while completely ignoring mental and spiritual training. Only recently have Western studies begun to focus on the mental benefits of exercise. (It's been shown, for example, that exercise creates endorphins, hormones that make us feel good.) But we in the West do not encourage meditation or other calming forms of mental and spiritual exercise, which have also been shown to improve well-being and health.

In the East, for thousands of years, exercise has focused on achieving mental and spiritual health *through* the body, using breathing and postures, for example. Fitness practitioner Karen Faye maintains that posture is extremely important for organ alignment. Standing correctly—with ears over shoulders, and shoulders over hips, with knees slightly bent and head straight up—naturally allows you to pull in your abdomen. According to Faye, many people who balance baskets over their heads or do a lot of physical work with their bodies are noted for correct postures and low rates of osteoporosis.

Nor should we ignore the Aboriginal and Northern traditions known to improve mental health and well-being, such as traditional dances, active prayers that incorporate physical activity, circles that involve community and communication, and even sweat lodges, believed to help rid the body of toxins through sweating. These are all forms of wellness activities that you should investigate.

The Meaning of Aerobic

If you look up the word "aerobic" in the dictionary, what you'll find is the chemistry definition: "living in free oxygen." This is certainly correct; we are all aerobes—beings that require oxygen to live. Some bacteria, for example, are anaerobic; they can exist in an environment without oxygen. All that jumping around and fast movement in aerobic exercise is done to create faster breathing, so we can take more oxygen into our bodies.

Why are we doing this? Because the blood contains *oxygen*! The faster your blood flows, the more oxygen can flow to your organs. But when your health care practitioner tells you to "exercise" or to take up "aerobic exercise," he or she is not referring solely to "increasing oxygen" but to exercising the heart muscle. The faster it beats, the better a "workout" it gets (although you don't want to overwork your heart either).

Why we want more oxygen

When more oxygen is in our bodies, we burn fat (see below), our breathing improves, our blood pressure improves and our hearts work better. Oxygen also lowers triglycerides and cholesterol, increasing our high-density lipoproteins (HDL) or the "good" cholesterol, while decreasing our low-density lipoproteins (LDL) or the "bad" cholesterol. This means that your arteries will unclog and you may significantly decrease your risk of heart disease and stroke. More oxygen makes our brains work better, so we feel better. Studies show that depression is decreased when we increase oxygen flow into our bodies. Ancient techniques such as yoga, which specifically improve mental and spiritual well-being, achieve this by combining deep breathing and stretching, which improves oxygen and blood flow to specific parts of the body.

With Type 2 diabetes, more oxygen in the body increases your cells' sensitivity to insulin, causing your blood-glucose levels to drop. More oxygen can also improve the action of insulin-producing cells in the pancreas. As you continue aerobic exercise, your blood sugar levels will become much easier to manage. You can also use exercise to decrease blood sugar levels in the short term, over a 24-hour period. People who are taking oral hypoglycemic pills may find that their dosages need to be lowered or that they no longer need the medication.

Exercise has been shown to dramatically decrease the incidence of many other diseases, including cancer. Some research suggests that cancer cells tend to thrive in an oxygen-depleted environment. The more oxygen in the bloodstream, the less hospitable you make your body to cancer. In addition, since many cancers are related to fat-soluble toxins, the less fat on your body, the less fat-soluble toxins your body can accumulate.

Burning fat

The only kind of exercise that will burn fat is aerobic exercise because *oxygen burns fat*. If you were to go to your fridge and pull out some animal fat (chicken skin, red-meat fat or butter), throw it in the sink and light it with a match, it would burn. What makes the flame yellow is oxygen; what fuels the fire is the fat. That same process goes on in your body. The oxygen will burn your fat, however you increase the oxygen flow in your body (through jumping around, increasing your heart rate or employing an established deep-breathing technique).

Of course, when you burn fat, you lose weight, which can also cause your body to use insulin more efficiently and lower your blood sugar levels. It may also cause your doctor to lower your dosage of oral hypoglycemics or stop your medication altogether.

The Western definition of aerobic

In the West, an exercise is considered aerobic if it makes your heart beat faster than it normally does. When your heart is beating fast, you'll be breathing hard and sweating and will officially be in your "target zone" or "ideal range" (the kind of terms that turn many people off).

There are official calculations you can do to find this target range. For example, it's recommended that by subtracting your age from 220, then multiplying that number by 60 percent, you will find your "threshold level," which means your heart should be beating X beats per minute for 20 to 30 minutes. If you multiply the number by 75 percent, you will find your "ceiling level," which means your heart should not be beating faster than X beats per minute for 20 to 30 minutes. But this is only an example. If you are on heart medications (drugs that slow down your heart, known as beta-blockers), you'll want to make sure you discuss what "target" to aim for with your health professional.

Finding your pulse

You have pulse points all over your body. The easiest ones to find are those on your neck, at the base of your thumb, just below your earlobe or on your wrist. To check your heart rate, look at a watch or clock and begin to count your beats for 15 seconds. Then multiply by 4 to get your pulse.

Borg's rate of perceived exertion (RPE)

This doesn't refer to the Borg on *Star Trek*, but to the Borg Scale of Perceived Exertion. This is a way of measuring exercise intensity without finding your pulse, and because of its simplicity, it is now the recommended method for judging exertion. The Borg scale goes from 6 to 20. Extremely light activity may rate a 7, for example, while a very, very hard activity may rate a 19. Exercise practitioners recommend that you do a "talk test" to rate your exertion, too. If you can't talk without gasping for air, you may be working too hard. You should be able to carry on a normal conversation throughout your activity. What's crucial to remember about RPE is that it is extremely individual; what one person judges a 7 another may judge a 10.

Other ways to increase oxygen flow

This will come as welcome news to people who have limited movement due to joint problems, arthritis or other diabetes-related complications ranging from stroke to kidney disease. You can increase the flow of oxygen into your bloodstream without exercising your heart muscle by learning how to breathe deeply through your diaphragm. Many yoga-like programs and videos can teach you this technique, which does not require you to jump around. You would be increasing the oxygen flow into your bloodstream, which is better than doing nothing at all to improve your health, and gain many health benefits, according to a myriad of wellness practitioners.

An "aerobic" activity versus active living

The term "aerobic activity" means that the *activity* causes your heart to pump harder and faster, and causes you to breathe faster, which increases oxygen flow. Activities such as cross-country skiing, walking, hiking and biking are all aerobic.

But you know what? Exercise practitioners hate the terms "aerobic activity" or "aerobics program" because it is not about what people do in their daily life. Health promoters are replacing these terms with the words "active living" because that's what becoming un-sedentary is all about. There are many ways you can adopt an active lifestyle. Here are some suggestions:

- If you drive everywhere, pick a parking space farther away from your destination so you can work some daily walking into your life.
- If you take public transit everywhere, get off one or two stops early so you can walk the rest of the way to your destination.
- Choose stairs more often over escalators or elevators.
- Park at one side of the mall and walk to the other.
- Take a stroll after dinner around your neighbourhood.
- Volunteer to walk the dog.
- On weekends, go to the zoo or get out to flea markets, garage sales and so on.

What About Muscles?

Forty percent of your body weight is made from muscle, where sugar is stored. The muscles use this sugar when they are being worked. When the sugar is used up, the muscles, in a healthy body, will drink in sugar from your blood. After exercising, the muscles will continue to drink in glucose from your blood to replenish the glucose that was there before exercise.

But when you have insulin resistance, glucose from your blood has difficulty getting inside your muscles; the muscles act like a brick wall. As you begin to use and tone your muscles, they will become more receptive to the glucose in your blood, allowing the glucose in. Studies show that the muscles specifically worked out in a given exercise take up glucose far more easily than another muscle in the same body that has not been worked out.

Doing weight-bearing activities is also encouraged because it builds bone mass and uses up calories. Building bone mass is particularly important; as Karen Faye tells me, "If you want a strong house, you need a strong frame!" Women who are vulnerable to osteoporosis (loss of bone mass) as a result of estrogen loss after menopause (unless they are on hormone-replacement therapy) will benefit from these activities. The denser your bones, the harder they are to break or sprain. As we age, we are all at risk for osteoporosis unless we've either been building up our bone mass for years or are maintaining current bone mass. For information on osteoporosis, call the Osteoporosis Society of Canada, listed at the back of this book.

By increasing muscular strength, we increase flexibility and endurance. For example, you'll find that the first time you ride your bike from home to downtown, your legs may feel sore. Do that same ride ten times, and your legs will no longer be sore. That's what's meant by building endurance. Of course, you won't be as out of breath either, which is another way of building endurance.

Hand weights or resistance exercises (using rubber-band products or pushing certain body parts together) help increase what's called "lean body mass"—body tissue that is not fat. That is why many people find their weight does not drop when they begin to exercise. Yet as your muscles become bigger, your body fat decreases.

Sugar and muscle

When you think "muscle," think "sugar." Every time you work any muscle in your body, either independent of an aerobic activity or during an aerobic activity, your muscles use up glucose from your bloodstream as fuel. People with high blood sugar prior to muscle toning will find that their blood sugar levels are lower after the muscle has been worked.

On the downside, if you have normal blood sugar levels prior to working a muscle, you may find that your blood sugar goes too low after you exercise *unless* you eat something; this should be carbohydrates. In fact, your muscles prefer to use carbohydrates rather than fat as fuel. When your muscles use up all the sugar in your blood, your liver will convert glycogen (excess glucose it stores up for these kinds of emergencies) back into glucose and release it into your bloodstream for your muscles to use.

To avoid this scenario, eat before and after exercising if your blood sugar level is normal. How much you eat prior to exercising largely depends on what you're doing and how long you're going to be doing it. The general rule is to follow your meal plan, eating smaller, more frequent meals throughout the day to keep your blood sugar levels consistent.

Athletes without diabetes will generally consume large quantities of carbohydrates before an intense workout. In fact, it's a known strategy in the athletic world to eat 40–65 g of carbohydrate per hour to maintain blood glucose levels to the point where performance is improved. It's also been shown that consuming glucose, sucrose, maltodextrins or high-fructose corn syrup during exercise can increase endurance. After a training session, athletes will typically consume more carbohydrates to replenish their energy and carry on throughout the day.

Athletes who have Type 1 diabetes do exactly the same thing, except they must be more careful about timing their food intake with insulin to avoid either too low or high blood sugar.

If your blood sugar is low, don't exercise at all as it may be life-threatening. Do not resume exercise until you get your blood sugar levels under control.

Exercises That Can Be Hazardous

These are activities, such as wrestling or weightlifting, that can worsen diabetes eye disease. In addition, they are short but very intense. As a result, unless you fuel up ahead of time, they will force your body to use glycogen (see Chapter 1), which is the stored glucose your liver keeps handy. When you have diabetes, it's not a great idea to force your liver to give up that glycogen. This can actually increase your blood pressure and put you at risk for other health problems, including hypoglycemia. To avoid this, you'll need to eat some carbohydrates prior to these exercises, which will provide enough fuel for the muscles.

LET'S GET PHYSICAL

More than 50 percent of all people with diabetes exercise less than once a week, and 56 percent of all diabetes-related deaths are due to heart attacks. This is terrible news, considering how beneficial and life-extending exercise can be. Reports from the United States show that one out of three American adults are overweight, a sign of growing inactivity. But, as mentioned earlier, the fitness industry has done an excellent job of intimidating inactive people. Some people are so put off by the health club scene, they become even more sedentary. This is similar to diet failure, where you become so demoralized that you "cheat" and binge even more.

If you've been sedentary most of your life, there's nothing wrong with starting off with simple, even leisurely activities such as gardening, feeding the birds in a park or a few simple stretches. Any step you take to be more active is a crucial and important one.

Experts also recommend that you find a friend, neighbour or relative to get physical with you. When your exercise plans include someone else, you'll be less apt to cancel plans or make excuses for not getting out there. Whoever you choose, teach this person how to recognize hypoglycemia just in case. (See Chapter 14.)

Things to Do Before "Moving Day"

1. **Choose an activity that's right for you:** Whether it's walking, chopping wood, jumping rope or folk dancing—pick something you enjoy. You don't have to do the same thing each time either. Vary your routine to avoid monotony. Just make sure that whatever activity you choose is continuous for the duration. Walking for two minutes, then stopping for three, isn't continuous. It's also important to choose an activity that doesn't aggravate a pre-existing problem, such as eye problems. Lowering your head in a certain way (as in touching your toes) or straining your upper body can increase blood pressure and/or aggravate eye problems. If foot problems are a concern, perhaps an activity that doesn't involve walking, such as canoeing, is better. And so on.

2. **Choose the frequency:** Decide how often you're going to do this activity. (Twice, three, or four times a week? Or once a day?) Try not to let two days pass without doing something. And pick a duration. If you're elderly or ill,

even a few minutes is a good start. If you're sedentary but otherwise healthy, aim for 20 to 30 minutes.

3. **Choose the intensity level that's right for you:** This is easy to do if you're using an exercise machine of some kind by just setting the dial. If you're walking, the intensity would mean how fast you are planning to walk, or how many hills you will be incorporating into your walk. In other words, how fast do you want your heart to beat?

4. **Work your activity into your meal plan:** Once you decide what kind of exercise you'll be doing and for how long, see your dietitian about incorporating your exercise needs into your current meal plan. You may need a small snack prior to and after exercise if you're planning to be active longer than 30 minutes. If you are overweight, you do not need to consume extra calories before exercising unless your blood sugar level is low.

5. **Tell your doctor what you're doing:** Your doctor may want to monitor your blood sugar more closely (or want you to do so) or adjust your medication. Don't do anything without consulting your doctor first.

Think Like a Cat

Ever watch a cat in action? Cats will never do anything before stretching. If stretching *is* your exercise, that's just fine; but if it's not the focus of your activity, do some stretching before and after you get really active to reduce muscle tightness.

When Not to Exercise

Everyone can and should exercise, but your diabetes may get in the way at times, especially if you're taking insulin. So here are some alarm bells to listen for; if they go off, skip your exercise and do what you have to do to get back on track:

- Keep track of where you're injecting insulin. Insulin injected into an arm or leg that is being worked out will use up the insulin faster. Any signs of low blood sugar mean STOP!
- Check your blood sugar after 30 minutes to make sure it's still normal. If it's low, eat something before you resume exercising. (Blood sugar below 4 mmol/L is low; anything that's 3 mmol/L or less means you should stop exercising or not start exercising at all.)

- If your blood sugar level is high, exercise will bring it down, but if it's greater than 14 mmol/L, check your urine for ketones and don't exercise. When your body is stressed, the blood sugar level can go even higher.

Exercise Parental Duties

Obesity in childhood and adolescence is at an all-time high in North America. For example, the American National Health and Nutrition Examination Survey III (NHANES III) revealed that 21 percent of people 12 to 19 were obese, while as many as 40 percent of people in that age group were physically unfit. It wasn't until 1995 that the Dietary Guidelines for Americans even recommended physical activity. If you have Type 2 diabetes, unless you can encourage your children to adjust their lifestyles early, they will be at high risk for Type 2 diabetes as well. Old habits die hard—something you're learning the hard way. By making sure that your children appreciate the value and benefits of getting physical, you can help them avoid going through what you are. In fact, why don't you encourage your children to exercise right along with you?

TABLE 8.1

Suggested Activities

More Intense	Less Intense
Skiing	Golf
Running	Bowling
Jogging	Badminton
Stair-stepping or stair-climbing	Cricket
Trampoline	Sailing
Jumping rope	Swimming
Fitness walking	Strolling
Race walking	Stretching
Aerobic classes	
Roller skating	
Ice skating	
Biking	
Weight-bearing exercises	
Tennis	
Swimming	

Source: Courtesy, Karen Faye, LPN, A.F.F.A. fitness practitioner.

PART 2

People in
Special Circumstances

Chapter 9

IF YOU'RE AN ABORIGINAL CANADIAN

● ● ● ● ● ● ● ● ● ●

It's not possible to write a book about Type 2 diabetes without addressing the impact of this disease on Canada's Aboriginal population. Since I originally began writing about diabetes in Aboriginal Canada in 1997, things have not changed, but only worsened. There are even higher numbers of cases of Type 2 diabetes and an alarming number of Type 2 diabetes in younger age groups, including children. As stated earlier, among Aboriginal people in Canada the rate of diabetes is five times that of non-Natives, which is one of the highest rates of diabetes worldwide.

The terms "Aboriginal" or "Native people" refer to people whose ancestors are indigenous to Canada. Those registered as "Indian" under the Indian Act were once referred to as "status" or "treaty Indians" but today are known as "people of the First Nations," with full political representation by the Assembly of First Nations. Over the last three decades as many as 40 percent of these people have moved off the reserves into large urban communities. The term "non-status Indians" refers to Aboriginal people who are not registered as Indians under the Indian Act. This group is politically represented by the Council of Aboriginal Peoples. The Métis, Aboriginal people of both French and Aboriginal ancestry, are represented by the Métis National Council. The Inuit people in Canada, who live in the Northwest Territories and northern Quebec, are represented by the Inuit Tapirisat of Canada, while the Inuit in what is now Nunavut are represented by the Kivalliq Inuit Association.

This chapter may read more like a history textbook than a health book, but it's not possible to understand the explosion of Type 2 diabetes in Canada's Aboriginal population without some history.

Thirty-one percent of all Aboriginal people over the age of 15 have a chronic health problem. According to extremely conservative estimates, overall, Type 2 diabetes affects 6 percent of Aboriginal adults, compared with 2 percent of all non-Native adults. But on many reserves, such as Akwesasne, Quebec, near Cornwall, Ontario, *more than 75 percent of residents older than 35 have diabetes*, up from 50 percent in 1989. Because the symptoms of diabetes can be vague and develop slowly, many Aboriginal people have the disease but do not realize it. For every known case of diabetes among Aboriginal people, at least one goes undiagnosed. And when you consider that Type 2 diabetes was not a recognized health problem in this community until the 1940s, this is a staggering increase.

Aboriginal Canadians also suffer more end-stage renal disease (ESRD), a common complication of diabetes, discussed in Chapter 19, than non-Native Canadians. Chronic renal failure among Native people is 2.5 to 4.0 times higher than in the general Canadian population, mostly due to Type 2 diabetes. The United States reports similar statistics.

The Native population is most at risk for this disease because of thrifty genes, which are discussed in Chapter 2 as well as further on in this chapter. Centuries of living off the land, eating seasonally and indigenously, bred metabolisms that weren't able to adapt to nutrient excess and a sedentary lifestyle. Yet prior to contact with Europeans, Canada's Aboriginal people were leading the kind of healthy lifestyle that may ultimately prevent diabetes from developing in the first place.

PRE-EUROPEAN CANADA

Aboriginal history in Canada is broken down into two periods: the pre-European or precontact period, and the postcontact period. We refer to the meeting of European and Aboriginal societies as "first contact." Europeans failed miserably in their first contact mission because they interfered, took over and ruined a culture, with both health and environmental consequences for *all* peoples.

At the time of their first contact with Europeans, Aboriginal people enjoyed good health. Infections were rare, fevers were unheard of, while mental, emotional and physical vigour was status quo. For any ailment, a common remedy was to enter a smoke house and "sweat it out." (Today, natural medicine gurus such as Dr. Andrew Weil highly recommend weekly sweats in saunas or steam baths.)

Before being exposed to European food, Aboriginal people lived on the ideal diet of seasonal foods native to Canada. Eating foods seasonably indigenous to the land is a concept widely written about in several disease-prevention health books, particularly by Eastern nutritionists, such as Mushio Kushi, the founder of macrobiotics. In pre-European Canada, there was no cholera, typhus, smallpox, measles, cancer or skin problems, while fractures were also rare. Mental illness among Aboriginal people during this time was also unheard of. Interestingly, more than 500 drugs used in pharmaceuticals today were originally used by Native people.

The Diseases

As European ships arrived in Canada, they brought with them a smorgasbord of strange and new bacteria and viruses, causing terrible epidemics among Native people. (This is not unlike what happens to Europeans when they go into Africa and Asia and are exposed to micro-organisms to which they have no immunity.) Many European explorers and settlers were weak and sick when they first met Aboriginal people because they'd survived a long voyage in crowded, unsanitary ships with both contaminated drinking water and food that had gone bad. Nevertheless, thousands of Aboriginal people got sick and died from infections they caught from Europeans. Influenza, measles, polio, diphtheria, smallpox and other diseases were brought to Canada from the public health disaster areas of Europe—*slums*! In a sense, the result was genocide as Native people died by the thousands during the 18th and 19th centuries. And thus began an incredible transformation: Healthy people became steadily unhealthy as more Europeans came to Canada. Sources of food and clothing from the land diminished, while centuries of a traditional economy dissolved. And worst of all, once-mobile, active people were confined to small plots of land with limited natural resources and poor sanitation. *Fit people became unfit.* Amid this physical deterioration, centuries of spiritual practices and beliefs were actually outlawed as Christianity took over. With ceremonial and spiritual activity banned (elders and healers were prosecuted by Christians for engaging in unlawful spiritual ceremonies), self-respect and cultural pride began to disappear.

The early 20th century was one of the worst periods in Canadian Aboriginal history. Epidemics and disease were rampant, and the Canadian government responded with feeble attempts to improve Native people's health. From the end of the 19th century to the middle of the 20th, semitrained RCMP agents, missionaries and officers tried to administer health care. By 1930, the first nursing station was opened on a Manitoba reserve. Fearing the spread of tuberculosis from Aboriginal communities into the general population, by 1950 the Canadian government was operating 33 nursing stations, 65 health centres and 18 small regional hospitals for registered Indians and Inuit. Virtually all providers of health and social services for Native people were non-Native—people who had no knowledge of Aboriginal healing skills, herbal medicines or other traditional treatments.

From disease to diseased environment

As waters became polluted and environmental raping of resources continued, the diseases changed from infectious to chronic. "Country food," traditional food indigenous to Canada, such as wild game, fish, root vegetables and fruit, whale meat and blubber (now known to contain omega-3 oils, which are linked to low levels of heart disease and cholesterol and hence are protective foods), became inherently more unavailable, forcing Aboriginal people to eat the processed, refined foods of Europeans. Cut off from their habitat, fishing, hunting, ceremonies and indigenous food supply, and exposed to infections, alcohol and overprocessed foods high in fat and sugar, Aboriginal people developed poor eating habits, and became obese and inactive. The main risk factors for Type 2 diabetes are obesity, poor eating habits and physical inactivity.

On the Akwesasne reserve, for example, diabetes exploded in the population as Mohawks turned to fast food after their traditional diet of perch became contaminated with PCBs. Yellow perch was the staple of the Mohawk diet for centuries until the 1950s, when the St. Lawrence Seaway was constructed and became polluted by industry. In 1980, scientists deemed the perch unsafe for human consumption. What's happened on Akwesasne has happened all over North America. Today, there's a project in place to raise healthy perch in tanks to replenish the once-healthy and traditional diet. Similar projects are springing up all over the country and are crucial in helping to contain the Type 2 diabetes epidemic among Native people.

The issue of cash crops

Cash crops have further deteriorated indigenous food supplies. By the early 20th century, chemical agriculture and factory farming revolutionized food production, a practice that has had a detrimental effect on the traditional Aboriginal diet. Canada's corn production over the last 40 years is a good example of the nutritional perils of overfarming.

Corn used to be the grain staple of Canada's Aboriginal people in the Gananoque region, and was an industry controlled by them until the introduction of hybrid corn during the 1930s and early 1940s. Hybrid corn replaced the open-pollinated varieties that naturally flourished in Ontario. Before 1960, corn was a fairly minor crop in Canada, mostly limited to Ontario. But because of new technology and the development of better-yielding and earlier-maturing hybrids, corn boomed throughout the 1960s and 1970s, transforming itself from a regional crop into a cash crop as it became the most popular feed grain for livestock (beef, pork and poultry). By 1980, more than 30 percent of Ontario's 3.5 million ha (8.6 million acres) of cultivated farmland was seeded annually to corn. But corn is also used to make paper and cardboard, automobiles, clothing, absorbents (in diapers and sanitary napkins), non-petroleum-based plastics and even ethyl alcohol. The problem with this type of farming is that corn soon became the *only* crop on several farms, causing a number of environmental problems. The soils in which corn was planted each year became overworked and nutrient-poor, leading to crop failures and unstable farm income. Corn rootworm, a pest common to one type of corn, became rampant in the 1970s and early 1980s, necessitating the use of pesticides. But the more pesticides were used, the more resistant the pests became, and the more exotic the pesticide concoctions became. Soon, these pesticides were detected in rivers and streams, getting into fish and groundwater, destroying important sources of food in that region and beyond.

The Impact of Poverty

Because poverty is also rampant among Aboriginal people, the food supply is further diminished. In 1990, 54 percent of Aboriginal people surveyed had a total annual income below $10,000. The proportion of single-parent families among Aboriginal people was at least 19 percent in 1986, compared to 13 percent in the non-Native population. Grocery bills are therefore a problem. Affordable items tend to be quick-energy, low-nutrient foods.

Food Availability and Familiarity

Another problem is the cost involved in transporting fresh vegetables and fruits to remote locations, where many Aboriginal people reside. Shipping costs and poor supplier selection aggravate matters. There is a real problem in understanding how to shop for Western food, too. Reading labels and interpreting ingredients creates so much confusion that grocery shopping tours are now being conducted by volunteers. In the Sandy Lake Project, for example, people are shown how to walk down grocery aisles, select food and read labels. Projects regarding health food choices labelling are also being initiated.

Planting vegetable gardens that can provide natural foods to communities sounds like a good idea, but in many communities, gardening is associated with a time when gardening was done out of necessity, when White culture killed off Native hunting, and so it is not a desired activity.

Meanwhile, a lack of familiarity with European food preparation aggravates matters, too. In the same way that most Europeans would be unfamiliar with whale blubber recipes, many Aboriginal people are not up on their lasagna or pot-roast recipes. Cooking methods for imported foods are also unfamiliar to many Aboriginal people. Therefore, high-protein, low-fat foods and quality game meats (much lower in fat than livestock-raised meats, high in iron and vitamin C) have become replaced with starches, fats, sugar and alcohol. As mentioned above, the traditional diet of Aboriginal people was far superior to today's. Today's diet, coupled with a sedentary lifestyle, is shown not only to increase the incidence of obesity—and hence diabetes—but to increase blood pressure and dental problems. Aboriginal people also boast an impressive list of heart diseases, cancer, infant morbidity and mortality in higher frequencies than non-Aboriginal Canadians.

Genetics

To our genes, 200 years is an exceedingly short amount of time to ask our immune systems and metabolisms to adjust. Aboriginal people have not built up an immunity to "overnutrition" the way many non-Native Canadians have. Europeans, for the most part, haven't lived nomadically for thousands of years and have therefore developed metabolisms to adjust to more sedentary lifestyles in response to urbanized living.

This is why it is said that Aboriginal people have an inherited tendency toward diabetes, known as thrifty genes. Because Aboriginal people lived seasonably on indigenous diets for so many centuries, their bodies are still behaving as though they were living in 17th-century Canada.

HEALING ABORIGINAL COMMUNITIES

As I have stressed throughout this book, diet is one of the most crucial aspects in managing Type 2 diabetes. Yet Aboriginal people with Type 2 diabetes often do not understand the Canadian Diabetes Food Choice Values and symbols or the concept of meal planning. That's because the role of food is different in Aboriginal culture. For one thing, there are strong cultural beliefs that equate health and prosperity with being overweight. The more central problem is that many Aboriginal people do not have information about the cost and availability of many of the foods recommended in these meal plans.

The traditional Aboriginal diet consisted mostly of high-protein game meat with very few vegetables. In fact, fruits and vegetables are not usually available in the small stores on most reserves. And if they are, they are so expensive that nobody buys them.

As a result, projects such as the Northern Food, Tradition and Health Kit, which encourages traditional foods for health and well-being, were developed for the Northwest Territories. This kit is far more relevant for people with diabetes in this culture and was developed by the Nutrition Section, Department of Health, Government of the Northwest Territories, after elders and Northern educators requested it. The kit incorporates traditional regional foods, cooking and preserving practices. Food items include small land mammals, sea mammals, three kinds of fish, sea urchins, fish eggs, birds, wild greens, berries and bannock. Pictures of the foods are in an accompanying booklet to increase comprehension, while a resource booklet provides a lot of background information, worksheets, posters and various other components to promote cultural pride in Northern foods and food preparation.

Traditional Healers

Treating diabetes in the Aboriginal population is not possible within the current Western framework. Many Aboriginal people with Type 2 diabetes usually do not follow a doctor's orders regarding medication, diet and exercise. But it's not because there's a problem with the patient; there is a problem with the way Western medicine is *communicating* with that patient.

Aboriginal people approach their health from a cultural perspective; the health of the culture and community is reflected in the individuals of that community. Therefore, telling an Aboriginal person to "work out" every day is not as effective as planning, say, a community walk. Health and wellness programs must be connected to the health and wellness of the community and environment. Western-trained health care providers are beginning to recognize that they are woefully unequipped to deliver health care to the Aboriginal community. In fact, Aboriginal doctors and nurses have clearly identified that the diabetes educational and prevention materials available to their patients are not culturally relevant. Individual self-care can only take place if there is *community* self-care.

Nor does the West provide health care services in accordance with the Circle of Life or the Medicine Wheel, which has guided the health and wellness of Aboriginal Canadians for generations. In fact, the Circle of Life is a far more progressive and sophisticated approach to health than Western medicine. It incorporates physical, emotional, social and spiritual aspects of health. The premise of the Circle of Life is that good health occurs when there is balance and harmony within the self, society and natural environment. When there is no harmony, there is ill health.

The West is only beginning to see that harmony and stress affect wellness; Aboriginal Canadians already know this instinctively. Therefore, the role of spirituality is central to Aboriginal health, while traditional healing methods and therapies can make an enormous contribution to managing diabetes in the Aboriginal population.

The majority of traditional healers went underground when they were persecuted by Canadian governments and the Christian Church for using ceremonies, herbal treatments and other Native therapies. By the 1960s, healers were almost wiped out. In the 1980s, some members of the Peguis First Nation community in Manitoba began exploring their cultural roots, and a new movement began to bring back the practices of traditional medicine. Today, in the decade of alternative medicine, traditional healing is encouraged by Western health care providers. Now, traditional healers come under the Non-Insured Health Benefits Program for Aboriginal people. There is a movement for traditional healers to be recognized by the College of Physicians and Surgeons in each province. It is hoped that healing centres and lodges will be accessible in urban, rural and reserve settings to all Aboriginal people, and that they will deliver integrated health and social services.

Aboriginal/Community Diabetes Programs

The most recent trend in treating Aboriginal people with Type 2 diabetes is to combine Western medicine with Northern traditions. Right now, professional organizations such as the Native Physicians Association in Canada (NPAC), Native Psychologists in Canada (NPC) and the Aboriginal Nurses Association of Canada (ANAC) play a crucial role in marrying the West and North. The NPAC includes over 100 physicians of Aboriginal ancestry; most members are women working in primary care, who are actively involved in Aboriginal health.

In Ontario, underserviced Aboriginal people with diabetes now have the Northern Diabetes Health Network, a special program that funds local initiatives in diabetes education. In the James Bay region (the Mushkegowuk Council), there is now a coordinator and dietitian, as well as four diabetes educators who are all Aboriginal Canadians and who tailor education for the community. That means that culturally appropriate questions such as "Did you have any bannock [a traditional bread] today?" will be asked of patients.

The Diabetic Education Program for Native People is based on the Standards and Guidelines of the Canadian Diabetes Association and includes a cultural component throughout.

The Sioux Lookout Diabetes Program (SLDP) serves Ojibway and Cree First Nations people from 30 remote communities in northwestern Ontario—many of which can be reached only by plane. This program is establishing a registry of people with diabetes within the community and, by 1994, had a staff that included a coordinator, two Native diabetes educators, a nurse educator, five dietitians and support staff. These professionals travel to the communities to provide education; in the past, the communities were expected to come to one out-of-the-way hospital for education.

Such community diabetes programs involve the community's input with respect to educational materials. Instead of pictures of people in aerobics classes, these materials show people doing familiar activities such as chopping wood. The materials are also translated into the community's first language—Cree rather than English or French.

The SLDP program is a model for other Aboriginal programs across North America. Health care providers, chiefs and councils, and people with diabetes welcome these community-relevant programs.

Healing Circles are also used to explain blood sugar monitoring in a blood-letting ceremony. Walking groups have also been started in a few communities; during these events the whole community, not just one individual, becomes more active. Other culture-specific programs involve elders in diabetes education, who remind their community about traditions of food patterns and fitness. Traditional feasts are also used to teach diabetes education, using only traditional foods without any "Western" foods.

These programs have proven beyond a doubt that Aboriginal people can learn to manage their diabetes when gaps created through language barriers are closed; when diet and activity are better suited to the cultural environment of Aboriginal communities; and when the intimidating Western health practitioner is removed. The issue of preventing diabetes is becoming more accepted as we look at diet and other lifestyle factors that trigger Type 2 diabetes in those who are genetically predisposed. Restoring Canada's lands and waters to their natural state, replenishing Canada's indigenous food supply and eating seasonal and more natural foods will help to heal all Canadians, while improving our spiritual and psychological health. Thousands of years of Aboriginal wisdom about food preservation, natural medicines, roots, herbs and spiritual healing already exist. This information is precious to anyone living in this climate and habitat. If we can learn to reduce the incidence of Type 2 diabetes in our Aboriginal population, perhaps we can help reduce the incidence of this disease in all Canadians.

Chapter 10

IF YOU'RE OBESE

• • • • • • • • • • •

At least 80 percent of those with Type 2 diabetes weigh 20 percent more than they should for their height and age—the technical definition of "obese." But when people go to their doctors, diabetes educators or dietitians, they will be given meal plans, lists of what and what not to eat, diabetes "codes" from the Canadian or American diabetes associations, and so on. The problem is much deeper than simply eating too much food. The key to losing weight for many is to examine *why* they got fat to begin with.

Many obese people say that they've "dieted themselves up" to their present weight. Obesity is the strongest risk factor for developing Type 2 diabetes. Basically, the longer you've been obese, the more you are at risk. Amazingly, diabetes experts have noted that when their patients lose just 2 kg (5 lb.), the body actually begins to use insulin more effectively. But the sentence "eat sensibly and exercise" just doesn't hold any weight for most people battling theirs.

This chapter will help you understand *why* we eat so much in North America, and why we're getting fatter in spite of "low-fat" culture. Part of the story is understanding where the modern diet came from. After all, you didn't create the modern diet; you were born into it. In fact, the root word of "diet" comes from the Greek *diatta*, meaning "way of life." Since controlling your diet and weight are the tools to managing Type 2 diabetes, let's start with understanding *how* diet and lifestyle became linked to Type 2 diabetes to begin with.

THE GOOD TIMES DISEASE

Type 2 diabetes is referred to as the "good times disease" partly because of the work of Dr. Bouchardat, a French physician in the 1870s, who noticed that his diabetic patients seemed to do rather well in war. When their food was rationed, the sugar in the urine of Dr. Bouchardat's diabetic patients disappeared. It was at this point that a connection between food *quantity* and diabetes was made. This observation paved the way for special low-carbohydrate diets as a treatment for diabetes, but it seemed to be effective only in eliminating sugar from the urine in "milder" diabetes, which was what Type 2 diabetes was called before the disease was better understood.

Economies and Scales

Bouchardat's observations were confirmed throughout Europe a few decades later. Many European countries experienced a significant drop, not just in "mild" diabetes, but in a number of obesity-related diseases during the First and Second World Wars, when meat, dairy food and eggs became scarce in large populations. Wartime rations forced people to survive on brown bread, oats and barley meal, and home-grown produce.

Had it not been for the Depression, we in North America may have seen an increase in Type 2 diabetes much earlier than we did. The seeds of sedentary life were already planted in the 1920s, as consumer comforts, mainly the automobile and radio, led to more driving, less walking and more sedentary recreation. The Depression interrupted what was supposed to be prosperous times for everyone. It also intercepted obesity and all diseases related to obesity, as the people in most industrialized nations barely ate enough to survive.

The Depression years, which ended in Canada when Britain declared war on Germany in 1939, combined with six long years of war, led to an unprecedented yearning for consumer goods such as cars, refrigerators, stoves, radios and washing machines. As the boys marched home, they were welcomed with open arms into civilian bliss. By 1948, university enrolment had doubled over the previous decade, leading to an explosion in desk jobs and the commuter economy that exists today. The return of the veterans led to an unprecedented baby boom, driving the candy, sweets and junk-food markets for decades to come. Moreover, a sudden influx of money from Victory Bond investments and veterans' re-establishment grants coincided with the first payments of government pensions and family allowances. Never before had North Americans had so much money.

Manufacturers and packaged-goods companies were looking for better ways to compete and sell their products. The answer to their prayers arrived in the late 1940s with the cathode ray tube: television. In the end, television would become the appliance most responsible for dietary decline and sedentary lifestyle as it turned into a babysitter that could mesmerize the baby boom generation for hours.

The Diet of Leisure

Naturally, after the war, people wanted to celebrate. They gave parties, they drank wine. They smoked. They went to restaurants. More than ever before, our diets began to include more high-fat items, refined carbohydrates, sugar, alcohol and chemical additives. And as people began to manage large families, easy-fix meals in boxes and cans were being manufactured in abundance and sold on television to millions.

The demand for the diet of leisure radically changed agriculture, too. Today, 80 percent of our grain harvest goes to feed livestock. The rest of our arable land is used for other cash crops such as tomatoes, sugar, coffee and bananas. Ultimately, cash crops have helped to create the modern Western diet: an obscene amount of meat, eggs, dairy products, sugar and refined flour.

Since 1940, chemical additives and preservatives in food have risen by 995 percent. In 1959, the Flavor and Extract Manufacturers Association of the United States (FEMA) established a panel of experts to determine the safety status of food flavourings to deal with the overwhelming number of chemicals that companies wanted to add to our foods.

One of the most popular food additives is monosodium glutamate (MSG), the sodium salt of glutamic acid, an amino acid that occurs naturally in protein-containing foods such as meat, fish, milk and many vegetables. MSG is a flavour enhancer that researchers believe contributes a "fifth taste" to savoury foods such as meats, stews, tomatoes and cheese. It was originally extracted from seaweed and other plant sources to function in foods the same way as other spices or extracts. Today, MSG is made from starch, corn sugar or molasses from sugar cane or sugar beets. MSG is produced by a fermentation process similar to that used for making products such as beer, vinegar and yogurt. While MSG is labelled Generally Recommended As Safe (GRAS) by the United States Food and Drug Administration (FDA), questions about the safety of ingesting MSG have been raised because food sensitivities to the substance have been reported. This fact notwithstanding, the main problem with MSG is that it arouses our appetites *even more*. MSG, widespread in our food supply, makes food taste better. And the better food tastes, the *more we eat.*

Hydrolyzed proteins are also used as flavour enhancers. These are made by using enzymes to chemically digest proteins from soy meal, wheat gluten, corn gluten, edible strains of yeast or other food sources. This process, known as *hydrolysis,* breaks down proteins into their component amino acids. Today, several hundred additive substances like these are used in our food, including sugar, baking soda and vitamins (see Chapters 6 and 7).

Of course, one of the key functions of food additives is to preserve foods for transport. The problem is, once we begin to eat foods that are not indigenous to our country, the food loses many of its nutrient properties. Refrigerators make it possible for us to eat tropical foods in Canada and Texas-raised beef in Japan. As a result, few industrialized countries eat "indigenously" any more.

Minimum wage, maximum fat

The legacy of the Western diet of leisure is that it has become cheaper to eat out of a box or can than off the land. In the developed Western world, where you find minimum wage, you also find maximum fat. At one time, fat was a sign of prosperity and wealth. Today, wealth is defined by thinness and fitness. Ironically, low-fat foods, diet programs and fitness clubs attract the segment of our population least affected by obesity. In fact, eating disorders tend to plague those who live in higher-income brackets.

In 1997, the Coalition for Excess Weight Risk Education, a Washington-based organization comprising the American Diabetes Association, the American Association of Diabetes Educators, the American Society for Clinical Nutrition, the North American Association for the Study of Obesity and four pharmaceutical manufacturers, issued statistics on obesity in the United States. The data can be used to interpret obesity patterns throughout the Western world. Based on a 33-city survey, the National Weight Report found that cities with high unemployment rates and low per capita income tended to have higher rates of obesity. Areas with high annual precipitation rates and a high number of food stores also contributed to obesity. (More rainy or snowy days lead to more snacking in front of the television set!) The study also revealed the following:

- Restaurant-rich New Orleans had the United States' highest obesity rate, where 37.5 percent of its adult residents were obese, while Denver, known for its outdoor living, had the lowest rate of obesity—only 22.1 percent of its residents were obese.

- Eating meals away from home and equating high-fat, fried food with a sense of "family" was most commonly reported among obese adults. (This suggests that our commuter society increases fast-food eating, while stress and a lack of emotional support lead people to eat for comfort rather than hunger.)
- Ethnic food (despite the fact that much of it can be lower in fat) tempted Cleveland, Ohio, residents (31.5 percent of Cleveland's adults are obese), while many people blamed their obesity on the cold climate, which made them crave meat, biscuits and French fries to help them fuel up.
- People in hot climates, such as Phoenix, Arizona, where 24.3 percent of its adult population is obese, reported that they gained weight when the weather got too hot for outdoor exercise. (This is a case for eating *seasonably*. Heavy foods in hot climates are unnecessary. This "eating on location" concept is discussed in detail in Chapter 7.)

Other statistics reveal that 35 percent of North American men and 27 percent of North American women are obese. Unfortunately, obesity, physical inactivity and dietary-fat intake are factors we have to look at when trying to understand why 6 percent of Canadian adults (the number is much higher in Aboriginal populations) between ages 18 and 74 currently have diabetes, and why 12 percent of Canadian adults, who were once diagnosed with *impaired glucose tolerance*, are now told they have diabetes (see Chapter 1).

DIETING YOUR WAY TO OBESITY

If you think the key to weight loss is avoiding fat, think again. There is new thinking about what many perceive to be the dangers of *low-fat dieting*. Not only do they *not* work according to many critics, but they promote insulin resistance. A low-fat diet is a diet in which most of your calories come from carbohydrates rather than protein or fat. Because carbohydrates convert into glucose quickly in the body, you eat, feel full, and then feel very hungry again. In order to feel satisfied and satiated, we must have some fat in our diets. But in addition to this, fat in our diets also triggers fat-burning compounds in our bodies. Years of conditioning us to "no fat" has made most people fatter and has dramatically increased our risk of developing Type 2 diabetes because of the amount of insulin we require to "clean up" the carbohydrates that convert so quickly into sugar (see Chapter 6 on meal planning). And higher insulin levels—get this—increase your appetite.

There is now a whole industry of diet books, promoting low- or no-carbohydrate diets, such as *Dr. Atkins' New Diet Revolution, Protein Power* and *The Zone.* But the diets promoted in these books are considered by many nutrition experts to be dangerous, too. The Dr. Atkins diet is dangerous because it is based on a huge amount of saturated fat, which is the major source of "bad cholesterol" in the diet. Regardless of how much weight you may lose on the Atkins diet, you are still at risk for heart disease because of the saturated fat and the high LDL (low-density lipids) levels. The Zone diet, according to some experts, has no scientific basis; the book claims that high carbs and insulin make you fat, when, in fact, it is calories from all sources of food that make you fat when you don't discharge the energy needed to burn them off. The best advice now is to limit carbohydrates in each meal to about 40 percent, and be sure to have about 30 percent protein and 30 percent of "helpful" fat (see below). Some carbohydrates convert into glucose faster than others. The Glycemic Index Table on page 84 can help you select slower-converting carbohydrates to balance your diet.

Why We Like Our Fat

Fat tastes good. Fat also *feels* good in our mouths. Foods that have the particular texture and taste of fat are more acceptable than foods that don't. This is why packaged-goods manufacturers describe their products as "smooth, creamy, moist, tender and rich." All the foods that boast these qualities—from ice cream to chocolate to cheese—give us that unique feeling of satiety and satisfaction that makes us feel good.

Eating is a sensual experience. When we enjoy our food, our brains produce endorphins, "feel good" hormones that are, ironically, also produced when we exercise. Eating fat is analogous to having a "mouth orgasm." To many of us, eating is an empty experience when food doesn't have the taste and texture of fat. And when we're in emotional pain or need, the texture and taste of fat become even more important. Bingeing or falling off the diet wagon is not due to "losing control" but to regaining lost "good feelings." Food, as millions of overeaters will tell you, is our friend. It's always there; it never lets us down.

The impact of "low-fat" products

Since the late 1970s, North Americans have been deluged with low-fat products. In 1990, the United States government launched Healthy People 2000, a campaign to urge manufacturers to double their output of low-fat products by the year 2000. Since 1990, more than 1,000 new fat-free or low-fat products have been introduced into North American supermarkets annually.

Current guidelines tell us that we should consume less than 30 percent of calories from fat, while no more than one-third of fat calories should come from saturated fat. According to U.S. estimates, the average person gets between 34 and 37 percent of his or her calories from fat and roughly 12 percent of all his or her calories from saturated fat. Data show that with regard to "absolute fat," the intake has increased from 81 g per day in 1980 to 83 g per day in the 1990s. Total calorie intake has also increased from 1,989 per day in 1980 to 2,153 calories per day. In fact, the only reason that data show a drop in the percentage of calories from fat is because of the huge increase in calories per day. The result is that as a population we weigh more today than in 1980, despite the fact that roughly 10,000 more low-fat foods are available to us now than in 1980.

Most of these low-fat products, however, actually encourage us to eat more. For example, if a bag of regular chips has 9 g of fat per serving (one serving usually equals five or six chips or one handful), you will more likely stick to that one handful. However, if you find a low-fat brand of chips that boasts "50 percent less fat" per serving, you're more likely to eat the whole bag (feeling good about eating "low-fat" chips), which can easily triple your fat intake.

Low-fat or fat-free foods trick our bodies with ingredients that mimic the functions of fat in foods. This is often achieved by using modified fats that are only partially metabolized, if at all. While some foods have the fat reduced by removing the fat (skim milk, lean cuts of meat), most low-fat foods require a variety of "fat copycats" to preserve the taste and texture of the food. Water, for example, is often combined with carbohydrates and protein to mimic a particular texture or taste, as is the case with a variety of baked goods or cake mixes. In general, though, the low-fat "copycats" are carbohydrate-based, protein-based or fat-based.

Carbohydrate-based ingredients are starches and gums that are often used as thickening agents to create the texture of fat. You'll find them in abundance in low-fat salad dressings, sauces, gravies, frozen desserts and baked goods. Compared to natural fats, which are at about 9 calories per gram, carbohydrate-based ingredients run anywhere from 0 to 4 calories per gram.

Protein-based low-fat ingredients are created by "doing things" to the proteins that make them behave differently. For example, by taking proteins such as whey or egg white and heating or blending them at high speeds, you can create the look and feel of "creamy." Soy and corn proteins are often used in these cases. You'll find these ingredients in low-fat cheese, butter, mayonnaise, salad dressings, frozen dairy desserts, sour cream and baked goods. They run between 1 and 4 calories per gram.

Low-fat foods that use fat-based ingredients tailor the fat in some way so that we do not absorb or metabolize it fully. These ingredients are found in chocolate, chocolate coatings, margarine, spreads, sour cream and cheese. You can also use these ingredients as low-fat substitutes for frying foods (you do this when you fry eggs in margarine, for example). Olestra, the new fat substitute just approved by the United States Food and Drug Administration (FDA), is an example of a fat substitute that is not absorbed by our bodies, providing no calories. Caprenin and salatrim are examples of partially absorbed fats (they contain more long-chain fatty acids; see Glossary) and are the more traditional fat-based low-fat ingredients. They are roughly 5 calories per gram.

There's no question that low-fat foods are designed to give you more freedom of choice with your diet, supposedly allowing you to cut your fat without compromising your taste buds. Studies show that taste outperforms "nutrition" in your brain. Yet many experts believe that in the long term low-fat products create more of a barrier to weight loss.

Researchers at the University of Toronto suggest that these products essentially allow us to increase our calories even though we are reducing our overall fat intake. For example, in one study, women who consumed a low-fat breakfast food ate more during the day than women who consumed a higher-fat food at breakfast.

The good news about low-fat or fat-free products is that they are, in fact, *lower in fat* and are created to substitute for the "bad foods" you know you shouldn't have but cannot live without. The boring phrase "everything in moderation" applies to low-fat products, too. Balancing these products with "good stuff" is the key. A low-fat treat should still be treated like its high-fat original. In other words, don't have double the amount because it's low-fat. Instead, have the same amount as you would of the original.

Chronic Dieting

The road to obesity is also paved with chronic dieting. It is estimated that at least 50 percent of all North Americans are dieting at any given time, while one-third of North American dieters initiate a diet at least once a month. The very act of dieting in your teens and 20s can predispose you to obesity in your 30s, 40s and beyond. This occurs because most people "crash and burn" instead of eating sensibly. In other words, they're chronic dieters. Because of unrealistic beauty standards, women are particularly vulnerable to chronic dieting.

The crash-and-burn approach to diet is what we do when we want to lose a specific amount of weight for a particular occasion or to be able to wear a particular outfit. The pattern is to starve for a few days and then eat what we normally do. Or we eat only certain foods (such as celery and grapefruit) for a number of days and then eat normally after we've lost the weight. Most of these diets do not incorporate exercise, which means that we burn up some of our muscle as well as fat. Then, when we eat normally, we gain only fat. And over the years, that fat simply grows fatter. The bottom line is that when there is more fat on your body than muscle, you cannot burn calories as efficiently. It is the muscle that makes it possible to burn calories. Diet it away, and you diet away your ability to burn fat.

If starvation is involved in our trying to lose weight, our bodies become more efficient at getting fat. Starvation triggers an intelligence in the metabolism; our body suddenly thinks we're living in a war zone and goes into "super-efficient nomadic mode," not realizing that we're living in North America. So, when we return to our normal caloric intake, or even a *lower*-than-normal caloric intake after we've starved ourselves, *we gain more weight.* Our bodies say, "Oh look— food! Better store that as fat for the next famine." Some researchers believe that starvation diets slow down our metabolic rates far below normal so that weight gain becomes more rapid after each starvation episode.

This cycle of crash or starvation dieting is known as the yo-yo diet syndrome, the subject of thousands of articles in women's magazines throughout the last 20 years. Breaking the pattern sounds easy: Combine exercise with a sensible diet. But it's not that easy if you've led a sedentary life most of your adult years. Ninety-five percent of the people who go on a diet gain back the weight they lost, as well as extra weight, within two years. As discussed further on, the failure often lies in psychological and behavioural factors. We have to understand why we need to eat before we can eat less. The best way to break the yo-yo diet pattern is to educate your children early about food habits and appropriate body weight. Experts say that unless you are significantly overweight to begin with or have a medical condition, *don't diet*. Just eat well.

A HEALTHIER APPROACH TO A DIET

If you're contemplating a diet, you should also consider the following:

▶ What is a reasonable weight for you, given your genetic makeup, family history, age and culture? A smaller weight loss in some people can produce dramatic effects.

▶ Aim to lose weight at a slower rate. Too much too fast will probably lead to gaining it all back.

▶ Incorporate exercise into your routine, particularly activities that build muscle mass.

▶ Eat your vitamins. Make sure you're meeting the Canadian Recommended Nutrient Intakes (RNIs). Many of the popular North American diets of the 1980s, for example, were nutritionally inadequate (the Beverly Hills Diet contained 0 percent of the U.S. recommendation for vitamin B_{12}).

EATING DISORDERS AND COMPULSIVE EATING

The two most common eating disorders involve starvation. They are *anorexia nervosa* ("loss of appetite due to mental disorder") and bingeing followed by purging, known as *bulimia nervosa* ("hunger like an ox due to mental disorder"). People will purge after a bingeing episode by inducing vomiting, and abusing laxatives, diuretics and thyroid hormone. Eating disorders are most common in women, but men are also succumbing to impractical body standards and are prone to purging behaviours in particular.

Perhaps the most accepted weight-control behaviour is *overexercising*. Today, rigorous, strenuous exercise is used as a method of "purging" and has become one of the tenets of socially accepted behaviour today.

Binge-Eating Disorder

When we hear the term "eating disorder," we usually think about anorexia or bulimia. Many people, however, binge without purging. This practice is also known as binge-eating disorder (a.k.a. compulsive overeating). In this case, the bingeing is still an announcement to the world that "I'm out of control." Someone who purges after bingeing is hiding his or her lack of control. Someone who binges and never purges is *advertising* his or her lack of control. The purger is passively asking for help; the binger who doesn't purge is aggressively asking for help. It's the same disease with a different result. But there is one more layer when it comes to compulsive overeating that is considered to be controversial and is often rejected by the overeater: The desire to get fat is often behind the compulsion. Many people who overeat insist that fat is a consequence of eating food, not a *goal*. Many therapists who deal with overeating disagree and believe that if a woman admits that she has an emotional interest in actually being large, she may be much closer to stopping her compulsion to eat.

Furthermore, many women who eat compulsively do not recognize that they are doing so. The following is a typical profile of a compulsive eater:

- eating when you're not hungry
- feeling out of control when you're around food, either trying to resist it or gorging on it
- spending a lot of time thinking or worrying about food and your weight
- always desperate to try another diet that promises results
- having feelings of self-loathing and shame
- hating your own body
- obsessing with what you can or will eat, or *have* eaten
- eating in secret or with "eating friends"
- appearing in public to be a professional dieter who's in control
- buying cakes or pies as "gifts" and having them wrapped to hide the fact that they're for you
- having a "pristine" kitchen with only the "right" foods
- feeling either out of control with food (compulsive eating), or imprisoned by it (dieting)
- feeling temporary relief by "not eating"
- looking forward with pleasure and anticipation to the time when you can eat alone
- feeling unhappy because of your eating behaviour

The Issue of Hunger

Most people eat when they're hungry. But if you're a compulsive eater, hunger cues have nothing to do with when you eat. You may eat for any of the following reasons:

1. As a social event: this includes family meals or meeting friends at restaurants. The point is that you plan food as the "social entertainment." Most of us do this now and then, but often we do it when we're not even hungry.
2. To satisfy "mouth hunger," the need to have something in your mouth, even though you are not hungry.
3. To prevent *future* hunger: "Better eat now because later, I may not get a chance."
4. As a reward for a bad day or bad experience, or to reward yourself for a *good* day or good experience.
5. Because "it's the only pleasure I can count on!"
6. To quell nerves.
7. Because you're bored.
8. Because you're "going on a diet" tomorrow. (Hence, the eating is done now out of a real fear that you will be deprived later.)
9. Because food is your friend.

Twelve Steps to Change

Food addiction, like other addictions, can be treated successfully with a 12-step program. For those of you who aren't familiar with this type of program, I've provided the text of "The 12 Steps" in the box "The 12 Steps of Overeaters Anonymous, on page 155."

The 12-step program was started in the 1930s by an alcoholic who was able to overcome his addiction by essentially saying, "God, help me!" He found other alcoholics who were in a similar position and through an organized, non-judgemental support system, they overcame their addiction by realizing that "God" (a higher power, spirit, force, physical properties of the universe or intelligence) *helps those who help themselves*. In other words, you have to want the help. This is the premise of Alcoholics Anonymous—the most successful recovery program for addicts that exists.

People with other addictions have adopted the program, using Alcoholics Anonymous and its "12 Steps and 12 Traditions," the founding literature for Alcoholics Anonymous, as the model. Overeaters Anonymous substitutes the phrase "compulsive overeater" for "alcoholic" and "food" for "alcohol." The theme of all 12-step programs is best expressed through the Serenity Prayer, the first few lines being, "God grant me the serenity to accept the things I cannot change, the courage to change the things I can, and the wisdom to know the difference." In other words, you can't take back the food you ate yesterday or last year, but you can control the food you eat today instead of feeling guilty about yesterday.

Every 12-step program also has the 12 Traditions, which, essentially, is a code of conduct. To join an OA program, you need only take the first step. Abstinence and the next two steps are what most people are able to do in a 6- to 12-month period before moving on. In an OA program, "abstinence" means three meals daily, weighed and measured, with nothing in between except sugar-free or no-calorie beverages, and sugar-free gum. The food you eat is recorded and monitored with the help of keeping a diary. The program also advises you to get your doctor's approval before starting. Abstinence is continued through a process of taking one day at a time and having "sponsors"—people who call you to check in, and whom you can call when the cravings hit. Sponsors are recovering overeaters who have been there and who can talk you through your cravings.

OA membership is predominantly female; if you are interested in joining OA and are male, you may feel more comfortable in an all-male group. Many women overeaters overeat because they have been harmed by men, and their anger is often directed at the one male in the room; this may not be a comfortable position if you're a male overeater. For this reason, OA is divided into all-female and all-male groups.

THE 12 STEPS OF OVEREATERS ANONYMOUS

Step 1: I admit I am powerless over food and that my life has become unmanageable.

Step 2: I've come to believe that a Power greater than myself can restore me to sanity.

Step 3: I've made a decision to turn my will and my life over to the care of a Higher Power, as I understand it.

Step 4: I've made a searching and fearless moral inventory of myself.

Step 5: I've admitted to a Higher Power, to myself, and to another human being the exact nature of my wrongs.

Step 6: I'm entirely ready to have a Higher Power remove all these defects of character.

Step 7: I've humbly asked a Higher Power to remove my shortcomings.

Step 8: I've made a list of all persons I have harmed and am willing to make amends to them all.

Step 9: I've made direct amends to such people wherever possible, except when to do so would injure them or others.

Step 10: I've continued to take personal inventory and when I was wrong, promptly admitted it.

Step 11: I've sought through prayer and meditation to improve my conscious contact with a Higher Power, as I understand it, praying only for knowledge of its will for me and the power to carry that out.

Step 12: Having had a spiritual awakening as the result of these steps, I've tried to carry this message to compulsive overeaters and to practise these principles in all my affairs.

BIOLOGICAL CAUSES OF OBESITY

Eating too much high-fat or high-calorie food while remaining sedentary is certainly one biological cause of obesity. Furthermore, a woman's metabolism slows down by 25 percent after menopause, which means that unless she either decreases her calories by 25 percent or increases her activity level by 25 percent to compensate, she will probably gain weight. Other hormonal problems can also contribute to obesity, such as an underactive thyroid gland (called hypothyroidism), which is very common in women over 50.

But since diet and lifestyle changes are so difficult, there is an interest in finding genetic causes for obesity. Discovering there are genetic causes would mean that obesity is *beyond our control* and is something we've inherited, which would probably be comforting for many people. Now that we are in the midst of the Human Genome Project, a project that intends to map every gene in the human body, efforts are underway to find the "obesity gene" or "fat gene," but few scientists believe that obesity is *simply* genetic. In other words, there are so many environmental and social factors that can "trip" the obesity "switch" that finding a specific gene for obesity is about as worthwhile as finding the "anger gene" or "crime gene."

Some Theories

An important theory about why we get fat concerns insulin resistance. It's believed that when the body produces too much insulin we will eat more to try to maintain a balance. This is why weight gain is often the first symptom of Type 2 diabetes. But then we have to ask what causes insulin resistance to begin with; many researchers believe that it is triggered by obesity, so it becomes a "chicken or egg" puzzle.

There are also many theories regarding the function of fat cells. Are some people genetically programmed to have more, or "fatter," fat cells than others? No answers here yet.

What about the brain and obesity? Some propose that obesity is "all in the head" and has something to do with the hypothalamus (a part of the brain that controls messages to other parts of the body) somehow malfunctioning when it comes to sending the body the message "I'm full." It's believed that the hypothalamus may control "satiation messages."

To other researchers, the problem has to do with some sort of "defect" in the body that doesn't recognize hunger cues or satiation cues, but the studies in this area are not conclusive.

What about the fat hormone?

A study reported in a 1997 issue of *Nature Medicine* showed that people with low levels of the hormone leptin may be prone to weight gain. In this study, people who gained an average of 22 kg (50 lb.) over three years started out with lower leptin levels than people who maintained their weight over the same period. Therefore, this study may form the basis for treating obesity with leptin. Experts speculate that 10 percent of all obesity may be due to a leptin resistance. Leptin is made by fat cells and apparently sends messages to the brain about how much fat our bodies are carrying. Like other hormones, it's thought that leptin has a stimulating action that acts as a thermostat of sorts. In mice, adequate amounts of leptin somehow signalled the mouse to become more active and eat less, while too little leptin signalled the mouse to eat more while becoming less active.

Interestingly, Pima Indians, who are prone to obesity and who are also at highest risk for Type 2 diabetes in the United States, were shown to have roughly one-third less leptin in blood analyses than the general population. Human studies of injecting leptin to treat obesity are in the works right now, but to date have not been shown to be effective.

Right now, researchers are working on using leptin as a prevention drug for Type 2 diabetes. Not only does leptin block the formation of fat in body tissues, but it apparently lowers blood sugar levels, too. It's believed that leptin somehow improves the function of insulin-producing cells in the pancreas, which helps the body to use insulin more effectively. Since you won't find leptin on your drugstore shelves just yet, you're going to have to be your own fat hormone and do the difficult work of losing some weight.

Drug Treatment for Obesity

Drug treatment for obesity has an awfully shady history. Women have been especially abused by the medical system. Throughout the 1950s, 1960s and even 1970s, women were prescribed thyroxine, which is thyroid hormone, to speed up their metabolisms. Unless a person has an underactive thyroid gland or no thyroid gland (it may have been surgically removed), this is a very dangerous medication that can cause heart failure. Request a thyroid function test before you accept this medication.

Amphetamines or "speed" were often widely peddled to women as well by doctors, but these drugs, too, are dangerous, and can put your health at risk.

One of the most controversial antiobesity therapies was the use of fenfluramine and phentermine (Fen/Phen). Both drugs were approved for use individually more than 20 years ago, but since 1992, doctors have tended to prescribe them together for long-term management of obesity. In 1996, U.S. doctors wrote a total of 18 million monthly prescriptions for Fen/Phen. And many of the prescriptions were issued to people who were not obese. This practice is known as "off-label" prescribing. In July 1997, the United States Food and Drug Administration and researchers at the Mayo Clinic and the Mayo Foundation made a joint announcement warning doctors that Fen/Phen can cause heart disease. On September 15, 1997, "Fen" was taken off the market. The Fen/Phen lesson: Diet and lifestyle modification are still the best pathways to wellness. More bad news has surfaced about Fen/Phen wreaking havoc on serotonic levels, a finding that only reinforces the message that in light of the safety concerns regarding current antiobesity drugs, diet and lifestyle modification are still considered the best approach to wellness.

Approved antiobesity pills

In 2000, Canada approved an antiobesity pill that blocks the absorption of almost one-third of the fat people eat. One of the side effects of this new prescription drug, called orlistat (Xenical), causes rather embarrassing diarrhea when the fat content in your meal exceeds 20 percent. To avoid the drug's side effects, simply avoid fat! The pill can also decrease absorption of vitamin D and other important nutrients, however.

Orlistat is the first drug to fight obesity through the intestine instead of the brain. Taken with each meal, it binds to certain pancreatic enzymes to block the digestion of 30 percent of the fat you ingest. When they combined it with a sensible diet, people on orlistat lost more weight than those not on orlistat. This drug is not intended for people who need to lose a few pounds; it is designed for medically obese people. The safety of orlistat for people with diabetes is under debate. Although in studies orlistat was found to lower cholesterol, blood pressure and blood sugar levels (as a result of weight loss), it can lead to pancreatitis (inflammation of the pancreas, discussed in Chapter 1) and inflammation of the gallbladder.

Another obesity drug, sibutramine, was approved for use in Canada in 2001. Sibutramine is meant for people whose body mass index (BMI) registers at 27 or higher. This is generally people who weigh more than 20 percent of their ideal weight. To calculate your BMI, you can visit www.4meridia.com.

Sibutramine's safety for people with Type 2 diabetes is debatable. Anyone with high blood pressure (see Chapter 2) is cautioned against taking sibutramine, because sibutramine can significantly raise your blood pressure.

If you're taking medications for depression, thyroid problems, seizures, glaucoma, osteoporosis, gallbladder disease, liver disease, heart disease or stroke prevention (see Chapter 15), kidney disease (see Chapter 19), migraines or Parkinson's disease, you are also cautioned against taking sibutramine and should discuss with your doctor whether the drug is safe. Also, many nutritional supplements, such as tryptophan, are not recommended with sibutramine, so please disclose to your doctor all non-prescription, over-the-counter medications as well as all herbal and nutritional substances you're taking if you're considering sibutramine.

Smoking and Obesity

Obviously, no health care provider will "prescribe" nicotine or smoking to you as a "weight loss" drug, but many people (especially women) will take up the habit anyway as a tool to weight loss or, worse, revisit the habit long after they've quit.

Smoking satisfies "mouth hunger," the need to have something in your mouth. It also causes withdrawal symptoms that can drive people to eat. If you need to lose weight, also smoke and have Type 2 diabetes, something has got to give! Smoking will restrict small blood vessels, which can put you at risk for a host of complications associated with Type 2 diabetes (see Part 3). The best way around this problem is to ask your health care team for some information on credible smoking-cessation programs. There are, unfortunately, no easy answers to the dilemma of weight loss versus quitting smoking. Most health care providers will assess your current risk of heart disease and/or stroke, and help you prioritize your lifestyle changes. For more on quitting smoking, see Chapter 2.

Chapter 11

TYPE 2 DIABETES, FERTILITY AND PREGNANCY

● ● ● ● ● ● ● ● ● ●

This chapter offers you information that is difficult to find because there is such a "splintered" market when it comes to pregnancy and diabetes. This chapter is designed for two specific groups of women: The first group is already diagnosed with Type 2 diabetes, has delayed having children (probably for social reasons) but nevertheless is planning a pregnancy or is already pregnant. A good many of the women in this group may also have been dealing with infertility or may be undergoing assisted reproductive technology. Many women in their mid- to late 40s, for example, have more options regarding pregnancy as a result of egg donation. Therefore, the old belief that "women with Type 2 diabetes are too old to have babies and don't need this information" is being radically revised. In fact, there has been an upsurge in what is called "postmenopausal pregnancy" as a direct result of new fertility treatments. What you need to know about fertility treatments and diabetes is therefore discussed, as well as how Type 2 diabetes often affects fertility. And of course, everything you need to know about managing Type 2 diabetes *during* pregnancy is discussed, too, under the section "Being Pregnant," on page 167.

The second group of women reading this chapter will not have been diagnosed at all with Type 2 diabetes, but instead will have been diagnosed with *gestational diabetes,* which means "diabetes during pregnancy." Gestational diabetes is not the same disease as Type 2 diabetes, even though it usually *behaves* the same way. It is a condition that occurs during pregnancy where your body is resistant to the insulin it makes, but it can often be managed through dietary changes and meal planning. And it often disappears after pregnancy. Gestational diabetes, however, is often a "warning" that unless lifestyle and dietary habits change between pregnancies or *after* childbirth, Type 2 diabetes may be "in the cards" after all. If this is the reason you're reading this chapter, go directly to the section on gestational diabetes on page 170. Finally, if you have Type 1 diabetes, this is *not* the book for you, although you may indeed find certain sections of this chapter helpful.

GETTING PREGNANT

You have Type 2 diabetes, but you still want to get pregnant. What do you need to do in order to have a healthy baby, while staying healthy yourself?

The first step is to *plan ahead*! Get yourself under tight control through diet, exercise and frequent blood sugar monitoring. If you are taking oral medication for your diabetes, you must stop; these medications cannot be taken during pregnancy. You must either discuss managing your diabetes through diet and exercise alone, or must go on insulin during your conception phase and pregnancy. If you have to go on temporary insulin, review Chapter 5 for some "getting started" information, as well as useful tables that will explain what kinds of insulins are available. However, be forewarned: You must be able to *handle* taking insulin and going through a fairly radical change in your lifestyle habits, as well as being able to "handle" another huge lifestyle change—having a baby! Please have a frank discussion with your partner and doctor prior to making this decision.

Experts recommend that you should ideally plan your pregnancy three to six months in advance of conception, so that you can make sure that your glycosylated hemoglobin levels (known as HbA_{1c} levels—see Chapter 3) are within normal ranges during this period. A normal level means that your diabetes is well managed, therefore the risk of birth defects is low. (This is a risk in the early stages of pregnancy if you have high blood sugar.) The following tests prior to getting pregnant are also recommended:

- eye exam (to rule out diabetes eye disease)
- blood pressure and urine test to check your kidney function
- a gynecological exam (this should include a pelvic exam, breast exam, Pap test and screening for vaginal infections or sexually transmitted diseases)
- a general checkup to rule out heart disease or other circulatory problems

Obesity

Regardless of your diabetes, obesity may be a sign that your pregnancy will become high risk. For the record, the definition of "obese" means that you weigh at least 20 percent more than you should for your height and age. In the United States, roughly 32 million women (one-sixth of the population) fit this definition, and 40 percent of these women are young. As if you didn't have enough to worry about, there is some more bad news. A recent study showed that women who are obese prior to conceiving are 60 percent more likely to have a Caesarean delivery than women of average weight. If you are obese with your first pregnancy, the news is even worse: You're 64 percent more likely to require a Caesarean section (also referred to as C-section). And the heavier you are, the more likely you are to have that C-section.

This is not a conspiracy. It just so happens that when you're obese *prior* to the pregnancy, the odds of a number of complications *during* pregnancy increase, including gestational diabetes, discussed further on.

Experts strongly suggest that the only way to combat this problem is to help women achieve a normal weight prior to conceiving, which would lead to a marked decrease in C-section deliveries. In fact, the current first-time Caesarean delivery rate of 20 to 25 percent is blamed on this obesity issue. If all women were of normal weight for their ages and heights, experts muse that the C-section rate in the United States would drop to roughly 12 percent for first-time Caesareans and 3 percent for repeat C-sections. An obstetrician is recommended if you were obese prior to conceiving.

Having Sex

Getting pregnant means having sex (usually!). But if you're a woman with diabetes, the act of having sex can interfere with blood sugar levels since it is, after all, an *activity*. Therefore, many experts recommend that you treat sexual activity as any other activity and plan for it accordingly as a physical exercise of sorts. The risk of developing low blood sugar, or hypoglycemia, is actually not uncommon with sexual activity and diabetes. You may need to eat after sex, or eat something beforehand to ward off low blood sugar.

There is also the opposite problem: *no desire* for sex. This can occur because of vaginal infections (see Chapter 16), or because of changing hormones if you are approaching menopause. Studies that looked specifically at the effect diabetes has on women and sexuality found that loss of libido was often caused by high blood sugar; vaginal infections, and resulting pain or itching during intercourse; the sheer fear of pain or itching during intercourse; as well as nerve damage, which affects blood flow to the female genitalia, and hence, can interfere with pleasure, sensation and orgasm.

Many women with diabetes also report that they feel more unattractive as a result of their diabetes. They are concerned with not just their own perform-ance, but their ability to please their partners. Fears of a "low blood sugar attack in the sack" are particularly common. The only way to avoid feelings of unat-tractiveness or fears is openness with your partner. Discussing these issues with a sex therapist or counsellor may also be a valuable experience.

Who Should Not Get Pregnant?

If your diabetes has affected your kidneys (see Chapter 19), then pregnancy is not in your best interests. You will need to weigh your desire to procreate against the risks of dying from kidney failure. By controlling your diabetes during pregnancy, it is still possible to give birth to a healthy child even when *you* have kidney disease, but it is unlikely that you yourself will live to see that child's fifth birthday. Since people with diabetic kidney disease do not do well on dialysis, pregnancy will put your life in danger, unless you have a kidney transplant. I recommend that any woman with diabetic kidney disease contem-plating pregnancy rent the film *Steel Magnolias*. It may give you a different perspective.

Infertility and Diabetes

And, then, of course, there are those of you who want to get pregnant, but cannot. This section may shed some light on a common problem affecting many women with Type 2 diabetes. It is a condition known as polycystic ovarian syndrome (PCO), which is also a classic female infertility problem in the general population.

What happens in PCO is that your body secretes far too much androgen, the male hormone, which counteracts your ovaries' ability to make enough proges-terone necessary for a normal cycle. Androgen levels interfere with your FSH (follicle-stimulating hormone), which you need to trigger progesterone. So your follicles never develop but turn into small, pea-sized cysts on your ovaries. Your ovaries can then enlarge. Because your androgen levels are out of whack, you can develop male characteristics: facial hair, hair on other parts of your body (this happens in 70 percent of the cases and is called *hirsutism*) or even a balding problem. Acne is another typical symptom because of an increase in androgen, as is obesity (although women who have a normal weight or are thin can also have this syndrome.) Your periods will also be irregular and, as result, you might be at greater risk for developing *endometrial hyperplasia,* a condition in which your uterine lining thickens to the point of becoming precancerous. (If you have endometrial hyperplasia, either progesterone supplements will be given to you to induce a period, or a dilatation and curettage may be required to get rid of the lining.) Because of your high levels of androgens, you may also be at an increased risk of cardiovascular disease. Diet can help reduce the onset of heart problems.

You can treat PCO with natural progesterone therapy or oral contraceptives.

Sometimes, women with normal cycles for many years may develop PCO later in life. In this case, they will suddenly develop irregular cycles (called *secondary amenorrhea*) out of the blue.

It's recently been discovered that insulin resistance and polycystic ovary syndrome go hand-in-hand, but it's been long known that low blood sugar prevents progesterone receptors from working properly in the body, causing progesterone deficiency, which can lead to PCO. Women with insulin resistance are either at risk for, or have been diagnosed with, Type 2 diabetes. Women who are obese (many of whom are also insulin-resistant) can be also predisposed to PCO because their fatty tissues produce estrogen, which can confuse the pituitary gland.

Lowering insulin in women with polycystic ovarian syndrome seems to help restore menstrual cycles and lower male hormone levels. Oral hypoglycemic agents used to treat Type 2 diabetes are now being used to treat PCO, although these agents must be stopped once you become pregnant. Only about half the women diagnosed with PCO have insulin resistance, however. Before you're placed on an insulin-lowering drug, ask your doctor about how diet and exercise can help your body use insulin more efficiently.

In general, PCO is hereditary and is more common among women of Mediterranean descent. It's also uncommon to develop PCO later in life, although it can happen. Generally, a PCO woman will begin to experience menstrual irregularities within three or four years after her menarche (first period). About 4 percent of the general female population suffer from this, which accounts for half of all hormonal disorders affecting female fertility.

Why are estrogen levels normal in PCO women?

Normal estrogen levels come as a surprise to women with PCO. In normally fertile women, estrogen is made from the follicles. In this case, however, your body converts the *androgens* into estrogen. If you're obese, estrogen will also be stored in fat cells. This constant estrogen level really confuses the hypothalamus, which assumes that high estrogen levels are present because of a developing egg inside the follicle. The hypothalamus will then tell the pituitary to slow down the release of FSH. Without FSH, your follicles won't mature and won't burst and hence you won't ovulate.

Reversing infertility

To reverse infertility in women with PCO, doctors will use the fertility drug clomiphene citrate in tablet form. You'll start clomiphene citrate around day 5 of your cycle, and then go off the tablet at about day 10. If you've had long bouts of amenorrhea, your period will first be induced via a progesterone supplement before starting on clomiphene citrate. An average dosage of clomiphene citrate in this case ranges between 25 and 50 mg. Roughly 70 to 90 percent of all PCO women on clomiphene will ovulate, but pregnancy rates really vary; 30 to 70 percent of PCO women on clomiphene will conceive.

If you're still not ovulating after taking clomiphene citrate, human chorionic gonadotropin (HCG) may be added to your hormonal "diet" during the luteal phase of your cycle (in other words, roughly one week after your last dose of clomiphene citrate).

If this regimen fails, you'll graduate to a very potent fertility drug, human menopausal gonadotropin (HMG, Pergonal or Metrodin). This drug is *pure* FSH, made from the urine of menopausal women. (During menopause, FSH naturally soars in the body to compensate for tired ovaries.)

Prior to starting HMG, you'll need to have a hysterosalpingogram, a procedure that checks whether your Fallopian tubes are clear. You may also need a pelvic ultrasound to rule out other structural abnormalities. PCO women don't do as well on HMG as they do on clomiphene citrate. While 70 to 80 percent will ovulate with HMG, only 20 to 40 percent will conceive. While taking HMG, you'll also need to be monitored through blood tests (to check estrogen levels) and ultrasound (to check follicle growth).

For more information on the side effects, costs and risks associated with fertility drugs and other fertility treatments, consult my book *The Fertility Sourcebook*.

I do urge any woman with diabetes, however, to consult her diabetes specialist prior to going on *any* fertility drugs. Estrogen can raise blood sugar levels, and you need to know how these drugs will affect your *blood sugar*, not just your ovaries.

Other treatments for PCO

In many PCO women, weight loss is considered the "cure," just as it often is for insulin resistance. However, when infertility is a concern and your birthdays are coming "fast and furious," weight loss alone may not be a realistic short-term treatment since it's a slow, time-consuming process. If you have PCO and are being treated with fertility drugs, you may be able to reverse your infertility through natural weight loss for future pregnancies. Your diabetes educator or a dietitian can help you with meal planning, which will not only help you control your diabetes, but may help you get pregnant.

If the ovaries have large cysts on them, some fertility specialists may want to attempt cauterizing the ovary (in about eight to ten small spots) through laproscopic surgery. This procedure is still considered experimental, but roughly 62 percent of PCO women who have this surgery go on to conceive, and when the surgery is combined with fertility drug therapy, the pregnancy rates are as high as 80 percent.

In some PCO women, androgens are also produced in the adrenal glands. Under these circumstances, your doctor may want to put you on a corticosteroid to suppress the adrenal gland, lowering the production of androgens. This will help induce ovulation as well.

Bromocriptine, which suppresses prolactin, will be given to 15 to 20 percent of all PCO women. The high levels of estrogen associated with PCO commonly cause hyperprolactenemia, meaning "too much prolactin," which can interfere with fertility.

A hairy situation

Women who have had diabetes for long periods of time may notice hirsutism, or overgrowth of hair. Apparently, some studies show that prolonged use of insulin can trigger higher levels of testosterone, which can cause facial hair growth. This is also one of the unpleasant symptoms of PCO. Typically, this hair growth appears on the face, navel or breasts, and many women will want to treat this problem. For more information about hair removal, consult my book *Women and Unwanted Hair*, available through most on-line bookstores such as Chapters.ca or Amazon.com.

Other causes of infertility

There are many other causes of female-factor and male-factor infertility that are completely unrelated to blood sugar. For the record, roughly 80 percent of all female-factor infertility is caused by structural problems in which the Fallopian tubes become blocked. This could be due to pelvic inflammatory disease, a condition that erupts when bacterial infections (from a sexually transmitted disease or bacteria entering during pelvic surgery or previous childbirth) travel up the reproductive tract, causing tubal scarring and inflammation. Endometriosis is another cause of tubal blockage. For more information on other causes of infertility, refer to my book *The Fertility Sourcebook*.

BEING PREGNANT

When you're diagnosed with Type 2 diabetes *prior* to becoming pregnant, this section is for you. This means you have what's known as *pre-existing diabetes* (diabetes before pregnancy). If you have developed diabetes *during* pregnancy, see the separate section on page 170 on gestational diabetes (diabetes during pregnancy).

So long as your blood glucose levels are normal throughout your pregnancy and you have normal blood pressure, you are "allowed" to be pregnant, and you and your baby should be fine. Nevertheless, there are some concerns unique to women with Type 2 diabetes.

For example, if you have Type 2 diabetes, statistics say that you're probably in worse shape than your Type 1 counterparts. First, you don't have the years of practice Type 1 women do at monitoring blood sugar levels. Second, if you were taking oral hypoglycemic agents prior to your pregnancy, you may not have learned to be as strict with your diet as you should be—something you *cannot* afford during pregnancy. But since these pills cannot be taken during pregnancy (they cause birth defects), your doctor will switch you over to insulin before you conceive, which puts you in the difficult predicament of "learning" a whole new disease. The danger of taking oral hypoglycemic agents during pregnancy is that the drug crosses the placenta and gets into the baby's bloodstream, which can cause very low blood sugar in the fetus. Insulin, however, does not cross the placenta and is safe during pregnancy.

Unfortunately, unless you became an expert on your diabetes *prior* to conceiving, you're in for a bumpy ride. In fact, the early weeks in pregnancy are so critical that if your blood sugar levels were not under control *three to six months prior to your pregnancy*, you should seriously ask your practitioners whether they advise continuing the pregnancy.

During the first three months of pregnancy the fetus is developing its brain, nervous system and other body organs. It's also during this time that your blood sugar levels are most vulnerable because of hormonal changes, vomiting as a result of morning sickness, and/or fatigue.

Staying in Control

No matter what type of diabetes you have, every diabetes book will tell you that a healthy pregnancy depends on how well *you* manage your disease. If you can keep your blood sugar levels as close to normal as possible throughout your pregnancy, then, as most books will also tell you, your chances of a healthy baby are as good as a non-diabetic woman's. The only way to do this is to carefully plan out your meals, exercise and insulin requirements with your doctor if, in fact, you do require insulin during your pregnancy. If you do, your insulin requirements will continue to increase as your pregnancy progresses. Keep in mind that the state of pregnancy means that your blood sugar levels are usually lower than they are for women who are not pregnant. Therefore, what's considered to be in the "normal range" for non-pregnant women will be different values than what is considered "normal" for pregnant women. Consult your doctor about what the normal range should be for you.

When you lose control

If you lose control of your blood sugar levels in the first eight weeks of pregnancy, your baby is at risk for birth defects. High blood sugar levels may interfere with the formation of your baby's organs, causing heart defects or spina bifida (open spine). Once your baby's organs are formed, the risk of birth defects from high blood sugar levels disappears, but new problems surface.

High blood sugar levels will cross the placenta and feed the baby too much glucose, causing the baby to make extra fat and therefore grow too big and fat for its gestational age. This condition is called macrosomia, which is defined as birth weight greater than 4,000 g, or greater than the 90th percentile babies.

In addition, the baby is at risk for becoming lethargic and developing a malfunctioning metabolism in utero, which can lead to stillbirth. This problem is solved when you regain control of your blood sugar levels. Babies with macrosomia are usually not able to fit through the birth canal; they often sustain damage to their shoulders (the shoulders get stuck) during a vaginal birth. So, if your baby is too big, you will need a Caesarean section.

The extra glucose that gets into the baby also causes the baby's pancreas to make extra insulin. Then, after birth, the baby's body needs time to adjust to normal glucose levels (since the placenta is gone), and this can cause the baby to suffer from hypoglycemia, or low blood glucose levels. These babies are also at higher risk for breathing problems and are at a higher risk for obesity later in life, as well as developing Type 2 diabetes.

Your baby may also develop jaundice after birth, which is very common for all newborns, but tends to happen more frequently in babies born to mothers with diabetes. Newborn jaundice is caused by a buildup of old or "leftover" red blood cells that aren't clearing out of the body fast enough. However, breast-feeding is the best cure for newborn jaundice. Consult my book *The Breastfeeding Sourcebook* for more information about this.

FIVE STEPS TO GOOD GLUCOSE

1. Use a home blood glucose monitor to test your blood sugar levels. Pregnancy can mask the symptoms of low blood glucose so you cannot rely on how well you "feel." The goal is to get your blood glucose levels to copy those of a non-diabetic pregnant woman, *which would be lower than in a non-diabetic, non-pregnant woman.*

2. Ask your doctor *when* you should test your blood glucose levels. During pregnancy, it's common to test up to *eight times per day,* especially after eating.

3. Record your results in a journal you keep handy. Take the journal with you when you go out, especially to restaurants.

4. In a *separate* journal, keep track of when you're exercising and what you're eating.

5. Check with your doctor or diabetes educator before you make any changes to your diet or insulin plan whatsoever. And, no, midwives and doulas are *not* the appropriate practitioners to rely on for this information!

YOUR DIABETES PRENATAL TEAM

A healthy pregnancy also depends on a good prenatal team that can help you stay in control. In the same way that you would handpick various skill sets for a baseball team, you must do the same for this team. So here are the specialists to look for:

1. An endocrinologist or internist who specializes in diabetes and diabetic pregnancies.

2. An obstetrician who specializes in high-risk pregnancies, particularly diabetic pregnancies. You may wish to use a *perinatologist*, a doctor who exclusively specializes in high-risk pregnancies.

3. A neonatologist (a specialist for newborns) "waiting in the wings" or a good pediatrician who is trained to manage babies of diabetic moms.

4. A nutritionist or registered dietitian who can help you plan a realistic diet and insulin plan during your pregnancy.

5. A diabetes educator who is available to answer questions throughout your pregnancy.

6. For additional support, a midwife or doula.

GESTATIONAL DIABETES

Gestational diabetes refers to diabetes that is first diagnosed during the 24th to 28th week of pregnancy. If you had diabetes prior to your pregnancy (Type 1 or Type 2), it is known as *pregestational diabetes*, which is a completely different story, in that the risks to the fetus exist throughout pregnancy.

Technically, gestational diabetes means "high blood sugar (hyperglycemia) first recognized during pregnancy." Three to 12 percent of all pregnant women will develop gestational diabetes between weeks 24 and 28 of their pregnancies. The symptoms of gestational diabetes are extreme thirst, hunger or fatigue, but many women do not notice these symptoms.

What Is GDM?

During pregnancy, hormones made by the placenta can block the insulin the pancreas normally makes. This forces the pancreas to work harder and manufacture three times as much insulin as usual. In many cases, the pancreas isn't able to keep up, and blood sugar levels rise. Gestational diabetes is therefore a common pregnancy-related health problem and is in the same league as other pregnancy-related conditions that develop during the second or third trimesters, such as high blood pressure.

Since pregnancy is also a time in your life when you're gaining weight, some experts believe that it is the sheer weight gain that contributes to insulin resistance, as the pancreas cannot keep up with the new weight and, hence, new "demand" for insulin. It's akin to a small restaurant with only ten tables suddenly being presented with triple the number of customers. It will be understaffed and unable to accommodate the new demand for "tables."

GDM, Type 2 diabetes, can be managed through diet and blood sugar monitoring. However, recent research on California women with gestational diabetes showed that only one-third were able to control their condition through diet and blood sugar monitoring. Therefore, insulin may be necessary if your GDM cannot be controlled. GDM will usually disappear once you deliver, but it recurs in future pregnancies two out of three times. In some cases, GDM is really the unveiling of Type 2 or even Type 1 diabetes *during* pregnancy.

If you are genetically predisposed to Type 2 diabetes, you are more likely to develop Type 2 in the future if you developed gestational diabetes.

Moreover, if you have GDM, you're more at risk for other pregnancy-related conditions, such as hypertension (high blood pressure), pre-eclampsia and polyhydramnios (too much amniotic fluid). And if you're carrying more than one fetus, your pregnancy is even more at risk. Therefore, it's wise to seek out an obstetrician if you have GDM. In very high-risk situations, a perinatologist (an obstetrician who specializes in high-risk pregnancies) may have to be consulted.

Diagnosing GDM

GDM is diagnosed through a test known as *glucose screening*. Obviously, if you've already been diagnosed with Type 2 diabetes, you will not need to be screened for diabetes during pregnancy. Candidates for glucose screening are women who are worried about developing diabetes during pregnancy because they believe they have risk factors (see Chapter 2), have a family history of gestational diabetes or have a personal history of gestational diabetes from a previous pregnancy.

Who should be screened?

The symptoms of gestational diabetes are extreme thirst, hunger or fatigue, all of which can be masked by the normal discomforts of pregnancy. Therefore, all women should be screened for GDM during weeks 24 to 28 of their pregnancy (see glucose screening section above). This is particularly crucial if

- you are of Aboriginal, African or Hispanic descent
- your mother had GDM
- you previously gave birth to a baby with a birth weight of more than 4 kg (9 lb.)
- you've miscarried or had a stillbirth
- you're over 25 years of age
- you're overweight or obese (20 percent above your ideal weight)
- you have high blood pressure

Some doctors believe it isn't necessary to screen a woman for GDM if she has no symptoms or any of the risk factors above; the attitude is that universal screening can create unnecessary anxiety. However, U.S. studies show that by screening only women with risk factors, almost half of all gestational diabetes are missed.

Since blood sugar levels rise steadily throughout pregnancy, it's entirely possible to have normal blood sugar levels at week 24 and high levels at week 28, which is why many physicians feel that universal screening produces more problems than it catches. Many feel that the anxiety it creates in women who have high blood sugar levels is an issue worth considering. And some doctors wonder if even selective screening (meaning screening only those women with risk factors) reduces the problem of macrosomic babies (fat, glucose-gorged babies).

Jelly beans versus cola

The good news is that a new jelly bean glucose test is being made available in some areas instead of the nauseating cola-like beverage now used, which causes nausea, vomiting, abdominal pain, bloating and profuse sweating. Apparently by eating 18 jelly beans and having blood glucose tested an hour later, gestational diabetes is just as accurately rooted out as it was with the old, horrid cola. Furthermore, the jelly beans did not cause any side effects other than a mild headache or nausea in a tiny percentage of women. If you are going to have your blood glucose tested, show your doctor this passage and ask for the jelly beans! Many women may be worried that a history of gestational diabetes means they will eventually develop Type 2 diabetes. If you developed (or will develop) gestational diabetes during pregnancy, consider yourself put on alert. Approximately 20 percent of all women with gestational diabetes develop Type 2, presuming no other risk factors. If you are genetically predisposed to Type 2 diabetes, a history of gestational diabetes can raise your risk of eventually developing the disease. Gestational diabetes develops more often in women who were overweight prior to pregnancy, and women who are over 35 because gestational diabetes increases with maternal age.

Treating GDM

The treatment for GDM is controlling blood sugar levels through diet, exercise, insulin, if necessary, and blood sugar monitoring. To do this, you must be under the care of a pregnancy practitioner (obstetrician, midwife, etc.), a diabetes specialist and a dietician! Guidelines for nutrition and weight gain during a diabetic pregnancy depend on your current health, the fetal size and *your* weight.

At least 80 percent of the time, gestational diabetes disappears after delivery. Unfortunately, it is destined to come back in subsequent pregnancies 80 to 90 percent of the time unless you get yourself in good physical shape between pregnancies. And experts report that each subsequent bout of gestational diabetes is more severe than the previous one.

Treating Low Blood Sugar in Pregnancy

Many women with gestational diabetes will find they have episodes of low blood sugar, which is not harmful to the fetus, but very unpleasant for the mother. The thinking is that it's better to risk low blood sugar (hypoglycemia) in pregnancy to avoid high blood sugar (hyperglycemia), which is damaging to the fetus. Treating low blood sugar is the same in pregnancy as at any other time. Review Chapter 4 for details.

SPECIAL DELIVERY

About one in four babies is delivered by Caesarean section. A Caesarean section is a surgical procedure that is essentially abdominal delivery. The procedure, as the name suggests, dates back to Julius Caesar, who, as legend tells us, was born in this manner. Whether Caesar's truly was a Caesarean birth is hotly debated among historians, but what historians *do* know is that the abdominal delivery dates back to Ancient Rome. In fact, Roman law made it legal to perform a Caesarean section *only* if the mother died in the last four weeks of pregnancy. The procedure therefore originated *only as a means to save the child.* Using the procedure to save the *mother* was not even considered until the 19th century, under the influence of two prominent obstetricians, Max Sanger and Eduardo Porro.

Women who have diabetes during pregnancy (pre-existing or gestational) are at a higher risk of requiring a Caesarean section than the general pregnant population. That's because they can give birth to very large babies, who may not be able to fit through the birth canal. What you need to do prior to your due date is to have a frank discussion with your pregnancy health care provider and ask him or her about what situations would warrant a Caesarean section.

This procedure is considered major pelvic surgery that usually involves either a spinal or epidural (a type of local anaesthetic). A vertical or horizontal incision is made just above your pubic hairline. Then the surgeon (usually) cuts horizontally through the uterine muscle and eases out the baby. Sometimes, this second cut is vertical, known as the "classic incision." It is this second cut, into the uterine muscle, that will affect whether you can have a VBAC (vaginal birth after Caesarean) or not. With a horizontal cut, women have gone on to have normal second vaginal births; with the classic cut, the scar is less stable and will mean that for *you* "once a C-section, always a C-section" is a reality.

In some instances, you'll know in advance whether you need to have a Caesarean section. Your pelvis may be clearly too small or you may have irreparable scarring on your cervix from previous pelvic surgery that will prevent dilation. Or an emergency may arise that requires the fetus to be taken out immediately.

A Dozen Good Reasons to Have a C-Section

Below are 12 legitimate reasons why a Caesarean section may be performed.

1. When a vaginal delivery, even with intervention, is risky. *Note: You may fall into this category if your baby is large.*
2. A prolonged labour (caused by failure to dilate, failure for the labour to progress, too large a head and several other reasons).
3. A failed induction attempt. (Labour induction sometimes fails, and when the baby is overdue, a Caesarean is the next alternative.)
4. When the baby is in a breech position.
5. Placental problems.
6. Fetal distress.
7. Health problems in the mother that prevent normal vaginal delivery.
8. A history of difficult deliveries or stillbirth.
9. When the baby is in a transverse lie (horizontal position).
10. When the mother has primary genital herpes or other sexually transmitted diseases, such as genital warts, chlamydia or gonorrhea, which are in danger of being passed on to the newborn via vaginal delivery.
11. When the mother is HIV positive.
12. A multiple birth.

Unnecessary versus Necessary Caesareans

There are, of course, many unnecessary Caesarean sections performed. Most second Caesareans are not necessary, for instance, if the uterine cut was horizontal. Another common practice is to perform a C-section when a woman fails to go into labour after being induced. Reasons for being induced usually have to do with progressing past the due date. In this case, if the fetus isn't in distress, you may want to wait or get a second opinion regarding a C-section. In a U.S. study, situations in which a C-section was performed depended more on the *doctor* than on any other single factor; the rate of C-sections varied from 19 to 42 percent according to the individual doctor's preference. This is a huge discrepancy. What it boils down to is the *doctor's* definition of what constitutes an emergency. No competent doctor will delay a C-section if he or she thinks that the labour is endangering the baby's or the mother's health.

Again, to avoid an unnecessary procedure, consult with your practitioner and midwife *before* the third trimester. Find out what situations truly warrant a

C-section, and whether you're a VBAC (pronounced vee-back) candidate. If you're experiencing a difficult or high-risk pregnancy or will be having a multiple birth, you *may* be more likely to have the procedure than a woman with a low-risk pregnancy.

AFTER THE BABY IS BORN

The question that may be at the top of your mind after you give birth is whether your diabetes is "gone." This is a valid question only for women who have had gestational diabetes. In this case, the only way to tell is to have another glucose tolerance test when you get your first postpartum menstrual period (if you're breast-feeding), or alternatively, six weeks after childbirth. If the test results are normal, then your diabetes is, indeed, gone—but should not be forgotten. It's a warning to you that you better "shape up" between pregnancies, or forever after. Otherwise future bouts of gestational diabetes or Type 2 diabetes in later years could come back to haunt you. Of course, there are some other issues that will surface for mothers who have (or had) diabetes.

If your test results show continuing high blood sugar, it's probably safe to assume that you have Type 2 diabetes that has just revealed itself during your pregnancy. In this case, your diabetes is a permanent health condition that was simply diagnosed during pregnancy or perhaps was even triggered by it.

Should You Breast-feed?

Yes. Next question.

Why Was I Told *Not* to Breast-feed?

Ignorant practitioners may tell you that you can't breast-feed if you've had diabetes. *This is completely false!* If your diabetes is well controlled and you've given birth to a healthy baby, breast-feeding is the normal way to feed your baby and does not place your baby at risk for the numerous, undisputed and well-documented health problems associated with babies fed with cow's milk. Stick to your "pregnancy rules" and keep self-monitoring your blood sugar levels so you can adjust your diet and exercise routine to your new levels of hormones. Estrogen levels affect blood sugar levels; when they rise, your blood sugar rises; when they drop—which is what happens during breast-feeding as a result of the hormone prolactin—blood sugar levels may drop, which could mean you may need to eat more while breast-feeding to keep up your levels. If you had gestational diabetes, this natural drop in blood sugar levels is nature's way of helping you bounce back to health faster if you breast-feed. If you need to take insulin to control high blood sugar after childbirth, your baby doesn't care! Insulin cannot be ingested, so even if it "crosses" into the breast milk, it will have zero effect on the baby. Remember, if insulin could be ingested, you wouldn't need to inject it in the first place!

Furthermore, several studies show that breast-fed babies have lower incidences of both Type 1 diabetes and Type 2 diabetes later in life.

If you have high blood sugar in the days and/or weeks following childbirth, your milk will be much sweeter than usual. That's not dangerous per se to the baby; the baby has his or her own functioning pancreas, which can produce the insulin she or he needs to handle the sweetness, but the baby could begin to put on too much weight and get fat as a result of the sweet milk. There may be cases when the sweetness is a "turn-off" to the baby and she or he may not be as receptive to the milk, which will cause problems with your milk supply, or cause engorgement, which is painful and can put you at risk for mastitis (inflammation in the breast, usually due to bacterial infection). In general, the main danger of high blood sugar during breast-feeding is to *you*; you'll want to control your diabetes so you can be as healthy and fit as possible. But this is the case for every woman—whether she has children or not, and whether she's breast-feeding or not. For more information about breast-feeding, consult my book *The Breast-feeding Sourcebook*.

Postpartum Blues and Diabetes

Many women will find the enormous lifestyle adjustment after childbirth tiring. They may be fatigued, stressed and overwhelmed and have all the other normal feelings that accompany the event of giving birth. Unfortunately, some women may also suffer from postpartum depression, which is characterized by a loss of interest in formerly pleasurable activities, changes in appetite, changes in sleep patterns (which happens after childbirth anyway), sadness and a host of other emotional and physical symptoms.

Just because you have diabetes does not mean that you can't develop another condition on top of it, such as postpartum depression. But keeping your blood sugar in check after childbirth will help to avoid a common problem of high or low blood sugar levels—and their associated mood swings—which may mask postpartum depression or vice versa. It's also recommended that you have your thyroid checked after childbirth to make sure that you are not also suffering from postpartum thyroid disease, which affects about 18 percent of the postpartum population and can be misdiagnosed as postpartum depression, too.

For more information on postpartum depression, consult my book *The Pregnancy Sourcebook*.

Diabetes never ceases to affect women in unique ways at different stages of their lives. The next chapter is the one to read after your baby graduates.

Chapter 12

MENOPAUSE AND TYPE 2 DIABETES

• • • • • • • • • • •

Menopause is a recent phenomenon in our society. Anywhere from 60 to 100 years ago, women simply died prior to menopause. Only in this century have women outlived their ovaries.

Menopause is a Greek term taken from the words *menos*, which means "month," and *pause*, which means "arrest"—the arrest of the menstrual cycle. It is a time in every woman's life when her ovaries are slowing down, running out of eggs and getting ready to retire. The process involves a complex shutting down of hormones that have nourished the menstrual cycle until this point. As a result, the normal hormonal fluctuations women are used to throughout their menstrual cycles become far more erratic and are responsible for the infamous "menopausal mood swings" that have created much of the negative mythology surrounding menopause in our culture.

Nevertheless, natural menopause and *menarche* (the first menstrual period) have a lot in common: They are both *gradual* processes that women ease into. A woman doesn't suddenly wake up to find herself in menopause any more than a young girl wakes up to find herself in puberty. However, when menopause occurs *surgically*—the by-product of an oopherectomy, ovarian failure following a hysterectomy or certain cancer therapies—it can be an extremely jarring process. One out of every three women in North America will not make it to the age of 60 with her uterus intact. These women may indeed wake up one morning to find themselves in menopause and, as a result, will suffer far more noticeable and severe menopausal symptoms than their natural menopause counterparts. It is because of *surgical* menopause that *hormonal replacement therapy* (HRT) and *estrogen replacement therapy* (ERT or "unopposed estrogen") have become such hotly debated issues in women's health. The loss of estrogen, in particular, leads to drastic changes in the body's chemistry that trigger a more aggressive aging process (discussed below).

Women with Type 2 diabetes have a little more to be concerned about than women without Type 2 diabetes. Estrogen loss increases *all* women's risk of heart disease, which is the major cause of death for postmenopausal women. But in postmenopausal women with diabetes, the risk of heart disease is two to three times higher than in the general female population. Furthermore, as estrogen and progesterone levels drop, women with diabetes can expect fluctuations in their blood sugar levels and possibly more episodes of low blood sugar (see Chapter 4). After menopause, women taking insulin may find that their insulin requirements have dropped by as much as 20 percent.

The purpose of this chapter is to discuss both the natural and surgical menopausal facts of life for women with diabetes, including the myths of menopause, the symptoms of menopause, the osteoporosis issue and the variety of health problems that women with diabetes face as they age. The benefits and risks of HRT and ERT are discussed below. Remember that your age, medical history and menopausal symptoms all need to be factored into the HRT or ERT decision and weighed against the health risks your diabetes poses.

NATURAL MENOPAUSE

When menopause occurs naturally, it tends to take place anywhere between the ages of 48 and 52, but it can occur as early as your late 30s or as late as your mid-50s. When menopause occurs *before* 45 it is technically considered "early menopause," but just as menarche is genetically predetermined, so is menopause. For an average woman with an unremarkable medical history, what she eats or the activities she engages in will *not* influence the timing of her menopause. However, women who have had chemotherapy or who have been exposed to high levels of radiation (such as radiation therapy in their pelvic area for cancer treatment) may go into earlier menopause. In any event, the average age of menopause is 50–51.

Other causes that have been cited to trigger an early menopause include mumps (in small groups of women, the infection causing the mumps has been known to spread to the ovaries, prematurely shutting them down) and specific autoimmune diseases, such as lupus or rheumatoid arthritis (some women with these diseases find that their bodies develop antibodies to their own ovaries and attack the ovaries).

The Stages of Natural Menopause

Socially, the word "menopause" refers to a process, not a precise moment in the life of your menstrual cycle, but medically, the word does *indeed* refer to one precise moment: the date of your last period. However, the events preceding and following menopause amount to a huge change for women both physically and socially. Physically, this process is divided into four stages:

1. **Premenopause:** Although some doctors may refer to a 32-year-old woman in her child-bearing years as "premenopausal," this is not really an appropriate label. The term "premenopause" ideally refers to women on the "cusp" of menopause. Their periods have just *started* to get irregular, but they do not yet experience any classic menopausal symptoms such as hot flashes or vaginal dryness. A woman in premenopause is usually in her mid- to late 40s. If your doctor tells you that you're premenopausal, you might want to ask him or her how he or she is using this term.

2. **Perimenopause:** This term refers to women who are in the thick of menopause—their cycles are wildly erratic, and they are experiencing hot flashes and vaginal dryness. This label is applicable for about four years, covering the first two years prior to the official "last" period to the next two years following the last menstrual period. Women who are perimenopausal will be in the age groups discussed above, averaging to about 51.

3. **Menopause:** This refers to your final menstrual period. You will not be able to pinpoint your final period until you've been completely free from periods for one year. Then you count back to the last period you charted, and *that* date is the *date of your menopause. Important: After more than one year of no menstrual periods, any vaginal bleeding is now considered abnormal.*

4. **Postmenopause:** This term refers to the last third of most women's lives and includes women who have been free of menstrual periods for at least four years to women celebrating their 100th birthday. In other words, once you're past menopause, you'll be referred to as postmenopausal for the rest of your life. Sometimes the terms "postmenopausal" and "perimenopausal" are used interchangeably, but this is technically inaccurate.

Used in a *social* context, however, nobody really bothers to break down menopause as precisely. When you see the word "menopausal" in a magazine article, you are seeing what's become acceptable medical slang, referring to women who are premenopausal and perimenopausal—a time frame that *includes* the actual menopause. When you see the word "postmenopausal" in a magazine article, you are seeing another accepted medical slang, which includes women who are in perimenopause and "official" postmenopause.

Recognizing premenopause or perimenopause

When you begin to notice the signs of menopause (discussed next), either you'll suspect the approach of menopause on your own, or your doctor will put two and two together when you report your "bizarre" symptoms. There are two very simple tests that will accurately determine what's going on and the stage of menopause you're in. Your FSH levels will dramatically rise as your ovaries begin to shut down; these levels are easily checked from one blood test. In addition, your vaginal walls will thin, and the cells lining the vagina will not contain as much estrogen. Your doctor will simply do a Pap-like smear on your vaginal walls—simple and painless—and then just analyze the smear to check for vaginal "atrophy"—the thinning and drying out of your vagina. In addition, as I'll discuss below, you need to keep track of your periods and chart them as they become irregular. Your menstrual pattern will be an additional clue to your doctor about whether you are pre- or perimenopausal.

Signs of Natural Menopause

There are really just three classic *short-term* symptoms of menopause: erratic periods, hot flashes and vaginal dryness. All three of these symptoms are caused by a decrease in estrogen. As for the emotional symptoms of menopause, such as irritability, mood swings, melancholy and so on, they are actually caused by a *rise in FSH*. As the cycle changes and the ovaries' egg supply dwindles, FSH is secreted in very high amounts and reaches a lifetime peak—as much as 15 times higher; it's the body's way of trying to "jump-start" the ovarian engine. This is why the urine of menopausal women is used to produce human menopausal gonadotropin (HMG), the potent fertility drug that consists of pure FSH.

Decreased levels of estrogen can make you more vulnerable to stress, depression and anxiety because estrogen loss affects REM sleep. When we're less rested, we're less able to cope with stresses that normally may not affect us.

Every woman entering menopause will experience a change in her menstrual cycle, discussed below. However, not all women will experience hot flashes or even notice vaginal changes. This is particularly true if a woman is overweight. Estrogen is stored in fat cells, which is why overweight women also tend to be more at risk for estrogen-dependent cancers. What happens is that the fat cells convert fat into estrogen, creating a type of estrogen reserve that the body will use during menopause and that can reduce the severity of estrogen loss symptoms.

Erratic periods

Every woman will begin to experience an irregular cycle before her last period. Cycles may become longer or shorter with long bouts of amenorrhea. There will also be flow changes, where periods may suddenly become light and scanty, or very heavy and crampy. The impact of suddenly irregular "wild" cycles can be disturbing, however, because menstrual cycle changes may also signify other problems, discussed throughout previous chapters. That's why it's imperative to chart your periods and try to sort out your own pattern of "normal" irregular cycles. It's also crucial to bring your chart to your gynecologist to confirm your suspicions that you are indeed entering menopause. If you're not entering menopause, you'll need to isolate the cause of your cycle changes.

Of course, since you can go into menopause earlier than you might have anticipated, irregular cycles may not always be on your list of suspected causes behind your sudden cycle changes. Is there any way you can predict more accurately when your own menopause might occur? Yes. If you can, try to find out how old your mother was when she went into menopause. If she's no longer living, you might try to ask other women still alive who were close to her, or your father if he's still living. Although most women can expect their menopause in their 50s, women who go into earlier menopause will usually have a family history of earlier menopause. Periods will generally become erratic approximately two years before the final period. However, some women may experience a longer premenopausal process than others.

Hot flashes

Roughly 85 percent of all pre- and perimenopausal women experience what's known as "hot flashes." They can begin when periods are either still regular or have just started to become irregular. The hot flashes usually stop between one and two years after your final menstrual period. A hot flash can feel different for each woman. Some women experience a feeling of warmth in their face and upper body; some women experience hot flashes as a simultaneous sweating with chills. Some women feel anxious, tense, dizzy or nauseous just before the hot flash; some feel tingling in their fingers or heart palpitations just before. Some women will experience their hot flashes during the day; others will experience them at night and may wake up so wet from perspiration that they need to change their bedsheets and/or nightclothes.

Nobody really understands what causes a hot flash, but researchers believe that it has to do with mixed signals from the hypothalamus, which controls both body temperature and sex hormones. Normally, when the body is too warm, the hypothalamus sends a chemical message to the heart to cool off the body by pumping more blood, causing the blood vessels under the skin to dilate, which makes you perspire. During menopause, however, it's believed that the hypothalamus gets confused and sends this "cooling off" signal at the wrong times. A hot flash is not the same as being overheated. Although the skin temperature often rises between 1 and 3°C (4 and 8°F), the internal body temperature drops, creating this odd sensation. Why does the hypothalamus get so confused? Decreasing levels of estrogen. We know this because when synthetic estrogen is given to replace natural estrogen in the body, hot flashes disappear. Some researchers believe that a decrease in leutinizing hormone (LH) is also a key factor, and a variety of other hormones that influence body temperature are being looked at as well. Although hot flashes have no health risks, they are disquieting and stressful symptoms. Certain groups of women will experience more severe hot flashes than others:

- Women who are in surgical menopause (discussed further below).
- Women who are thin. When there's less fat on the body to store estrogen reserves, estrogen loss symptoms are more severe.
- Women who don't sweat easily. An ability to sweat makes extreme temperatures easier to tolerate. Women who have trouble sweating may experience more severe flashes.

Just as you must chart your periods when your cycles become irregular, it's also important to chart your hot flashes. Keep track of when the flashes occur, how long they last and rate their intensity from 1 to 10. This will help you determine a pattern for the flashes and allow you to prepare for them in advance, which will reduce the stress involved in the flashes to begin with. It's also crucial to report your hot flashes to your doctor, just as you would any changes in your cycle. Symptoms of hot flashes can also indicate other health problems, such as circulatory problems and so on.

You can lessen your discomfort by adjusting your lifestyle to cope with the flashes. The more comfortable you are, the less intense your flashes will feel. Once you establish a pattern by charting the flashes, you can do a few things around the time of day your flashes occur. Some suggestions:

- Avoid synthetic clothing, such as polyester, because it traps perspiration.
- Use only 100 percent cotton bedding if you have night sweats.
- Avoid clothing with high necks and long sleeves.
- Dress in layers.
- Keep cold drinks handy.
- If you smoke, cut down or quit. Smoking constricts blood vessels and can intensify and prolong a flash. It also leads to severe complications from diabetes, discussed in Chapter 13.
- Avoid "trigger" foods such as caffeine, alcohol, spicy foods, sugars and large meals. Substitute herbal teas for coffee or regular tea.
- Discuss with your doctor the benefits of taking vitamin E supplements. Evidence suggests that it's essential for proper circulation and the production of sex hormones.
- Exercise to improve your circulation.
- Reduce your exposure to the sun; sunburn will aggravate your hot flashes because burnt skin cannot regulate heat as effectively. (The sun is discussed on page 203.)

A variety of conventional and alternative therapies can reduce the severity of hot flashes. For more information, consult my book *Women of the '60s Turning 50*.

Vaginal changes

Estrogen loss will also cause vaginal changes. Since it is the production of estrogen that causes the vagina to continuously stay moist and elastic through its natural secretions, the loss of estrogen will cause the vagina to become drier, thinner and less elastic. This may also cause the vagina to shrink slightly in terms of width and length. In addition, the reduction in vaginal secretions causes the vagina to be less acidic. This can put you at risk for more vaginal infections, particularly if you have high blood sugar. As a result of these vaginal changes, you'll notice a change in your sexual activity. Your vagina may take longer to become lubricated, or you may have to depend on lubricants to have comfortable intercourse.

Estrogen loss can affect other parts of your sex life as well. Your libido may actually increase because testosterone levels can rise when estrogen levels drop. (The general rule is that your levels of testosterone will either stay the same or increase.) However, women who *do* experience an increase in sexual desire will also be frustrated that their vaginas are not accommodating their needs. First, there is the lubrication problem: More stimulation is required to lubricate the vagina naturally. Secondly, a decrease in estrogen means that less blood flows to the vagina and clitoris, which means that orgasm may be more difficult to achieve or may not last as long as it normally has in the past. Other changes involve the breasts. Normally, estrogen causes blood to flow into the breasts during arousal, which makes the nipples more erect, sensitive and responsive. Estrogen loss causes less blood to flow to the breasts, which makes them less sensitive. And finally, since the vagina shrinks as estrogen decreases, it doesn't expand as much during intercourse, which may make intercourse less comfortable, particularly since it is less lubricated.

Mood swings

Mood swings can be an especially tricky symptom of both menopause and fluctuating blood sugar levels. Many women with diabetes struggle with severe mood swings, which can make controlling blood sugar more difficult. While anger and depression can be symptoms of low blood sugar, anxiety and irritability can be symptoms of high blood sugar. Factor in hormonal changes during menopause, and your moods can be severely affected. Unfortunately, depression and irritability can lead women to poor control of their diabetes. Frequent monitoring of your blood sugar levels and sticking to your meal plan can help to prevent drastic mood swings.

Menopause and Blood Sugar

As you approach menopause, you'll want to revisit your blood sugar monitoring habits. That's because menopause often masks the symptoms of low or high blood sugar and vice versa. For example, hot flashes (or sweating), moodiness and short-term memory loss are also associated with low blood sugar. Experts recommend that before you decide that "you're low" and bite into that chocolate bar, you may want to test your blood sugar first to see if your symptoms are caused by sugar or hormones. Otherwise, ingesting more sugar than you need could cause high blood sugar unnecessarily.

That said, many women find that because estrogen and progesterone levels are dropping, they are experiencing more frequent and severe episodes of low blood sugar as a result. As mentioned a few times in this book, estrogen can trigger insulin resistance; the loss of estrogen will therefore have the opposite effect, causing insulin to be taken up more quickly by the body, which could result in low blood sugar. An easy way to remember how estrogen levels affect blood sugar is to simply note that when estrogen is up, so is blood sugar; when estrogen is down, so is blood sugar. Therefore, high estrogen levels = high blood sugar; low estrogen levels = low blood sugar.

The only way to cope with these fluctuations is to try to eliminate other causes of blood sugar fluctuations, such as stress, deviating from meal and exercise plans and so on. If you're on oral hypoglycemic agents, you may need to adjust your dosages around the time of menopause to compensate for less resistance to insulin as your hormone levels drop. (Although if you go on hormone replacement therapy, you may need to readjust your dosages again.)

Women who have persistent high blood sugar levels may find the normal menopausal symptoms, such as vaginal dryness, for example, exacerbated. In this case, by gaining more control over blood sugar levels, they may find their menopausal symptoms are less severe.

SURGICAL MENOPAUSE

Surgical menopause is the result of a bilateral oophorectomy, the removal of both ovaries before natural menopause. Surgical menopause can also be the result of ovarian failure following a hysterectomy or following cancer therapy, such as chemotherapy or radiation treatments. A bilateral oopherectomy is often done in conjunction with a hysterectomy, or sometimes as a single procedure, when ovarian cancer is suspected, for example.

Bilateral Oopherectomy Symptoms

If you've had your ovaries removed after menopause, you won't be in "surgical menopause." You won't feel any hormonal differences in your body, although you may experience some structural problems. If you've had your ovaries removed before you've reached natural menopause, you'll wake up from your surgery in *post*menopause. Once the ovaries are removed, your body immediately stops producing estrogen and progesterone. Your FSH will skyrocket in an attempt to "make contact" with ovaries that no longer exist. Unlike women who go through menopause naturally, women wake up after a bilateral oopherectomy in immediate estrogen "withdrawal." It's that sudden: One day you have a normal menstrual cycle, the next, you have none whatsoever. This can cause you to become understandably more depressed, but you'll also *feel* the physical symptoms of estrogen loss far more intensely than a woman in natural menopause. That means that your vagina will be *extremely* dry, your hot flashes will feel like sudden violent heat waves that will be very disturbing to your system and of course your periods will cease altogether instead of tapering off naturally. The period that you had prior to your surgery will have been your last, so you won't even experience pre- or perimenopause, just postmenopause. That means you'll need to begin estrogen replacement therapy (ERT) *immediately* following surgery to prevent these sudden symptoms of menopause. As discussed below, if you no longer have your uterus, you'll be on estrogen only or unopposed estrogen. If you still have your uterus, you'll be placed on estrogen and progesterone hormone replacement therapy (HRT) for the reasons explained in the HRT/ERT section below. Any short-term menopausal symptoms will be alleviated by HRT/ERT. Prior to going on HRT/ERT, your doctor will perform a vaginal smear and a blood test to detect your FSH levels, which will indicate how much estrogen you need. Dosages will vary from woman to woman, so don't compare notes with your friends and wonder why "she's taking only X amount" when you're taking Y amount. ERT and HRT is discussed further on in the chapter.

If you've had just one ovary removed

If the blood supply leading to your ovary was not damaged during your surgery, you should still be able to produce enough estrogen for your body. If you begin to go into ovarian failure, the symptoms will depend on how fast the ovary is failing; you may experience symptoms more akin to natural menopause or you may experience sudden symptoms mirroring the surgical menopause experience.

Ovarian Failure Resulting from Cancer Therapy

Chemotherapy and radiation treatments that involve the pelvic area may throw your ovaries into menopause. As above, you may experience a more gradual menopausal process, or you may be overwhelmed by sudden symptoms of menopause. This depends on what kind of therapy you've received and the speed at which your ovaries are failing. Before you undergo your cancer treatment, discuss how the treatments will affect your ovaries and which menopausal symptoms you can expect.

HORMONE REPLACEMENT THERAPY AND DIABETES

The average Canadian woman will live until age 78, meaning that she will live one-third of her life after her menopause. In a survey of the general Canadian population, 11 percent of those between 65 and 74 reported having diabetes. Since heart disease is a major complication of Type 2 diabetes, and women are more prone to heart disease as a result of estrogen loss after menopause, the current recommendation is for women with Type 2 diabetes to seriously consider hormone replacement therapy after menopause. Right now, the Women's Health Initiative (WHI) is studying 25,000 postmenopausal women, many of whom have diabetes. The results of this study (expected by 2003) are expected to present more concrete facts regarding the perceived benefits of HRT on postmenopausal women with Type 2 diabetes.

Many women, of course, will also be concerned about their risk of breast cancer. Taking estrogen can stimulate or trigger the growth of an estrogen-dependent breast cancer cell (that is, a breast cancer cell that "feeds" or thrives on the hormone estrogen). Current studies show that these types of cancers are far more treatable than other kinds of breast cancers. And, as I'll discuss further on, since many more women die of a heart attack than breast cancer—particularly if they have Type 2 diabetes—preventing heart disease, as well as fractures from osteoporosis, is considered beneficial. Nevertheless, you have some thinking to do if you're considering hormone replacement therapy, so here are the facts you need to make a more informed choice.

What Is HRT?

Hormone replacement therapy (HRT) in the medical community usually refers to estrogen and progestin, a synthetic progesterone, which should not be confused with natural progesterone. Natural hormone therapy (see page 200) can be obtained through a compounding pharmacy, which means that the pharmacy prepares the therapy from scratch.

Progesterone or progestin is given to postmenopausal women who still have their uterus to prevent the lining from overgrowing and becoming cancerous.

Estrogen replacement therapy (ERT) refers to estrogen only, which is given to women after surgical menopause who no longer have a uterus. Both HRT and ERT are "prophylactic" therapy and a "cure" for the menopausal symptoms discussed above. They are designed to replace the estrogen lost after menopause, and hence

1. prevent or even reverse the long-term consequences of estrogen loss (osteoporosis, skin changes, vaginal thinning and dryness and a list of other symptoms) and
2. treat the short-term symptoms of menopause such as hot flashes and vaginal dryness.

Therefore, you have the choice of taking HRT or ERT as either a short-term therapy or a long-term therapy. However, some risks are involved with HRT and ERT that you'll need to weigh against the benefits.

The Benefits

What exactly is estrogen responsible for in our bodies? In addition to protecting our bones and maintaining our reproductive organs, estrogen also helps to maintain appropriate levels of high-density lipoprotein (HDL), which keeps our arteries clear of plaque, preventing them from clogging and causing heart attacks and strokes. By raising HDL, known as the "good cholesterol," the "bad" cholesterol (the low-density lipoproteins that cause fatty substances to *collect* in the arteries, causing arteriosclerosis) drops. Estrogen also helps protect us from rheumatoid arthritis. It's our ovaries, of course, that make estrogen, but other sources of estrogen come from androstenedione (a hormone) and testosterone, which are converted by our tissues into a form of estrogen called *estrone*, a weaker form of estrogen than the kind our ovaries produce. Obese women have estrone in greater amounts. Although this may prevent any severe menopausal symptoms, estrone is *not* considered a potent enough form of estrogen to protect against osteoporosis or heart disease.

Thirty years ago, all women, regardless of whether they still had a uterus, were placed on pure estrogen hormone without any progesterone. This is known as "unopposed estrogen therapy" because in a natural cycle the progesterone "opposes" the estrogen and counterbalances high estrogen levels, preventing you from becoming "estrogen toxic" at far higher dosages than what's given today. This created several problems. First, women experienced side effects, similar to those caused by the early oral contraceptives: nausea, dizziness, bloating and so on. Second, women who went into menopause naturally tended to develop endometrial hyperplasia (overgrowth of the uterine lining), which often became uterine cancer. Finally, both surgical and natural menopause recipients of this estrogen therapy were considered at higher risk of developing estrogen-dependent cancers, such as breast cancer and ovarian cancer.

Today, all women who have gone through menopause naturally and who decide to go on HRT will be given estrogen *and* progesterone. The progesterone, of course, triggers the uterine lining to shed regularly, *preventing endometrial hyperplasia*, which is what predisposes women on unopposed estrogen (i.e., those with a uterus and who are taking only estrogen) to uterine cancer. Estrogen and progesterone *together* also mirror the normal menstrual cycle and help prevent the side effects normally felt with solo estrogen. The estrogen levels now are much lower than they were in the past; current HRT doses are about ten times lower than the average combination oral contraceptive.

If you're in surgical menopause, you won't need any progesterone because you're not at risk for endometrial hyperplasia any more, but because your menopausal symptoms will be more severe, your need for estrogen may be greater. Since the estrogen doses are so much lower now, you'll likely not experience any short-term side effects from the estrogen.

What to expect in the short term

Generally, HRT/ERT will begin to relieve your estrogen-loss menopausal symptoms within days of starting the therapy. Your hot flashes will disappear, your vagina will become moist again and will lubricate on its own during sex, and your vagina's acidic environment will be restored, preventing yeast and other vaginal infections from plaguing you. However, if you change your mind and go off the therapy, your symptoms will return in a far more severe form!

What to expect in the long term

Your HDL levels will be maintained and you won't experience any severe bone loss, which can put you at risk for fractures and breakages. However, research shows that HRT is more effective than ERT in preventing osteoporosis.

As for heart disease, roughly half a million North American women die of heart disease every year. Statistics show that heart attack rates are much lower in premenopausal women than in postmenopausal women. Men who suffer heart attacks and are in the same age group as premenopausal women outnumber those women by a vast degree. However, 10 to 15 years after menopause, women equal men in heart attacks. To date, most of the research shows that estrogen will *protect* women from heart disease.

But it's also important to review these studies in the proper context. First, the women who are selected for these studies are generally upper middle class and educated: two major factors that appear to decrease the risk of heart disease anyway! Second, women who take estrogen are usually healthier and more willing to make other lifestyle changes that will lower their risk, such as changing their diet or not smoking.

Some animal research has revealed that the progesterone added to HRT may have the *opposite* influence on HDL as estrogen. What you might want to do if you decide to go on HRT for strictly the heart benefit is to have your cholesterol level checked before you start HRT so you have a baseline, then get your levels checked after you've been on HRT for about three months. If there's no improvement in your cholesterol levels, you may want to review your decision with your doctor.

However, the heart benefits seen with estrogen occur only if the estrogen is taken orally, not in patches or vaginal creams. In order for the estrogen to work its magic with HDL, it needs to be metabolized in the liver.

Finally, estrogen will not counteract a poor diet and lifestyle. If you smoke, drink excessively, are under tremendous stress, eat copious amounts of the wrong foods (you know the ones) or come from a family with a history of heart attacks, don't expect estrogen alone to shield you from heart disease.

Don't expect miracles

If your decision for going on ERT or HRT is based on cosmetic reasons ("Gee, I won't get any wrinkles with hormone therapy!") you're in for a big surprise: Hormone or estrogen replacement therapy *does not prevent wrinkles*. Estrogen can cause you to retain water, which can make your skin puffier, making your wrinkles less noticeable. However, the majority of women have wrinkles because of heredity, excessive or accumulative sun exposure, smoking and drinking excessive amounts of alcohol. Estrogen can also cause skin dryness, rashes and permanent brown blotches on your skin (harmless skin decoloration known as hyperpigmentation).

Estrogen therapy will not prevent weight gain, another myth that has been passed down through the estrogen folklore. Weight gain has to do with our metabolism slowing down as we age, something that estrogen cannot prevent or reverse.

Some women may want to take estrogen to keep their breasts full and shapely; this is not a good reason to go on HRT. Although estrogen promotes cell growth in the breasts, and while the retention of body fluid can make breasts swell and become fuller, your breasts can also become more tender and painful. Taking HRT to keep your breasts full is not recommended because of the health risks.

The Risks

The risk that we hear about most regarding the estrogen issue is uterine cancer. Today, this is no longer a risk! Here's why: In the past, as discussed earlier, unopposed estrogen was given to both women who still had a uterus and women who were without one. Of course, if you don't have a uterus, there is no risk of uterine cancer. But what about the women who had one? Well, a funny thing happened: Doctors *forgot* about the uterus, ignoring the fact that the female body is very smart. When it detects estrogen in the body, it says, "Oh, look— estrogen again! Better start preparing the endometrium for a baby!" And guess what? There's no progesterone to trigger the lining to shed, and certainly no baby, so the lining just keeps growing until you wind up with endometrial hyperplasia, overgrowth of the uterine lining and eventually uterine cancer. When the uterine cancer rate began to increase in uterus "owners" on unopposed estrogen, the medical community realized its mistake, remembered the uterus and the importance of progesterone and, today, will not administer unopposed estrogen to any woman with a uterus.

Just for the record, women in natural menopause who take nothing have a one in 1,000 risk of uterine cancer; women with a uterus on unopposed estrogen increase their risk to anywhere from four to eight in 1,000. What if you were once on unopposed estrogen in the past and have your uterus? This is still in debate. It seems that once you go off the estrogen, your uterine cancer risk drops. However, a Boston University School of Medicine study, using 1,217 women, revealed that the risk of cancer may not drop until you've been off the estrogen for as long as ten years.

With HRT and the added progesterone to the estrogen therapy, the risk of uterine cancer decreases: It's lower in women on HRT than in women on nothing. As for the risk of breast cancer and HRT, refer to page 198.

The risks you don't read about ...

It might interest you to know that you can *triple* your chances of developing gallbladder disease on ERT or HRT. However, gallbladder disease is easily prevented by removing the gallbladder, which is one of the most common surgeries performed.

If you have fibroids, they may grow larger on HRT. Estrogen also causes fluid retention, which has been known to exacerbate *existing* conditions such as asthma, epilepsy, pre-existing heart disease, kidney disease and sometimes migraine headaches.

The Forms of HRT and ERT

You can take estrogen in a number of ways. The most common estrogen product is called Premarin, which uses a synthesis of various estrogens that are derived from the urine of pregnant horses. That way the estrogen mimics nature more accurately. Premarin is taken from "pregnant mare's urine"—*pre* (pregnant), *mar* (mare's) and *in* (urine). Premarin is a brand name for this type of replacement estrogen and comes in either pills, patches (transdermal) or vaginal creams. Other common, synthetic forms of estrogen include micronized estradiol, ethinyl estradiol, esterified estrogen and quinestrol.

As a short-term therapy, you may need only the vaginal cream to help with vaginal dryness or bladder problems. As a long-term therapy, you'll need the pill form if you want to protect yourself from heart disease. Estrogen can also be "worn." In this case, it's placed in a small plastic patch around the size of a silver dollar, worn on the abdomen, thighs or buttocks, and changed twice weekly.

When estrogen is in patch or cream form, it goes directly to the bloodstream, bypassing the liver, and hence does not affect HDL or protect against heart disease. Some women also have an allergic reaction to the skin patch and get a rash. If you're one of them, you can investigate taking the estrogen in other forms.

Finally, you can also have estrogen injected. Each shot lasts between three and six weeks, but this method is expensive and inconvenient because the dosages aren't as flexible with hormone therapy taken in pill form. Women react differently to synthetic forms of estrogen; some do better on different chemical recipes. So if you don't do well on Premarin, see if estradiol, for example, is better for you, or vice versa. Don't just give up and go off the HRT or ERT altogether; explore all the estrogen possibilities. Dosages are discussed below.

Progestins

Progestin is a synthetically produced progesterone (as opposed to natural progesterone from plant sources); there are dozens of brands. Progestins are taken in separate tablets along with estrogen. Together, the estrogen and progestin you take is called HRT. HRT can be administered two ways: *cyclically* or *continuously*. Taking HRT cyclically is very similar to taking an oral contraceptive because the hormones more closely mirror a natural cycle. The first day you start is considered day 1 of your mock "cycle." You take estrogen from days 1 to 25; you then add the progesterone from days 14 to 25. Then you stop all pills and bleed for two or three days, just as you would on a combination oral contraceptive. This vaginal bleeding is called "withdrawal bleeding," which is lighter and shorter than a normal menstrual period, lasting only two or three days, just like a period on a combination oral contraceptive. In fact, if the bleeding is heavy or prolonged for some reason, this is a warning that something's not right and you should get it checked.

In addition, you may experience "breakthrough bleeding"—spotting during the first three weeks after you begin HRT. This kind of bleeding is again similar to what happens on a combination oral contraceptive. This bleeding usually goes away after a few months, but report it anyway. You may need to switch to a lower dose of estrogen or take a higher dose of progestin. Once your mini-period of withdrawal bleeding is finished, you simply start the cycle again. Many women can't tolerate cyclical HRT because they feel as though they should be *rid* of their periods by now and not have to deal with pads and tampons ever again. However, it is believed that cyclical HRT offers slightly better heart protection.

When HRT is taken continuously, you simply take one estrogen pill and one progestin pill each day. When you do it this way, the progesterone *counteracts* the estrogen; no uterine lining is built up, so there's no withdrawal bleeding that needs to happen.

The appropriate dosages

Every woman requires a different dosage of estrogen and progestin, but you will always be placed on the lowest possible dosage of either one and may have the dosage increased gradually if necessary. If your estrogen dosage is too high, you'll experience side effects similar to those seen with estrogen oral contraceptives: headaches, bloating and so on.

Before you determine how much estrogen you'll need, it's crucial to first determine how much your body is still producing, which can be measured by your doctor. This really depends on your weight, menopausal symptoms and a hundred other things.

Estrogen

Estrogen tablets come in dosages of 0.3 mg, 0.625 mg, 0.9 mg or 1.25 mg. The strength of the dosage you take will be determined by why you're taking estrogen. For women who are in a high-risk category for osteoporosis, the most common starting dosage is 0.625 mg. But for women who just want short-term relief from their menopausal symptoms, such as hot flashes, starting at 0.3 mg is more usual. If you forget to take your estrogen tablet one day, don't worry about it. You will not need to double up the way you would with birth control pills. The only reason you even double up then is to avoid pregnancy. Obviously, pregnancy, in this case, is not a concern any more. It's important, however, that once you begin the estrogen, you continue to take it daily without a noticeable break (a noticeable break being more than two days). Studies show that when you stop your estrogen, you can suffer from far more severe hot flashes and insomnia than you did before you started the estrogen.

If you're not taking estrogen orally and are on the vaginal estrogen cream, you can use the cream for about three weeks on and one week off. Women who opt for the vaginal cream have decided on estrogen for short-term relief of vaginal dryness and thinning, as well as relief from urinary incontinence, another postmenopausal problem, discussed below. But vaginal cream does not relieve hot flashes or offer any protection for osteoporosis or heart disease. Using the vaginal creams occasionally, the way you would a lubricant, for example, will do you no good. Again, every woman is different, as are brands and dosage measurements in each brand. Make sure you discuss how much estrogen you're getting per application with either your doctor or pharmacist.

As for skin patches, they contain either 4 or 8 mg of estrogen. The 4 mg patch releases .05 mg of estrogen daily; the 8 mg patch releases twice that amount. You'll need to change the patch twice a week. Some doctors recommend that you wear the patch for three weeks, then take a one-week break from the patch before you start again. Obviously, you'll need to discuss this with your doctor and decide what's right for you. Again, women who take the patch will not derive any HDL benefits, but they will be protected from bone loss and menopausal symptoms. In fact, the patch delivers a more continuous flow of estrogen than the pills because there is no fluctuation in dosage. With pills, it's impossible to be as constant since the timing of taking the pill can fluctuate.

The androgen strain

ERT or HRT medications sometimes contain androgens, male hormones. Doctors will prescribe androgens to improve your libido if you're experiencing problems. This may indeed be appropriate, but it's important to *know what you're getting*! If your androgen dosage is too high, you can develop male features, such as increased body hair, a deeper voice and shrinking breasts. These symptoms do not magically vanish once you go off the androgens. Some studies also show that added androgens may have a negative effect on blood cholesterol, actually *increasing* heart disease risk. This may explain why men on estrogen derive no HDL benefits!

Common side effects

If you're taking cyclical progestins with your estrogen because you still have your uterus, bleeding is *not* a side effect! The whole point of adding progestin to your estrogen is to trigger withdrawal bleeding and get your uterine lining to routinely shed. However, if you're taking continuous progestins with your estrogen, bleeding is not the norm and should be checked.

A common side effect of estrogen will be fluid retention, because estrogen will decrease the amount of salt and water excreted by kidneys. This excess water is retained by legs, breasts and feet, which can swell. Because of the fluid retention, you may weigh more. Nausea is another common side effect, also seen with oral contraceptives. You may experience nausea during the first two or three months of your therapy; it should just disappear on its own. Some women find that taking their dosages at night (for pills) may remedy this problem. Decreasing the dosage is also an option.

Some other side effects reported include headaches, facial skin colour changes called *melasma*, more cervical mucus secretion, liquid secretion from breasts, change in curvature of cornea, jaundice, loss of scalp hair and itchiness. Again, these side effects vary and depend on the brand you're taking, the dosage, your medical history and so on.

Finally, a minor side effect estrogen causes is a vitamin B6 deficiency, which is also seen with oral contraceptives. Symptoms of this deficiency are vague and include fatigue, depression, loss of concentration, loss of libido or insomnia. This is easily remedied by taking a vitamin B6 supplement!

Are You an HRT or ERT Candidate?

Again, HRT or ERT is not for everyone. Some women make better candidates than others. Here's a guide that may help you make the decision:

- Do you suffer from severe hot flashes that don't respond to natural remedies, outlined above?
- Are your vaginal changes causing painful intercourse, urinary tract infections or vaginitis, which does not respond to natural remedies, such as lubricants (sexual stimulation will also cause more lubrication)?
- Are you in a high-risk category for endometrial cancer? If so, taking progestin to trigger withdrawal bleeding will lower your risk.
- Are you in a high-risk group for heart attacks or strokes? If so, ERT or HRT will lower your risk.
- Are you in a high-risk group for developing osteoporosis? Again, ERT or HRT will lower your risk.

Women who shouldn't be on ERT or HRT

- Women with endometrial cancer or a history of endometrial cancer should not be on unopposed estrogen ERT. Again, if you still have a uterus, you'll be placed on HRT (estrogen and progesterone), which lowers your cancer risk anyway.
- Women with breast cancer. You shouldn't be on either ERT or HRT if you have (or have a history of) breast cancer.
- Women who have had a stroke. Neither ERT nor HRT is recommended.
- Women who have a blood clotting disorder. Neither ERT nor HRT is recommended.
- Women with undiagnosed vaginal bleeding. Neither therapy is recommended.
- Women with liver dysfunction. You can be on the estrogen patch or vaginal cream to relieve your menopausal symptoms, but you shouldn't take any pills orally.

Women who should think twice about HRT or ERT

Women with Type 2 diabetes are encouraged to discuss whether they are candidates for HRT, given its protective effects against heart disease. However, you may need to think twice if you have the following *other* conditions:

- sickle cell disease
- high blood pressure
- migraines
- uterine fibroids
- a history of benign breast conditions such as cysts or fibroadenomas
- endometriosis
- seizures
- gallbladder disease
- a family history of breast cancer
- a past or current history of smoking

Common HRT Questions

Q. *What if I begin my estrogen therapy while I'm still perimenopausal and am still getting my period? Will estrogen delay or reverse menopause?*

A. Estrogen won't interfere with your natural menopause because your ovaries *will* run out of eggs with or without hormone treatment.

Q. *What if I just take progesterone?*

A. Remember, natural progesterone is not the same thing as synthetic progesterone, which is known as a progestin. Progesterone alone can relieve up to 80 percent of your menopausal symptoms—especially hot flashes—but it won't affect your vaginal changes.

Q. *So I can't go on and off hormone therapy the way I could with oral contraceptives?*

A. You shouldn't go on and off estrogen because it may cause either irregular uterine bleeding or hyperplasia. Moreover, any protection from bone loss or heart disease is negated by going on and off.

Natural Hormone Replacement Therapy (NHRT)

Many of you may have heard the media hype surrounding natural hormone replacement therapy (NHRT, which includes natural progesterone) versus conventional hormone replacement therapy (HRT). The difference is akin to breast milk and formula for a baby. NHRT is a combination of human estrogens and natural progesterone from botanical sources. HRT, on the other hand, is "factory-made" estrogen, much of which is derived from horse estrogen and a factory-made progesterone, called progestin. (As explained earlier, a manufactured progesterone is called a progestin.) Now, many reports and studies show that the symptoms of menopause are better controlled with NHRT with fewer side effects. Studies also show that the benefits of HRT—protection from heart disease and osteoporosis—are more dramatic and pronounced using NHRT.

What NHRT contains

When you go on NHRT, you're getting 60 to 80 percent estriol, 10 to 20 percent estrone and 10 to 20 percent estradiol, as well as natural human progesterone, DHEA (dehydroepiandrosterone), a natural androgen that turns into a natural testosterone in the body, something all women need to maintain sex drives. On HRT, you're getting 75 to 80 percent estrone, 6 to 15 percent equilin (a horse-derived estrogen) and 5 to 19 percent estradiol, progestin, a "factory-made" progesterone and sometimes anabolic steroids (see "The androgen strain" on page 197) if your libido needs a boost.

As you can see from the range of concentrations of various natural estrogens, it may take a while for you to find just the right dose of each kind of natural estrogen and progesterone, so you'll have to work with your doctor and experiment until you get it right. There is a perception that NHRT is perfect the first time you take it, but many women have to tinker with their "triple estrogens" before they find the right combination for them. A typical prescription for NHRT is often 10 percent estrone, 10 percent estradiol and 80 percent estriol, mixed with 25–30 mg of natural progesterone after menopause and 10–30 mg DHEA, which should (but doesn't always) convert into necessary amounts of testosterone. (If it doesn't, you may need to add a steroid to the mix of natural hormones if your libido is very low, which can be debilitating.)

Where do you find NHRT?

All the books and articles about the natural hormone therapy can mislead you into thinking that they are available everywhere. This is not so. You can't just walk into a health food store and buy natural estrogens or progesterones. They need to be prescribed by a doctor (although the doctor need not be an M.D.; several naturopathic doctors [N.D.s] are prescribing them, too). A pharmacist has to prepare a doctor's prescription for NHRT from scratch. This is known as a "compounding pharmacist." Not all pharmacies are compounding pharmacies, so ask your doctor or current pharmacist about where to go to get a prescription prepared. You can also call the International Academy of Compounding Pharmacists (IACP) or the Professional Compounding Centers of America, Inc. (PCCA) for the nearest compounding pharmacist in your area. Several Canadian compounding pharmacists are members of either or both organizations. You can reach the PCCA at 1-800-331-2498 or at www.compassnet.com/~iacp/. You can also contact Canada's leading natural pharmacy, Smith's Pharmacy, at 1-800-361-6624 or www.smithspharmacy.com.

Phytoestrogens

If you are uncomfortable with the idea of taking any kind of hormone replacement therapy, you may wish to consider the therapeutic benefits of phytoestrogens, or plant estrogens. Women are treating their symptoms with capsules of powdered herbs, such as licorice, burdock, wild yam, motherwort and dong quai (*Angelica sinensis*).

These herbs contain a multitude of chemicals, including estrogenic substances. Although phytoestrogens have been used in Asian cultures for centuries to treat hot flashes, they're just beginning to catch on in the West. The first controlled trial began in 1996 at Columbia-Presbyterian Medical Center in New York.

Many food sources, such as tofu and soy, contain such high concentrations of phytoestrogens that scientists believe it may account for the incredible lack of menopausal symptoms in Japan, which has a soy-heavy diet. Phytoestrogens in the blood of Japanese women are 10 to 40 times higher than in their Western counterparts, but Japanese women report hot flashes about one-sixth as often as Western women. Even the average vegetarian would not consume nearly as much soy as the average Japanese woman.

More interesting, plant hormones not only help prevent menopausal symptoms, but may protect you from breast cancer; breast cancer rates are dramatically lower in Japan than in the United States, but there may be other factors involved, such as child-bearing habits and low-fat diets. After menopause, high-fat diets can increase your risk of heart attack and stroke no matter how much estrogen you take. Meanwhile, bad habits, such as drinking coffee, drinking alcohol and smoking can all increase your risk of osteoporosis. Right now, most doctors will tell you to go ahead and add as much soy as you want to your diet. It may well help and it certainly can't hurt! For more information about alternative healing and therapies during perimenopause and menopause, consult my book *Women of the '60s Turning 50*.

BENEFITS AND RISKS OF HRT
(progesterone or progestin and estrogen)

Benefits

▶ Reduces bone loss during and after menopause.

▶ Reduces menopausal symptoms.

▶ Reduces the risk for heart disease by 40–50 percent.*

▶ Reduces thinning of vaginal tissue and associated discomforts.

*Note: Benefits are less clear when progesterone is added to the estrogen. Some studies suggest that the progesterone added to the estrogen may even cancel out the protection against heart disease.

Risks

▶ Is not effective for every woman.

▶ Can raise cholesterol levels.

▶ May have side effects such as depression and anxiety.

▶ Is not recommended for women with a high risk of breast cancer, or a history of severe blood clotting disorders.

Source: Laurinda M. Poirier, R.N., M.P.H., C.D.E., and Katharine M. Coburn, M.P.H., *Women & Diabetes Life Planning for Health and Wellness:* 133.

LONG-TERM EFFECTS OF ESTROGEN LOSS:
POSTMENOPAUSAL SYMPTOMS

The long-term effects of estrogen loss have to do with traditional symptoms of aging. One of the key reasons why women will choose HRT or ERT (discussed further on) is to slow down or even reverse these symptoms. Yet it's important to keep in mind that the long-term effects of estrogen loss will not immediately set in after menopause. These changes are subtle and happen over several years. Even women who experience severe menopausal symptoms will not wake up to find that they've suddenly aged overnight; these changes occur gradually whether you experience surgical or natural menopause.

Blood Sugar Levels

As stated above, decreasing levels of estrogen and progesterone in your bloodstream lead to decreased blood sugar levels as your body's responsiveness to insulin improves. As a result, you may need to adjust your diabetes medication or insulin regimen if you require insulin.

You may also need to adjust your meal and exercise plan because menopause slows down your metabolism. That means it will be easier to gain weight on fewer calories. The only way around this is to increase activity or decrease your calorie intake.

Skin Changes

As estrogen decreases, skin, like the vagina, tends to lose its elasticity; it too becomes thinner because it is no longer able to retain as much water. Sweat and oil glands also produce less moisture, which is what causes the skin to gradually dry, wrinkle and sag.

Good moisturizers and skin care will certainly help to keep your skin more elastic, but there is one known factor that aggravates and speeds up your skin's natural aging process, damaging the skin even more: *the sun*. If you cut down your sun exposure, you can dramatically reduce visible aging of your skin. The bad news is that much of the sun's damage on our skin is cumulative from many years of exposure. In fact, many researchers believe that when it comes to visible signs of aging, *estrogen loss is only a small factor.* For example, it's known that ultraviolet rays break down collagen and elastin fibres in the skin, which cause it to break down and sag. This is also what puts us at risk for skin cancer, the most notorious of which is melanoma, one of the most aggressive and malignant of all cancers.

Other sun-related problems traditionally linked to estrogen loss are what we call "liver spots"—light brown or tan splotches that develop on the face, neck and hands as we age. First, these spots have *nothing* to do with the liver; they are sun spots and are caused by sun exposure. They are also sometimes the result of HRT, known in this case as *hyperpigmentation.*

Currently, dermatologists are recommending sunblocks with a minimum of SPF 15. In fact, people are so concerned about sun damage that sunblock has become part of most North American women's daily cosmetic routine; women put it on as regularly as a daily moisturizer.

Women who have high blood sugar levels may find that their skin is drier and more scaly, while vaginal dryness may be more severe, than women with lower blood sugar levels. They may also notice that their nails are deteriorating more rapidly. Controlling blood sugar can reverse these effects.

The Osteoporosis Issue

Osteoporosis literally means "porous bones" and is perhaps the most feared condition in the postmenopausal community. Unfortunately, osteoporosis is not always preventable and is a classic symptom of aging. Normally, a healthy, unremarkable woman's bones will become less dense by her late 30s and 40s. By the time she reaches her 50s, she may begin to experience bone loss in her teeth and become more susceptible to wrist fractures. Gradually, the bones in her spine weaken, fracture and compress, causing upper back curvature and loss of height, known as a "dowager's hump." Osteoporosis is unfortunately more common in women because when their skeletal growth is completed, they typically have 15 percent lower bone mineral density and 30 percent less bone mass than men of the same age. Studies also show that women lose more trabecular bone (the inner, spongy part making up the internal support of the bone) and at a higher rate than men.

Women are prone to three types of osteoporosis: *postmenopausal, senile* and *secondary. Postmenopausal osteoporosis* usually develops 10 to 15 years after the onset of menopause. In this case, estrogen loss interferes with calcium absorption, and you begin to lose your trabecular bone three times faster than the normal rate of trabecular bone loss. You will also begin to lose parts of your *cortical* (the outer shell of the bone), but not as quickly as the trabecular bone.

Senile osteoporosis affects men and women. Here, you lose cortical and trabecular bone because of a decrease in bone cell activity that results from aging. Hip fractures are seen most often with this kind of osteoporosis. The decreased bone cell activity affects your capacity to rebuild bone in the first place, but is also aggravated by low calcium intake.

Secondary osteoporosis means that there is an underlying condition that has caused bone loss. These conditions include chronic renal disease, hypogonadism (an overstimulation of the sex glands), hyperthyroidism (an overactive thyroid gland), some forms of cancer, gastrectomy (removal of parts of the intestine that interfere with calcium absorption) and the use of anticonvulsants.

Right now, 1.5 million Canadians are affected by osteoporosis; one in four is a woman over age 50.

Fractured statistics

At least 30 million North American women over the age of 45 are affected by osteoporosis, while more than 500,000 postmenopausal women in the U.S. alone will have an osteoporosis-related fracture each year. These fractures usually involve the spine, hip or wrist. In Canada, the number of hip fractures linked to osteoporosis will have increased by 73.7 percent between 1987 and 2006.

Fractures lead to death 12 to 20 percent of the time as a result of pneumonia. As the rib cage moves forward toward the pelvis, gastrointestinal and respiratory problems increase. Meanwhile, at least 23 percent of all fractures lead to permanent disability after one year. Osteoporosis-related fractures of the wrist, usually the result of a fall on the outstretched hand, are painful and can require a cast for four to six weeks.

Women with diabetes who are suffering from other complications (see Part 3), such as nerve damage, poor vision or foot problems, are also more likely to fall and suffer a fracture.

What causes bone loss anyway?

Our bones are always regenerating (known as "remodelling"). This process helps to maintain a constant level of calcium in the blood, essential for a healthy heart, blood circulation and blood clotting. About 99 percent of all the body's calcium is in the bones and teeth; when blood calcium drops below a certain level, the body will take calcium from the bones to replenish it. But by the time we reach our late 30s, our bones lose calcium faster than it can be replaced. The pace of bone calcium loss speeds up for "freshly postmenopausal" women, who are three to seven years beyond menopause. The pace then slows once again, but as we age, the body is less able to absorb calcium from food. One of the most influential factors in bone loss is estrogen; it slows or even halts the loss of bone mass by improving our absorption of calcium from the intestinal tract, which allows us to maintain a higher level of calcium in our blood. And the higher the calcium levels in the blood, the less chance you have of losing calcium from your bones to replenish your calcium blood levels. In men, testosterone does the same thing for calcium absorption, but unlike women, men never reach a particular age when their testes stop producing testosterone. If they did, they would be just as prone to osteoporosis as women.

But estrogen alone cannot prevent osteoporosis. There is a long list of other factors that affect bone loss. One of the most obvious factors is calcium in our diet. Calcium is regularly lost in urine, feces and dead skin. We need to continuously account for this loss in our diet. The less calcium we ingest, the more we force our body into taking it out of our bones. Exercise also greatly affects bone density; the more we exercise, the stronger we make our bones. In fact, the bone mass we have in our late 20s and early 30s will affect our bone mass at menopause.

Finally, several physical conditions and external factors help to weaken our bones, contributing to bone loss later in life. These include the following:

- **Heavy caffeine and alcohol intake:** Because they are diuretics, they cause you to lose more calcium in your urine.
- **Smoking:** Research shows that smokers tend to go into earlier menopause, while older smokers have 20 to 30 percent less bone mass than non-smokers.
- **Women in surgical menopause who are not on ERT:** Losing estrogen earlier than you would have naturally increases your bone loss.
- **Diseases of the small intestine, liver and pancreas:** They prevent the body from absorbing adequate amounts of calcium from the intestine.
- **Lymphoma, leukemia and multiple myeloma:** These affect the blood and therefore calcium levels.
- **Chronic diarrhea from ulcerative colitis or Crohn's disease:** These conditions cause calcium loss through feces.
- **Surgical removal of part of the stomach or small intestine:** This affects absorption.
- **Hypercalciuria:** This is a condition in which one loses too much calcium in the urine.
- **Early menopause (before age 45):** The earlier you stop producing estrogen, the more likely you are to lose calcium.
- **Lighter complexions:** Women with darker pigments have roughly 10 percent

more bone mass than fairer women because they produce more *calcitonin*, the hormone that strengthens bones.

- **Low weight:** Women with less body fat store less estrogen, which makes the bones less dense to begin with and more vulnerable to calcium loss.
- **Women with eating disorders (yo-yo dieting, starvation diets, binge or purge eaters):** When there isn't enough calcium in our bloodstream through our diet, the body will go to the bones to get what it needs. These women also have lower weight.
- **A family history of osteoporosis:** Studies show that women born to mothers with spinal fractures have lower bone mineral density in the spine, neck and mid shaft.
- **High-protein diet:** This contributes to a loss of calcium in urine.
- **Women who have never been pregnant:** They haven't experienced the same bursts of estrogen in their bodies as women who have been pregnant.
- **Antacids with aluminum:** They interfere with calcium absorption.
- **Lactose intolerance:** Since so much calcium is in dairy foods, this allergy is a significant risk factor.
- **Teenage pregnancy:** When a woman is pregnant in her teens, her bones are not yet fully developed and she can lose as much as 10 percent of her bone mass unless she has an adequate calcium intake of roughly 2,000 mg during the pregnancy and 2,200 while breast-feeding.
- **Scoliosis:** Curvature of the spine.

Osteoporosis and diabetes

If you are overweight, as at least 80 percent of women with Type 2 diabetes are, you're less at risk for osteoporosis, but at greater risk of developing other health problems. If you have a history of chronic dieting or eating disorders, however, your risk of osteoporosis increases because you may have deprived yourself of vital nutrients in the past that are necessary for healthy bone density.

Regardless of your weight, however, high blood sugar levels can also increase your risk of osteoporosis, although high insulin levels—the nature of Type 2 diabetes—is conversely associated with a lower risk of osteoporosis.

Preventing osteoporosis

As boring and repetitive as it may sound, the best way to prevent osteoporosis is to ingest more calcium and increase your bone mass. This boils down to eating right and exercising. It's not enough to just take calcium supplements or eat high-calcium foods; you need to cut down on foods that have diuretic qualities to them: caffeine and alcohol. How much is "enough" calcium? According to the National Institutes of Health Consensus Panel on Osteoporosis, premenopausal women require roughly 1,000 mg of calcium a day; perimenopausal or post-menopausal women already on HRT or ERT need 1,000 mg; and peri- and post-menopausal women not taking estrogen need roughly 1,500 mg per day. For women who have already been diagnosed with osteoporosis, the panel recommends 2,500 mg of calcium a day. Foods that are rich in calcium include all dairy products (a 250 mL/8 oz. glass of milk contains 300 mg of calcium), fish, shellfish, oysters, shrimp, sardines, salmon, soybeans, tofu, broccoli and other dark green vegetables (except spinach, which contains oxalic acid, preventing calcium absorption). It's crucial to determine how much calcium you're getting in your diet *before* you start any calcium supplements; too much calcium can cause kidney stones in people who are at risk for them. In addition, not all supplements have been tested for absorbency. Dr. Robert Heaney, in his book *Calcium and Common Sense,* suggests that you test absorbency yourself by dropping your supplement into a glass of warm water, while stirring occasionally. If the supplement doesn't dissolve completely, chances are it won't be absorbed by your body efficiently. It's crucial to remember that a calcium supplement is in fact a supplement and should not replace a high-calcium diet. The dosage of your supplement would only need to be 400–600 mg per day, while your diet should account for the remainder of your 1,000–1,500 mg daily intake of calcium. Calcium is discussed more thoroughly in Chapter 7, which covers nutrition.

As for exercise, the best kinds of activities are walking, running, biking, aerobic dance or cross-country skiing. They are considered good ways to put more stress on the bones, increasing their mass. Carrying weights is also a good way to increase bone mass.

The most accurate way to measure your risk of osteoporosis is through a bone densitometry (or DEXA), which measures bone mass and provides you with a "fracture risk estimate." This test involves low-dose X-rays and takes about 30 minutes. For more information about osteoporosis, contact the Osteoporosis Society of Canada at 1-800-463-6842 (also listed at the back of this book).

OTHER POSTMENOPAUSAL CONCERNS

As you age, several health problems might plague you as a result of estrogen loss. Here is a brief overview.

Heart Disease

Ladies, if you have Type 2 diabetes, you must educate yourselves about the signs and symptoms of heart disease. Again, heart disease kills more postmenopausal women than lung cancer or breast cancer because estrogen loss increases the risk of coronary artery disease. If you have Type 2 diabetes, your risk increases two or three times. Other risk factors, such as smoking, high blood pressure, high cholesterol, obesity and an inactive lifestyle, will further increase your risk. In fact, the Nurses' Health Study, a study that looked at 120,000 middle-aged women, found that women who were obese had a two- to threefold increase in heart disease, particularly in women with "apple-shaped" figures (meaning abdominal or upper body fat).

Studies show that hormone replacement therapy, cholesterol-lowering drugs and lifestyle changes can significantly reduce your risk of heart disease. Women who are physically active have a 60 to 75 percent lower risk of heart disease than inactive women. For more information on women and heart disease, see Chapter 15 and my book *50 Ways Women Can Prevent Heart Disease*.

Breast Cancer

As you probably know, postmenopausal breast cancer is considered to be epidemic among women over 50. There are many reasons for this, all of which are discussed in my book *The Breast Sourcebook*. Women with Type 2 diabetes will probably be told that they should consider hormone replacement therapy to reduce their risk of heart disease, a disease they are two or three times more likely to suffer from than the average woman. Therefore, you may be concerned about breast cancer risk and HRT.

It's still not clear whether hormone replacement therapy increases your risk of breast cancer, but there's actually more consensus in the medical research community over this issue than many others. That's because the incidence of breast cancer in Western nations dramatically rises *anyway* after menopause whether you're on HRT or not, so it's not clear whether HRT really contributes to this increase. The current thinking seems to be that if you're on HRT, there's a slightly increased risk of developing breast cancer. If you do develop it, it's apparently a very treatable type of cancer that's estrogen-receptor positive, which means that your risk of dying from breast cancer is decreased.

If you add up all the data, you may want to rethink HRT if your risk of breast cancer is significant (due to other factors such as family history, for example), or if the risk of breast cancer significantly outweighs your risk of heart disease.

If you're on HRT and are diagnosed with breast cancer, you may be interested in a 1995 study done in Ottawa, Ontario, that found women on HRT had more difficulty battling breast cancer *once it was diagnosed.* However, a doctor will simply take you off hormone replacement therapy if a breast cancer is diagnosed, which completely eliminates the problem and restores your survival rate to that of the general population's. That said, many medical papers suggest that women undergoing breast cancer treatment can still be on HRT. It is not necessarily a conflict. If you have been diagnosed with breast cancer, discuss with your doctor whether you should continue HRT.

Your menstrual and pregnancy history

Unfortunately, your menstrual history can apparently affect your risk of breast cancer, but many experts disagree as to how significant a role it plays in the big picture. For example, one factor is what experts call "early menarche." Menarche refers to your first period; early menarche means that you got your first period prior to age 12. This somewhat trivial detail also means that you've been making estrogen longer than the average woman, which is why your menstrual history may influence your risk of breast cancer. Menarche levels can vary enormously. The average age of menarche is 12.8 in the United States and 17 in China. Some researchers say this is why breast cancer occurrence in China is one-third that of the United States. And even within China, provinces with later menarche tend to have lower rates of breast cancer.

Another factor is cycle length. If your cycles are either longer or shorter than average, your breast cancer risk increases by some estimates as high as 50 percent. (An average cycle is anywhere from 26 to 29 days.) It's believed that shorter or longer cycles indicate a hormonal imbalance at work, which *may* contribute to an increased breast cancer risk. Shorter cycles also indicate that you're making more estrogen than women with longer cycles.

Pregnancy history is a *huge* factor in determining your overall risk of breast cancer. In fact, according to a 1751 edition of the *Chambers Encyclopedia,* breast cancer is described as "a most dread disease, particularly of the celibate and barren." To a large extent, this is still true today. For example, according to the National Cancer Institute, lesbians are two to three times more likely to develop breast cancer than heterosexual women, while childless women are 50 percent more likely to develop breast cancer than women who have borne children when they were under 35. Curiously, if you bear your first child after 35, your pregnancy no longer offers you the same protection against breast cancer *unless you decide to breast-feed.*

Urinary Incontinence

Urinary incontinence means "involuntary urination." This condition tends to plague women with diabetes, as well as women who do a lot of sitting, have several children, have repeated urinary tract infections (UTIs), have diseases that affect the spinal cord or the brain (such as Parkinson's disease, multiple sclerosis or Alzheimer's disease), have a history of bladder cancer, or have had major pelvic surgery, such as a hysterectomy. As we age the muscles of our pelvic floor and abdomen get weaker and our urinary apparatus drops down. On top of this, less estrogen causes the urethra to thin and change, similar to the vaginal changes older women experience.

When we're younger, we have tremendous control over one particular muscle: the *pubococcygeal* muscle (a.k.a. the *levator ani muscle*). This muscle controls both our vaginal opening and the urinary opening. Normally, we feel the urge to urinate, but we hold it in until we get to the right place! When we get to the toilet, urine doesn't come out immediately. First we relax slightly, and then urinate. This "relaxing" prior to urination is the relaxing of the pubococcygeal muscle. We can also stop and start our streams. Anyone who's had to have a urinalysis has probably mastered this technique. Again, this ability to stop and start the stream is controlled by the same muscle. Sometimes after an orgasm, this muscle takes longer to kick in. We may try to urinate, feeling the urge to, but find we are unable to. But after the postorgasmic feeling wears off, we are once again in control of this muscle.

Urinary incontinence is categorized into four groups: stress incontinence, urge incontinence, overflow incontinence and irritable bladder. Stress incontinence occurs when urine leaks out during a sudden movement, such as a sneeze or cough, or even uncontrollable laughing. This can happen to women of all ages and is considered the most common form of incontinence. It happens when the urethra becomes stretched out from overuse caused by the habit of "holding it in" or simple aging.

Urge incontinence refers to a sudden, sometimes painful urge to urinate that is so unexpected and powerful you may not always be able to make it to the toilet. This is not seen in younger women and is almost exclusively a postmenopausal problem in women over 60.

Overflow incontinence occurs in only a small percentage of overall incontinence problems. Here, with no warning, urine suddenly overflows after you change your position (from sitting to standing, for example). You may lose just a few drops of urine or enough to require a maxi-pad. Sometimes these episodes are followed by the urge to urinate a few minutes later, but when you try, nothing comes out. This condition often precedes or accompanies a urinary tract infection (also see Chapter 16 on neuropathy). Causes of this type of incontinence are similar to the causes of UTIs.

Finally, an irritable bladder is a mishmash of the other three incontinence symptoms and UTIs. You'll need to see a urologist to sort out what's causing your bladder to behave so erratically.

Treating incontinence

Estrogen is very helpful as a treatment for incontinence because it restores the "lustre" of your urethra just as it restores the vagina. Estrogen in pill, cream or patch form will have the same beneficial effects.

Something known as the *Kegel exercise* is also very helpful in strengthening the pubococcygeal muscle. The Kegel exercise can be done in any position, anywhere, anytime: in an elevator, on the subway, in a movie theatre, while you're cooking, eating or lying down! First, you isolate the muscle that stops and starts your urinary stream. To isolate it, you can also insert your finger into your vagina and try to squeeze your finger with your vaginal opening. Once you've isolated the muscle, just squeeze five times and count five; squeeze five and count five. Or squeeze ten and count ten. Whatever. The key is to keep the muscles in shape. It's *that* simple, and it really helps. You can also do general exercises to firm up your abdomen and pelvis in conjunction with your Kegel exercises.

Being more conscious of your diet and medications is also important. For example, certain drugs for high blood pressure or heart disease, sedatives or tranquillizers can trigger bouts of incontinence. Ask your pharmacist about this. Some drugs or foods are diuretics, which will cause you to urinate more frequently. Caffeine and alcohol are classic diuretics you can easily cut out of your diet, for example. Fruit juice and spicy foods can also irritate the bladder.

Overweight women are also more likely to experience incontinence because the weight exerts more pressure on the bladder, causing the muscles and urethra to overwork themselves. Weight loss may help to resolve the problem. (See Chapters 7 and 10.)

More invasive treatments for incontinence involve surgery that lifts and tightens the pelvic floor, or using a *pessary*, a stiff, doughnut-shaped rubber device that needs to be fitted and sized, fits into the top of the vagina and holds it up slightly. It raises the neck of the bladder and helps to reposition it.

Some women may choose to just live with the problem and wear bladder-control products, maxi-pads or diaper-like products to avoid the embarrassment of incontinence.

PART 3

Type 2 Diabetes Complications

Chapter 13

PREVENTING COMPLICATIONS: WHAT THE STUDIES SHOW

● ● ● ● ● ● ● ● ● ● ●

At least 40 percent of all people with Type 2 diabetes will develop another disease as a result of their condition. Many of you reading this may already be affected by some of the conditions discussed in this section. The good news is that much of the bad news outlined in this section of the book can be prevented. By keeping your blood sugar levels as stable as possible as often as possible, losing some weight and quitting smoking, you're well on the way to an uncomplicated life with diabetes.

THE DIABETES CONTROL AND COMPLICATIONS TRIAL

In earlier chapters, I have made reference to a study known as the Diabetes Control and Complications Trial (DCCT). This study involved 1,441 people with Type 1 diabetes, who were randomly managed according to one of two treatment philosophies: "intensive" treatment (or tight control) and "conventional" treatment (medium control). Intensive treatments involve frequently testing your blood sugar, and adding a short-acting insulin that requires three to four injections daily, or one dose of longer-acting insulin. The goal of this type of management is to achieve blood sugar levels that are as normal as possible as often as possible. Conventional treatment involves controlling your diabetes to the point where you avoid feeling any symptoms of high blood sugar, such as frequent urination, thirst or fatigue, without doing very much, if any, self-testing.

The Results

The results of the DCCT were pretty astounding, so much so that the trial, planned for a ten-year period, was cut short—a rare occurrence in research trials. The DCCT results were unveiled in 1993 at the American Diabetes Association's annual conference.

The people who were managed with intensive therapy were able to delay microvascular complications 36 to 76 percent of the time. Microvascular complications include nerve damage and all of the problems associated with it (Chapter 16), eye damage (Chapter 17), tooth decay and gum disease (Chapter 18), kidney damage (Chapter 19) and foot complications (Chapter 20).

Specifically, eye disease was reduced by 76 percent, kidney disease by 56 percent and nerve damage by 61 percent. Frequent blood sugar testing and blood sugar control also reduced high cholesterol by 35 percent, which can reduce macrovascular complications such as heart and stroke (Chapter 15). *Those are very significant results*. Statistically, anything over 1 percent is considered "clinically significant." Wow! The overwhelming consensus among diabetes practitioners is that intensive therapy for people with either Type 1 or Type 2 diabetes prolongs health and greatly reduces complications.

The National Institute of Diabetes and Digestive and Kidney Diseases (NIDDK) in the United States reported comparable findings when they did a similar study. NIDDK research found that with intensive therapy, eye disease was still reduced by 76 percent, kidney disease by 50 percent, nerve disease by 60 percent and cardiovascular disease by 35 percent.

What the DCCT Means for Type 2 Diabetes

The DCCT did not look at blood sugar control and *macrovascular complications*—the cardiovascular complications (such as heart disease and stroke) for which people with Type 2 diabetes are most at risk—but it showed a significant reduction in cholesterol levels. A cholesterol-lowering drug can also achieve lower cholesterol, while blood pressure-lowering drugs can reduce the risk of heart attack and stroke, too (see Chapter 15).

For several years the DCCT was controversial with Type 2 specialists. Should people with Type 2 diabetes be counselled to *intensively* control their blood sugar or not? Many specialists said that losing weight and getting the diet under control are hard enough, and that asking people to self-test their blood sugar three to four times per day is too much for most people with Type 2 diabetes. In other words, what's the point of avoiding microvascular complications when you're about to drop dead from a massive heart attack or stroke? Nevertheless, many specialists felt that since the DCCT showed such overwhelming reductions in complications for Type 1, until more data was out, people with Type 2 diabetes should be intensively controlling their blood sugar.

THE BRITISH STUDY

In 1998, the results of a 20-year British study was published. Known as the United Kingdom Prospective Diabetes Study (UKPDS), it set out to determine whether blood sugar control reduces macrovascular complications in Type 2 diabetes, together with lowering blood pressure. Macrovascular complications are the cardiovascular complications, such as heart disease and stroke risk, as well as peripheral vascular disease problems, which have to do with poor blood flow to other body parts and can cause foot problems, impotence and sexual problems for women, as well as a host of other things.

The results show that frequent blood sugar testing can reduce the risk of blindness and kidney failure in people with Type 2 diabetes by 25 percent. In those Type 2 diabetics with high blood pressure, lowering blood pressure reduced the risk of stroke by 44 percent and heart failure by 56 percent. And, for every one percentage point reduction in the value of the HbA_{1c} test (see Chapter 5), there was a 35 percent reduction in eye, kidney and nerve damage, and an overall 25 percent reduction in deaths related to diabetes.

The bottom line is that the UKPDS shows that frequently self-testing your blood sugar can prevent long-term complications of diabetes for people with Type 2 diabetes, and by combining that strategy with a heart-smart lifestyle, you can live well with diabetes—without complications.

Chapter 14

PREVENTING HYPOGLYCEMIA

● ● ● ● ● ● ● ● ● ● ●

When you're diagnosed with Type 2 diabetes, whether your treatment revolves around lifestyle modification, oral hypoglycemic therapy or insulin therapy, you may experience an episode of low blood sugar. This is clinically known as *hypoglycemia*. Hypoglycemia can sometimes come on suddenly, particularly overnight. If left untreated, it can also result in coma, brain damage and death. Hypoglycemia is considered the official cause of death in about 5 percent of the Type 1 diabetes population. In the past, hypoglycemia was a more common problem among people with Type 1 diabetes. But since 40 to 50 percent of all people with Type 2 diabetes will eventually graduate to insulin therapy, the incidence of hypoglycemia has increased by 300 percent in this group. Moreover, hypoglycemia is a common side effect of oral hypoglycemic pills, the medication the majority of people with Type 2 diabetes take when they are first diagnosed.

This chapter will explain exactly what happens when you have low blood sugar, who's at risk, how to treat it and how to avoid it.

THE LOWDOWN ON LOW BLOOD SUGAR

Any blood sugar reading below 3.5 mmol/L is considered too low. A hypoglycemic episode is characterized by two stages: the warning stage and what I call the *actual* hypoglycemic episode. The warning stage occurs when your blood sugar levels *begin* to drop and can happen as early as a blood sugar reading of 6 mmol/L in people with typically higher than normal blood sugar levels. When your blood sugar drops to 3.5 mmol/L or less, you are *officially* hypoglycemic.

During the warning stage, your body responds by piping adrenaline into your bloodstream. This causes symptoms such as trembling, irritability, hunger and weakness, some of which mimic drunkenness. The irritability can simulate the rantings of someone who is drunk, while the weakness and shakiness can lead to the lack of coordination seen in someone who is intoxicated. For this reason, it's crucial that you carry a card or wear a bracelet that identifies that you have diabetes. (See "Your Diabetes ID Card" later in this chapter.) Your liver will also release any glucose it has stored for you, but if it doesn't have enough glucose to get you back to normal, there won't be enough glucose for your brain to function normally and you will feel confused, irritable or aggressive.

Once your blood sugar is 3.5 mmol/L and falling, you'll notice a more rapid heartbeat, trembling and sweating. As the levels become lower, your pupils will begin to dilate, you will begin to lose consciousness and you could perhaps experience a seizure. No one with diabetes is immune to hypoglycemia; it can occur in someone with long-standing diabetes just as much as in someone newly diagnosed. The important thing is to be alert to the warning signs, be prepared and try to avoid future episodes.

Who's at Risk?

Since hypoglycemia can be the result of too high an insulin dose, it is often called insulin shock (or insulin reaction). This is a misleading term, however, because it implies that only people who take insulin can become hypoglycemic. For the record, all people with Type 1 or Type 2 diabetes can become hypoglycemic. If you are taking more than one insulin injection a day, you are at greater risk of developing hypoglycemia. But hypoglycemia can be triggered just as easily by

- delaying or missing a meal or snack (see Chapter 6)
- drinking alcohol (see Chapter 6)
- exercising too long or too strenuously (without compensating with extra food) (see Chapter 8)
- taking too high a dose of an oral hypoglycemic agent (this can happen if you lose weight but are not put on a lower dose of your pill)

If you're taking pills

All people taking sulfonylureas (see Chapter 5 and further in this chapter) are vulnerable to hypoglycemia because this drug stimulates the pancreas to produce insulin. It is synonymous with taking an insulin injection. Furthermore, if you lose weight after you begin taking sulfonylureas, but don't lower your pill dosage, you could also experience hypoglycemic episodes. That's because losing weight will make your body more responsive to insulin.

Yet biguanides (see Chapter 5 and further on in this chapter) do not typically cause hypoglycemic episodes, since they work by preventing the liver from making glucose rather than stimulating anything to make insulin. Similarly, acarbose does not, by itself, cause hypoglycemia. It works by delaying the breakdown of starch and sucrose into glucose. That's not to say, however, that hypoglycemia can't happen to you if you're taking biguanides or acarbose; you can still develop it if you miss meals or snacks or overexercise without compensating for it, although this is rare.

As discussed in Chapter 5, your diabetes pills may also react with other medications. For example, some of the older oral hypoglycemic agents may work less or more effectively when combined with certain medications, including blood thinners (anticoagulants), oral contraceptives, diuretics, steroids, aspirin and various anticonvulsive and antihypertensive medications.

Another factor is the half-life of your oral medication. By knowing when the drug peaks in your body, you'll be able to prevent hypoglycemia from occurring. For example, tolbutamide is a short-acting oral hypoglycemic agent. It begins to work about an hour after you take it and lasts for about 12 hours, peaking between five and six hours after you ingest it.

Acetohexamide starts working about an hour after you take it, stays in your body for about 14 hours and peaks at about five hours. Glyburide goes to work in about 1.5 hours, stays in your body for 24 hours and peaks at about three hours. Finally, chlorpropamide has the longest half-life. It starts to work an hour after you take it, stays in your body for 72 hours and peaks within 35 hours.

Combination therapy

Roughly 40 percent of all people taking a combination of oral hypoglycemic agents experience hypoglycemic episodes, while 33 to 47 percent of people who combine insulin with sulfonylureas experience hypoglycemic episodes. These are higher odds than if you were taking only one oral hypoglycemic agent.

Recognizing the Symptoms

If you can begin to recognize the warning signs of hypoglycemia, you may be able to stabilize your blood sugar before you lose consciousness. Watch out for the adrenaline symptoms: initially hungry and headachy, then sweaty, nervous and dizzy. Those who live with you or spend a lot of time with you should learn to notice sudden mood changes (usually extreme irritability, "drunklike aggression" and confusion) as a warning that you are "low."

One of the best examples of hypoglycemia symptoms on film is in the movie *Steel Magnolias*, in which Julia Roberts portrays a woman with Type 1 diabetes opposite Sally Fields, who plays her mother. At the local beauty parlour, amidst happy chatter over Roberts's upcoming wedding, her character suddenly becomes aggressive and begins to verbally attack her mother, shaking all the while. The other customers look alarmed. Sally Fields realizes at once that Roberts is "low" and calmly takes over the situation. She grabs Roberts and calms people down. "It's all right, it's all right, she's just low. With all the excitement that's gone on, it's only natural. Get me some juice."

"I have a candy in my purse," pipes up a customer.

"No," insists Fields. "Juice is better, juice is better." Roberts becomes even more upset. Her reaction is sheer confusion and fright. Fields takes the juice and starts to feed her; Roberts, in confusion, spits it out and puts up a fight every step of the way. After Fields force-feeds her a little longer, Roberts starts to drink on her own and finally utters an intelligible sentence. "Oh, she's making some sense now," coos Fields. "Yes, she is. She's starting to make sense." In other words, Roberts's blood sugar is beginning to rise and the hypoglycemic symptoms that appeared out of nowhere are starting to dissipate. In this scene, Fields says "juice is better" because it is a more immediate source of glucose. But in fact, juice is *not* a good idea when someone is resisting it; in this case, it is better to use glucose gel rather than risk someone aspirating or inhaling the juice when it is force-fed.

Whether you notice your own mood changes or not, you, too, will feel "suddenly" unwell. This is a warning that your blood sugar is low. Reach for your snack pack (page 226). Not everyone experiences the same warning symptoms, but here are some signs to watch for:

- pounding, racing heart
- fast breathing
- skin turning white
- sweating (cold sweat in big drops)
- trembling, tremors or shaking

- goosebumps or pale, cool skin
- extreme hunger pangs
- light-headedness (feeling dizzy or that the room is spinning)
- nervousness, extreme irritability or a sudden mood change
- confusion
- feeling weak or faint
- headache
- vision changes (seeing double or blurry vision)

Some people will experience no symptoms at all. If you've had a hypoglycemic episode without any warning symptoms, it's important for you to eat regularly and to test your blood sugar. If you're experiencing frequent hypoglycemic episodes, it's important to find out why it keeps happening so you can adjust meal plans and activities accordingly. In some cases of long-standing diabetes and repeated hypoglycemic episodes, experts note that the warning symptoms may not always occur. It's believed that in some people, the body eventually loses its ability to detect hypoglycemia and send adrenaline. Furthermore, if you've switched from an animal to human insulin, warning symptoms may not be as pronounced.

"JUICE IS BETTER"

If you start to feel symptoms of hypoglycemia, stop what you're doing (especially if it's active) and have some sugar. Next, test your blood sugar to see what it reads. Eating some regular food will usually do the trick. If your blood sugar is below 3.5 mmol/L, ingest some glucose. If you can drink and swallow, Sally Fields was right: real fruit juice *is* better when your blood sugar is low. The best way to get your levels back up to normal is to ingest simple sugar; that is, sugar that gets into your bloodstream fast. Half a cup of any fruit juice or one-third of a can of a sugary soft drink is a good source of simple sugar. Artificially sweetened soft drinks are useless. *It must contain real sugar.* If you don't have fruit juice or soft drinks handy, here are some other sources high in simple sugar:

- two or three tablets of commercial dextrose, sold in pharmacies. If you're taking acarbose or combining it with an oral hypoglycemic agent or insulin, the only sugar you can have is dextrose (Dextrosol or Monoject), due to the rate of absorption.

- three to five hard candies (that's equal to about six Life Savers)
- 10 mL (2 tsp.) of white or brown sugar (or two sugar cubes)
- 15 mL (1 tbsp.) of honey

Once you've ingested enough simple sugar, your hypoglycemic symptoms should disappear within 10 to 15 minutes. Test your blood sugar ten minutes after having your sugar to see if your blood sugar levels are coming back up. If your symptoms don't go away, have more simple sugars until they do.

After a Low

If you've had a close call to the point where you experienced those adrenaline symptoms, be sure to have a snack or meal as soon as possible. If your next meal or snack is more than an hour away, eat half a sandwich or some cheese and crackers. That will ensure that your blood sugar levels don't fall again. Then check your blood sugar levels after you eat to make sure your levels are where they should be. Try to investigate the cause of your episode by asking yourself the following:

1. Did you miss a meal or eat late? (Were you at one of those dinner parties where you came on time but everybody else arrived an hour later?)
2. Did you eat less than normal? (Are you sick or upset over something?)
3. Did you give yourself the right amount of pills or insulin?
4. Did you do anything physically active that you didn't plan in the last hour or so? (For instance, did someone ask you to help move some heavy object from one side of the room to the other?)
5. Did you remember to compensate for any exercising you did with the appropriate amount of carbohydrates? (See Chapter 8.)

Glucagon

Most people will be able to treat their low blood sugar without becoming unconscious, but on rare occasions, it can happen. And if that's the case, it's too late for juice, soft drinks or any other kind of sugar. That's when something known as a Glucagon Kit comes in. Glucagon is particularly useful for people who have little or no warning symptoms of low blood sugar and have previously lost consciousness from low blood sugar.

Glucagon is a hormone injected under the skin. Like insulin, glucagon is destroyed by the digestive system when it's taken orally. Glucagon causes an increase in blood glucose concentration; it basically stimulates the body to make glucose. It does this by forcing the liver to convert all its glycogen stores into glucose almost immediately after it's injected. You'll need about 1 mg of glucagon to do the trick.

Glucagon will make you nauseous when you come to, so if glucagon is injected, it's crucial to ingest simple sugars as soon as you wake. The simple sugar will replace the glycogen your liver releases and will get rid of the nausea. Once you feel normal again, you should consume regular food. Get a prescription for a Glucagon Kit through your doctor, then purchase the kit at any pharmacy.

If you do not respond to glucagon, glucose will be administered intravenously in a hospital or ambulance.

People in states of starvation (anorexics) or who have chronic hypoglycemia will not benefit from glucagon, because in those cases there will be no glycogen stores in the liver ready for conversion into glucose. Injected under the skin, glucagon takes eight to ten minutes to work its wonders.

The Third Person

The Glucagon Kit is for another person to use, someone who has been shown how to administer the drug to revive you. This may be someone close to you who is likely to be with you when you lose consciousness. The kit should have all the necessary instructions regarding giving injections. But here are the instructions just in case. Photocopy these instructions and post them in a safe place:

1. Inject 1 mg of glucagon anywhere under the skin. (The abdomen or thighs are good spots.) For children five and under, .50 mg of glucagon is recommended.
2. Wait about ten minutes for the person to regain consciousness. Call 9-1-1 if he or she does not regain consciousness in 15 minutes.
3. After the person wakes up, immediately give her or him about half a cup of fruit juice or a third of a can of a sugary soft drink. The drink must contain sugar; artificially sweetened drinks will not work.
4. Continue feeding the drink to this person until he or she feels well enough to eat regular food.

For your wallet

Photocopy the following and carry it in your wallet (I, the author, give you permission) as soon as you finish reading this chapter:

To whom it may concern:

These instructions will help you assist this person with diabetes, who has passed out because his or her blood sugar is too low.

1. Give this person a form of simple sugar (juice, candies, table sugar, honey). If this person is unconscious, go to #2.
2. Do *not* give this person any food or drink or put anything in his or her mouth; he or she could choke.
3. Call 9-1-1 and say: "I'm with a person who has diabetes who has passed out from low blood sugar. I need someone to get here as soon as possible." Be sure to give a clear address with specific instructions about your location.

RECIPE FOR PREVENTION

The recipe for preventing hypoglycemia or low blood sugar is the same one for preventing high blood sugar: frequent blood sugar monitoring (Chapter 4), following your meal plan (Chapter 6), following an exercise plan (Chapter 8) and taking your medication as prescribed (Chapter 5). Any changes in your routine, diet, exercise habits or medication dosages should be followed by a period of very close blood sugar monitoring until your routine is more established.

Frequent episodes of hypoglycemia may also be a sign that your body is changing: You may be losing weight, thanks to those lifestyle changes you've made, and the dosage of pills that were prescribed to you when you weighed 86 kg (190 lb.) may be too strong now that you're down to 65 kg (145 lb.). Or you may be taking too high an insulin dose.

A Snack Pack

People with Type 1 or 2 diabetes should have a snack pack with them for emergencies or for unplanned physical activity. The pack should contain all the following:

- two or three boxes or cans of juice (in a pinch, you can substitute with two cans of a sweet soft drink—sweetened with real sugar)
- one package of dextrose tablets (alternatively, a bag of hard candies)
- some protein and carbohydrates (e.g., packaged cheese and crackers)
- a card that says "I have diabetes." (see page 228)
- glucagon, if you suffer from repeated episodes

Wear Your Bracelets

All people with diabetes ought to wear a MedicAlert bracelet or necklace, the most recognized medical alert "outerwear." The newer styles don't have that basic red lettering that announces to the world "I'm allergic or diabetic." The newer bracelets can be quite discreet, yet still have your medical information, personal ID number and a 24-hour emergency hotline number engraved on it. This crucial jewellery is yours for a one-time, upfront fee of $35. That will get you a lifetime membership in the Canadian MedicAlert Foundation, as well as a bracelet or necklace and free updates on your information. You can reach Canadian MedicAlert Foundation at 1-800-668-6381.

Tell People You Have Diabetes

A crucial word about dealing with hypoglycemia: Tell people close to you, or who work closely with you, that you have diabetes. You never know when you might experience symptoms: at a family function (weddings are notorious for delaying meals), at work and so on. If you tell people about the symptoms of hypoglycemia and instruct them on what to do, you'll have more bases covered in case you experience an episode.

YOUR DIABETES ID CARD

If you don't have the following information on you already, photocopy this section and put it in an obvious place in your wallet or on your person.

I have diabetes. If I am unconscious or if my behaviour appears unusual, it may be related to my diabetes or my treatment. I am not drunk. If I can swallow, give me sugar in the form of fruit juice, a sweet soft drink, candies or table sugar. Phone my doctor or the hospital listed below. Or phone 9-1-1 if I am unconscious.

Name _____

Address _____

_____

Phone number _____

Chief contact _____

Relationship _____

My doctor's name is: _____

He or she can be reached at (phone number): _____

after hours _____

My hospital: _____

My blood type is: ☐ A ☐ B ☐ AB ☐ O ☐ Rh+ ☐ Rh-

I wear: ☐ lens implants ☐ dentures ☐ contact lenses
☐ an artificial joint ☐ a pacemaker

I'm allergic to: _____

My health card/insurance number is _____

My group insurance number is _____

Source: Adapted from "Health Record for People with Diabetes," 1996, McNeil Consumer Products Company.

Chapter 15

DIABETES, HEART AND STROKE

● ● ● ● ● ● ● ● ● ● ●

The most important thing to grasp about diabetes complications is that there are two kinds of problems that can lead to similar diseases. The first kind of problem is known as a *macrovascular complication*. The prefix *macro* means "large"; the word *vascular* means "blood vessels"—the veins and arteries that carry the blood back and forth throughout your body. Put it together and you have "large blood vessel complications." A plain-language interpretation of "macrovascular complications" is "BIG problems with your blood vessels."

If you think of your body as a planet, a macrovascular disease would be a disease that affects the whole planet; it is body-wide, or systemic. Cardiovascular disease is a macrovascular complication that can cause heart attack, stroke, high blood pressure and body-wide circulation problems, clinically known as peripheral vascular disease (PVD). Peripheral vascular disease refers to "fringe" blood-flow problems and is part of the heart disease story. PVD occurs when blood flow to the limbs (arms, legs and feet) is blocked, creating cramping, pain or numbness. *In fact, pain and numbing in your arms or legs may be signs of heart disease or even an imminent heart attack.*

Macrovascular complications are caused, not only by too much blood sugar, but also by pre-existing health problems. People with Type 2 diabetes are far more vulnerable to macrovascular complications because they usually have contributing risk factors from way back when, such as high cholesterol and high blood pressure, both of which are discussed in Chapter 2. Obesity, smoking and inactivity can then aggravate those problems, resulting in major cardiovascular disease and leaving the individual at risk for heart attack or stroke. What people don't understand is that when the terms "heart disease" or "cardiovascular disease" are used, they refer to your risk of not just heart attack but *stroke.*

UNDERSTANDING HEART DISEASE

What to Expect When You Have a Heart Attack

A heart attack is clinically known as a myocardial infarction (MI). The myocardium is the clinical name for "heart muscle." An MI occurs when there is not enough, or any, blood supply to the myocardium, something that happens when one of the coronary arteries is blocked. A coronary artery supplies blood to the heart muscle. Roughly 90 percent of heart attacks are due to a blood clot. A variety of symptoms can occur during a heart attack. Men experience different symptoms than women. If you're a woman reading this, please see the section "Women and Heart Disease." If you're male, the following can be signs of a heart attack. You may experience only one of the symptoms below, or a combination:

- Feeling a crushing or compression in the chest, combined with pain. You may feel as though a heavy weight has been dropped on your chest.
- Feeling squeezed or constricted, as though a vice was gripping your chest.
- Feeling as though you're being choked or strangled, along with a sickening feeling in the chest. It may resemble a panic or anxiety attack and not feel like a heart attack.
- Burning and indigestion. This could be, in fact, heartburn, a common problem with people with diabetes. Many people believe their heartburn is a heart attack; many people also believe their heart attack is "only heartburn." Always see a doctor. If sweating, weakness, shortness of breath and a feeling of "impending doom" accompany the indigestion, it's probably a heart attack.
- Tearing, gripping pain. You feel as though your chest is being ripped apart.
- Mild discomfort in the chest. Clearly, this is a mild heart attack, but it is still a sign of a heart attack.
- Tingling, numbness or heaviness over the arm. This symptom is very common in women (see further on).
- A sharp, stabbing pain in the chest.

- Severe dizziness or weakness. This symptom may be confused with low blood sugar, but can also be a sign of heart attack.
- Nausea with chest pain. Without vomiting or diarrhea, this symptom is frequently a sign of a heart attack.
- Aching pain under the arm or breastbone.

Additional symptoms

As you can see from this list, the pain and discomfort can vary from severe to mild discomfort. When the above heart attack symptoms are accompanied by any of the following, call an ambulance or get to an ER: profuse sweating, difficulty breathing, "a feeling of impending doom" (this is described by almost all heart attack survivors as feeling very anxious and fearful quite suddenly), severe and sudden weakness, dizziness or lightheadedness, nausea and vomiting, restlessness, shortness of breath, coughing, sudden drop in blood pressure (which may cause the weakness and dizziness), slower heart rate (check your pulse) and chest discomfort.

Diagnostic tests that can confirm a heart attack include a manual exam (doctor examining you with a stethoscope), an electrocardiogram, an exercise stress test, an echocardiogram, as well as a myriad of imaging tests that may use radioactive substances to take pictures of the heart.

Heart attacks in women

Heart disease is currently the number one cause of death in postmenopausal women; more women die of heart disease than of lung cancer or breast cancer. Half of all North Americans who die from heart attacks each year are women.

One of the reasons for such high death rates from heart attacks among women is medical ignorance: Most studies looking at heart disease excluded women (see Introduction), which led to a myth that more men than women die of heart disease. The truth is, more men die of heart attacks before age 50, while more women die of heart attacks after age 50, as a direct result of estrogen loss. Moreover, women who have had oopherectomies (removal of the ovaries) prior to natural menopause increase their risk of a heart attack by *eight times*. Since more women work outside the home than ever before, a number of experts also cite stress as a huge contributing factor to increased rates of heart disease in women.

Another problem is that women have different symptoms than men when it comes to heart disease, and so the "typical" warning signs we know about in men—angina, or chest pains—are often never present in women. In fact, chest pains in women are almost never related to heart disease. For women, the symptoms of heart disease, and even an actual heart attack, can be much more vague, seemingly unrelated to heart problems. Signs of heart disease in women include some surprising symptoms, some of which are the same as in men, but some that are completely different:

- Shortness of breath and/or fatigue
- Jaw pain (often masked by arthritis and joint pain)
- Pain in the back of the neck (often masked by arthritis or joint pain)
- Pain down the right or left arm
- Back pain (often masked by arthritis and joint pain)
- Sweating (also have your thyroid checked—this is a classic sign of an overactive thyroid gland; also test your blood sugar as you may be low)
- Fainting
- Palpitations (ladies, again, have your thyroid checked, also a classic symptom of an overactive thyroid)
- Bloating (after menopause, this is a sign of coronary artery blockage)
- Heartburn, belching or other gastrointestinal pain (this is often a sign of an actual heart attack in women)
- Chest "heaviness" between the breasts (this is how women experience "chest pain"; some describe it as a "sinking feeling" or burning sensation; also described as an "aching, throbbing, or a squeezing sensation"; "hot poker stab between the chest" or feeling like your heart jumps into your throat)
- Sudden swings in blood sugar
- Vomiting
- Confusion

Clearly, there are lots of other causes for the symptoms on this list, including low blood sugar. But it's important that your doctor includes heart disease as a possible cause, rather than dismissing it because your symptoms are not "male" (which your doctor may refer to as "typical"). Bear in mind that if you're suffering from nerve damage, you may not feel a lot of these symptoms. Therefore, you should take extra care to be suspicious of anything that feels out of the ordinary.

If you're diagnosed with heart disease, the "cure" is prevention through diet and exercise, and protection through hormone replacement therapy (see Chapter 12). If you are premenopausal and if you have diabetes that is not well controlled, the high blood sugar will cancel out the protective effects of estrogen against heart disease even if your ovaries are still making estrogen. Therefore, stay alert to the symptoms above. Keeping your blood sugar levels in the normal range will help to restore estrogen's protective properties.

Recovering from a heart attack

You can recover from a heart attack, but the damage resulting from the heart attack greatly depends on how long the blood supply to the heart muscle was cut off. The longer the blood supply was cut off, the more damage you will suffer. We all know that a heart attack is a major cause of death, but it can also leave you with varying degrees of disability depending upon the severity of the attack. For example, roughly half of all heart attack survivors will continue to have heart-related problems, which include reduced blood flow to the heart—called ischemia—and chest pains. As a result, the lifestyle you once enjoyed will need to change: Your diet will need to be restricted to a "heart smart" diet (see Chapter 7), and you will need to find ways to reduce lifestyle stress and incorporate more activity into your routine. If you don't make these changes, the risk of repeated heart attacks will loom, which can greatly affect your quality of life. You may also feel more fatigued and winded after normal activities when recovering from a heart attack. Successful recovery greatly depends on the severity of the attack and lifestyle changes you make after the episode. The same medical strategies designed to prevent a first heart attack can also be used to avoid recurrent episodes.

How Can I Prevent Cardiovascular Disease?

The way to prevent heart disease and peripheral vascular disease is by modifying your lifestyle (stop smoking; eat less fat; get more exercise). Smoking, high blood pressure, high blood sugar and high cholesterol (called the "catastrophic quartet" by one diabetes specialist) will greatly increase your risk of heart disease.

Heart surgery

You can also reduce your risk of a heart attack or stroke by undergoing heart surgery, which ranges from minor surgical procedures such as angioplasty to major heart bypass surgery.

Angioplasty, also known as coronary balloon surgery, was developed in Zurich in 1977. This operation involves inserting a catheter through your skin into the coronary artery. The catheter has a balloon on the end, which is inflated once inside. The inflated balloon squashes the plaque that is blocking the artery, easing blood flow. The balloon also widens the artery by essentially stretching it. Several inflations may be necessary to do the trick, but it is successful about 70 percent of the time. As your blood flow improves, so does your overall health. There is about a 5 percent risk of having a heart attack during the procedure, which you must weigh. Also, about 25 percent of the time, the artery is too narrow for the catheter to fit or too clogged for angioplasty to work.

Laser angioplasty is the same procedure as above, except a laser is passed through the catheter and dissolves the plaque. This is a good way to handle very narrowed arteries or arteries that are too hardened with plaque for balloon angioplasty to work.

The first successful coronary artery bypass surgery was performed by a heart surgeon in 1967 in Cleveland. Since then, it has become a fairly standard surgery. Here, a vein from your leg is removed and connected to the aorta as it leaves the heart; the other end is connected to the coronary artery, just before the blockage. The vein acts as a bridge between the two, enabling the blood to flow, thus fixing the blood flow problem. The risk of a heart attack during this procedure is about 10 percent higher than with angioplasty, but after five years, 70 percent of bypass patients are still enjoying an active life and are free from any symptoms of heart disease. Not everyone is a good candidate for this surgery, however. If you're considering this option, you'll need to discuss the risks of undergoing the surgery in light of your overall health.

Lower blood pressure

High blood pressure is discussed on page 19 in Chapter 2, along with blood pressure-lowering drugs (also called antihypertensive medications).

Lower cholesterol

High cholesterol is discussed on page 16 in Chapter 2, along with cholesterol-lowering drugs.

Drugs that prevent platelet clumping

Sometimes confused with anticoagulants (blood thinners), drugs that prevent platelet clumping work by preventing the platelets from clumping due to "stickiness." The best-known drug in this category is aspirin. If you're male, there's clear evidence that taking a daily aspirin can help prevent a heart attack; if you're a woman, the effects of daily aspirin are less clear, so discuss this treatment with your doctor. Other drugs reduce platelet clumping, too, but aspirin is available over the counter. *Note: Anticoagulants, also called "blood thinners," are not as useful for preventing heart attacks as they are for preventing strokes. Anticoagulants dissolve clots.*

Quit smoking

This is discussed on page 22 in Chapter 2.

Reducing stress

There's no question about it: Stress can lead to heart disease. Generally, stress is defined as a negative emotional experience associated with biological changes that allow you to adapt to it. In response to stress, your adrenal glands pump out stress hormones that speed up your body: Your heart rate increases and your blood sugar levels increase so that glucose can be diverted to your muscles in case you have to run from a threatening situation. This is known as the "fight or flight" response. These hormones are technically called the catecholamines, which are broken down into epinephrine (adrenaline) and norepinephrine.

The problem with stress hormones in the 21st century is that the fight or flight response isn't usually necessary, since most of our stress stems from interpersonal situations rather than dangerous situations such as being chased by a predator. Occasionally, we may want to flee from a bank robber or mugger, but most of us just want to flee from our jobs or our kids! In other words, our stress hormones actually put a physical strain on our bodies and can lower our resistance to disease. Initially, stress hormones stimulate our immune systems. But after the stressful event has passed, it can suppress the immune system, leaving us vulnerable to a wide variety of illnesses and physical symptoms.

Hans Selye, considered the "father" of stress management, defined stress as the "wear and tear" on the body. Once we are in a state of stress, the body adapts to the stress by depleting its resources until it becomes exhausted. The wear and tear on our bodies is mounting; we can suffer from a host of stress-related ailments that include high blood pressure, high cholesterol and heart disease. Current statistics reveal that 43 percent of all adults suffer from health problems directly caused by stress, while 75 to 90 percent of all visits to primary care physicians are for stress-related complaints or disorders.

Managing your stress is no easy feat, particularly since there are different types of stress: acute stress (which can be episodic) and chronic stress. Acute stress results from an acute situation, such as a sudden, unexpected negative event, or from, for example, organizing a wedding or planning for a conference. When the event passes, the stress will pass. Acute stress is when you're feeling the pressure of a particular deadline or event, but there is an end to the stress. There are numerous symptoms of acute stress: anger or irritability, anxiety, and depression, tension headaches or migraines, back pain, jaw pain, muscular tension, digestive problems, cardiovascular problems and dizziness.

But acute stress can be what's known as "episodic," meaning that there is one stressful event after another, creating a continuous flow of acute stress. Someone who is always taking on too many projects at once is someone who suffers from *episodic* acute stress rather than simply acute stress. Workaholics and those with the so-called "Type A" personality are classic sufferers of episodic acute stress.

I sometimes refer to acute stress as the "good stress" because often good things come from this kind of stress, even though it feels "stressful" or bad in the short term. This is the kind of stress that challenges us to stretch ourselves beyond our capabilities, which is what makes us meet deadlines and invent creative solutions to our problems. Examples of "good" stress include taking on challenging projects; undergoing positive life-changing events (moving, changing jobs or ending unhealthy relationships); or confronting fears, illness or people who make us feel bad (this is one of those bad-in-the-short-term/good-in-the-long-term situations). Essentially, whenever a stressful event triggers emotional, intellectual or spiritual growth, it is a "good stress." It is often not the event as much as it is your *response* to the event that determines whether it is a "good" or "bad" stress. The death of a loved one can sometimes lead to personal growth because we may see something about ourselves we did not see before—new resilience, for example. So even a death can be a "good stress" though we grieve and are sad in the short term.

What I call the "bad stress" is known as chronic stress. Chronic or bad stress results from boredom and stagnation, as well as from prolonged negative circumstances. Essentially, when no growth occurs from the stressful event, it is "bad stress." When negative events don't seem to yield anything positive in the long term, but more of the same, the stress can lead to chronic and debilitating health problems. This is not to say that we can't get sick from good stress either, but when there is nothing positive from the stress, it has a much more negative effect on our health. Some examples of bad stress include stagnant jobs or relationships, disability from terrible accidents or diseases, long-term unemployment, chronic poverty, racism or lack of opportunities for change. These kinds of situations can lead to depression, low self-esteem and a host of physical illnesses.

In addition to acute and chronic stress, stress can be defined in even more precise ways:

- Physical stress (physical exertion)
- Chemical stress (when we're exposed to a toxin in our environment, including substance abuse)
- Mental stress (when we take on too much responsibility and begin worrying about all that has to be done)
- Emotional stress (when our feelings stress us out, such as anger, fear, frustration, sadness, betrayal or bereavement)
- Nutritional stress (when we're deficient in certain vitamins or nutrients, overindulged in fat or protein or experience food allergies)
- Traumatic stress (caused by trauma to the body such as infection, injury, burns, surgery or extreme temperatures)
- Psychospiritual stress (caused by unrest in our personal relationships or belief system, personal life goals and so on; in general, this is what defines whether we are happy)

The bottom line is this: *Stress makes us sick.* Stress management is a complex topic that I can't possibly cover here, but the principles of stress management involve reorganizing your priorities so you can reduce chronic stress as well as incorporate some "healing" strategies to help combat acute stress. Finding ways to downshift (work less, take more time off, reduce "e-stress," incorporate hands-on healing [get a massage!], eat better, exercise [see Chapter 8] and generally care for yourself through simple things such as getting enough sleep, for example) can dramatically reduce your current stress and improve your overall cardiovascular health.

Redford B. Williams, Jr., M.D., author of *The Trusting Heart,* documents that people with a Type A personality suffer from more heart disease than people who are calmer and more relaxed about life. The term "Type A personality" was coined in the early 1970s by researchers Meyer Friedman and Ray Rosenman.

Type A people tend to be driven, overachieving, very competitive, easily upset and/or angered by everyday occurrences and, ultimately, have a hostile personality.

According to Williams's research, hostility is bad for your heart. This sentiment is echoed by renowned health expert Deepak Chopra, who, in numerous public appearances, has stated the shocking statistic that more heart attacks are recorded Monday mornings (the most stressful morning of the week) than on any other day of the week.

Physiologically, anger and hostility will raise your blood pressure (hence the term "red-faced with anger"). Many cardiologists are starting to list hostility as a risk factor for heart disease, along with smoking, obesity, high blood pressure, high cholesterol and a sedentary lifestyle.

Consider the following tips for becoming less hostile:

- Get into the habit of stopping yourself when you have a hostile thought. In other words, next time you're stuck in traffic, instead of cursing, honking and trying to furiously lane-change, just *stop* getting upset and remind yourself that there's nothing you can do about the situation. Turn on the radio for some soothing music and "chill."
- Imagine the life of the person in front of you. If someone cuts in front of you in a line-up or in traffic, instead of raising your middle finger and yelling, ask yourself what's going on in that other person's life that caused him or her to cut you off. In other words, try to see that it's not personal.
- See the humour. Some situations are so ridiculous that laughing will get you further than ranting and raving. This includes things like terrible service, missing flight connections and so on.
- Look upon your hostility as a character flaw you can work on. Some people are too shy; some people are too passive; you get angry too quickly. Recognizing it and accepting it is a big step.

UNDERSTANDING STROKE

As mentioned earlier, cardiovascular disease puts you at risk for not just a heart attack, but a "brain attack" or stroke, which occurs when a blood clot (a clog in your blood vessels) travels to your brain and stops the flow of blood and oxygen carried to the nerve cells in that area. When that happens, cells may die or vital functions controlled by the brain can be temporarily or permanently damaged.

Bleeding or a rupture from the affected blood vessel can lead to a very serious situation, including death. People with Type 2 diabetes are two to three times more likely to suffer from a stroke than people without diabetes. About 80 percent of strokes are caused by the blockage of an artery in the neck or brain, known as an "ischemic stroke"; the remainder are caused by a burst blood vessel in the brain that causes bleeding into or around the brain.

Since the 1960s, the death rate from strokes has dropped by 50 percent. This drop is largely due to public-awareness campaigns regarding diet and lifestyle modification (quitting smoking, eating low-fat foods and exercising), as well as the introduction of blood pressure-lowering drugs and cholesterol-lowering drugs that have helped people maintain normal blood pressure and cholesterol levels (see pages 17 and 21).

Strokes can be mild, moderate, severe or fatal. Mild strokes may affect speech or movement for a short period of time only; many people recover from mild strokes without any permanent damage. Moderate or severe strokes may result in loss of speech, memory and paralysis; many people learn to speak again and learn to function with partial paralysis. How well you recover depends on how much damage was done.

A considerable amount of research points to stress as a risk factor for stroke. The section "How Can I Prevent Cardiovascular Disease?" on page 233 suggests ways to cut down on stress.

Signs of a Stroke

If you can recognize the key warning signs of a stroke, it can make a difference in preventing a major stroke or reducing the severity of a stroke.

Call 9-1-1 or get to Emergency if you *suddenly* notice one or more of the following symptoms:

- Weakness, numbness and/or tingling in your face, arms or legs, especially on one side of the body; this may last only a few moments
- Loss of speech or difficulty understanding somebody else's speech; this may last only a short time
- Confusion
- Severe headaches that feel different from any headache you've had before
- Feeling unsteady, falling a lot
- Trouble seeing in one or both eyes

If you have any of the signs of stroke above, it's important to get to the hospital as soon as possible. There are treatments that can reduce the severity of the damage caused by the stroke, making the difference between partial or severe disability and full recovery. For example, there are drugs that can dissolve clots, known as tissue-type plasminogen activators (TPA), such as reteplase or strep-tokinase, which are proteins, derived from bacteria. Plasminogen activators made from recombinant DNA technology are alteplase and anistreplase. Anticoagulants, such as coumadin, are drugs that can dissolve clots as well.

Common Disabilities Caused by Stroke

There's no question that stroke is responsible for a range of functional and physical disabilities, especially in people over 45. Depending on the severity of the stroke, your general health and the rehabilitation process involved, the following impairments may dramatically improve over time:

- Weakness or paralysis on one side of the body. This may affect the whole side or just the arm or leg. The weakness or paralysis is always on the opposite side of the body from where the stroke occurred. So if the stroke affected the right side of the brain, you will experience the weakness or paralysis on the left side of your body. Paralysis may affect the face, an arm, a leg or the entire side of the body. Walking, grasping objects and the ability to swallow can be consequences of one-sided paralysis.
- Muscle spasms or stiffness
- Problems with balance and/or coordination
- Problems understanding, speaking and writing in your first language (called aphasia). This is a common problem, affecting about 25 percent of stroke survivors. At least one-fourth of all stroke survivors experience language impairments. It can take two forms: problems comprehending others, or problems articulating their own words. Stroke survivors may be able to think clearly, but are unable to make the words "come out right," resulting in disconnected gibberish when they try to speak. The most severe form of aphasia is called global aphasia, which results in the loss of all language abilities: They are not able to understand or communicate in any language. There is also a form of very mild aphasia, called anomic aphasia, where language is mostly unaffected, except for a few words that may be forgotten selectively, such as names of people or particular kinds of objects.

- Inability to respond to bodily sensations on one side of the body (a.k.a. bodily neglect). This means that the ability to feel, touch, sense pain or temperature can be lost. There may be no recognition of the person's own limb—an arm or leg may not be "noticeable" any more.
- Pain, numbness or odd sensations (called paresthesia). Pain can be the result of damage to the nervous system (neuropathic pain). Stroke survivors who have a paralyzed arm, for example, may feel as though the pain is radiating outward from the shoulder (the lack of movement causes the joint to be fixed or "frozen"). Physical therapy can help to alleviate this. Pain can also result from a confused signal from the damaged brain, sending out pain to the side of the body that is not affected.
- Difficulty remembering, thinking, focusing or learning. Extremely short attention spans, combined with short-term memory loss, can make it difficult for stroke survivors to learn new tasks, make plans or engage in a complex discussion. Often the ability to connect a thought to an action is lost.
- Unawareness of the stroke's effects. A stroke survivor may be paralyzed on one side, but not acknowledge the paralysis and have no awareness of the impairment, or the fact that a stroke has taken place.
- Difficulty swallowing (called dysphagia)
- Urinary or bowel incontinence (bladder or bowel control). The ability to sense bladder or bowel urge may be lost, or simply the mobility required to go to the bathroom may be the obstacle. Incontinence becomes less severe with time. Physical therapists can help stroke survivors strengthen their pelvic muscles through special exercises. And by following a timed voiding schedule, incontinence may be solved. In other cases, people can learn to use catheters to prevent other incontinence-related health problems from developing.
- Fatigue
- Mood swings. Natural feelings of anger, anxiety and frustration can cause extreme mood swings or even personality changes in stroke survivors. Anger is frequently taken out on loved ones, family or friends.
- Depression. A mild depression can become a major depression when the stroke survivor loses all engagement and interest in life, doesn't maintain a healthy weight, doesn't sleep properly and/or exhibits other physical symptoms. Sometimes intervention with antidepressants is necessary if counselling is not effective due to language difficulties.

Recovering from Stroke

According to the National Stroke Association in the United States, 40 percent of all stroke survivors experience moderate to severe impairments that require special care, while 10 percent will need to be placed in a facility or nursing home; 25 percent of stroke survivors have only minor disabilities that enable them to care for themselves, while 10 percent will survive the stroke and completely recover with no long-term side effects. The remaining 15 percent of stroke sufferers die shortly after the stroke. But 14 percent of all stroke survivors, regardless of their level of recovery, will have another stroke.

Stroke survivors may recover in long-term care facilities within hospitals or a separate rehabilitation hospital. Many receive home care through outpatient programs or various institutions. The crucial part of stroke rehabilitation is timing: It should begin as soon as a stroke survivor is stable, which is often within 24 to 48 hours after a stroke. Early stroke rehabilitation doesn't imply a rigorous physical therapy program at all. Because paralysis or weakness on one side is so often the result of the stroke, it's important to get stroke survivors moving again by helping them change positions frequently while lying in bed, or having a physical therapist move stroke-impaired limbs (called "passive" range-of-motion exercises). Helping survivors progress to sitting up in bed or transferring them to a chair from a bed are all part of rehabilitation. Eventually, many may be able to stand, bearing their own weight, or walk with or without assistance. Early rehabilitation also includes helping stroke survivors with bathing, dressing and using a toilet.

The recovery team

There are many health care providers who may become involved in stroke recovery. The recovery team can include your primary care physician, health care specialists in physical medicine and rehabilitation, neurologists, internists, geriatricians (specialists in eldercare) and rehabilitation nurses, who specialize in nursing care for people with disabilities.

One of the most important steps in stroke recovery is receiving good physical therapy. Physical therapists help survivors learn to reuse their impaired limbs by teaching them how to compensate for their disabilities with other ways to move, or by preventing the impaired parts of the body to waste away further through non-use. An occupational therapist helps stroke survivors find new ways to complete self-directed tasks, such as cleaning, cooking, gardening, dressing and so on.

Another important recovery team member is the speech-language pathologist, who helps stroke survivors relearn language or develop new ways to communicate. They coach conversations by helping survivors develop prompts or cues to remember words; they may use sign language, symbol boards or computers as language aids. (Voice-synthesized products may be especially useful for people recovering from strokes.) Difficulties with swallowing can be improved through helping with swallowing reflexes, helping the stroke survivor to manipulate food with the tongue, or finding better eating positions, or encouraging different eating habits such as taking small bites and chewing slowly.

To help stroke survivors adjust to the emotional problems that may follow a stroke (such as despair or depression), social workers, psychologists or psychiatrists may also become involved with recovery.

Quality of Life Decisions After Stroke

For many stroke survivors, quality of life decisions are a factor in long-term care. Twenty-five years ago, stroke survivors who suffered from extreme impairments leaving them with no quality of life (meaning one cannot speak, eat, understand or move) were often kept alive through medical interventions, such as tube-feeding, force-feeding, IV or life-saving measures when pneumonia or heart failure occurred. This is now seen as futile and an act of prolonging death rather than preserving life.

Today, when there is no quality of life, families have the option of withdrawing medical treatment. If you are at high risk for stroke, you may wish to draft an advanced directive that tells your family members your wishes should you become incapacitated by stroke and left with no quality of life. In the case of stroke, withdrawal of medical treatment means that feeding is stopped (meaning that there is no tube feeding, no IV or forced feeding), and no life-saving interventions are introduced when breathing becomes laboured or the heart stops. Withdrawal of medical treatment is *not* the same thing as euthanasia or assisted suicide; in these cases, medical intervention is used to actually stop a life.

Preventing Another Stroke

Preventing another stroke involves the same strategies as preventing a heart attack recurrence (see page 233). Obesity, inactivity and especially *smoking* spell "ANOTHER STROKE" unless you make some lifestyle changes.

You're also at greater risk for another stroke if you have

- high blood pressure (hypertension),
- restricted blood flow (called ischemia),
- heart disease,
- celebrated your 65th birthday, or
- high cholesterol.

Cardiovascular disease (which leads to heart attack and/or stroke) is certainly the most common disease caused by macrovascular or large blood vessel complications. But most of the other notorious diabetes complications (eye disease, kidney problems, impotence, foot problems, etc.) result when restricted blood flow from macrovascular complications results in nerve damage, known as diabetic neuropathy, discussed in the next chapter.

MAKING SENSE OUT OF CARDIOVASCULAR DRUGS

Drug Category	Also Called	Used for	Common Types
antihypertensives	blood pressure-lowering drugs	lowering blood pressure	Diuretics *beta-blockers alpha-blockers centrally acting agent *calcium channel blockers ace inhibitors *vasodilators
antihyperlipidemic agents	cholesterol-lowering drugs	lowering cholesterol/ triglycerides	niacin statins fibrates resins
anticoagulants	blood thinners	preventing stroke; dissolving clots	warfarin
thrombolytic agents	clot busters	dissolving clots	plasminogen activators
platelet aggregation inhibitors	none	preventing heart attacks	ASA (aspirin)

*NOTE: These drugs are also used to relieve angina and palpitations.

Source: Compiled from the Compendium of Pharmaceuticals and Specialties, 2001.

Chapter 16

WHEN DIABETES GETS ON YOUR NERVES

● ● ● ● ● ● ● ● ● ● ●

A second type of diabetes complication is known as a *microvascular complication.* *Micro* means tiny, as in microscopic. Microvascular complications refer to problems with the smaller blood vessels (a.k.a. capillaries) that connect to various body parts. A plain-language interpretation of microvascular complications would be "Houston, we've got a problem." In other words, the problem *is* serious, but it's not going to affect the whole planet, just the spacecraft in orbit. Nerve damage (neuropathy) is a microvascular complication that targets body parts such as feet, eyes, genitals and skin. But unlike macrovascular complications (large blood vessel complications), you're not going to have a sudden life-threatening event such as heart attack or stroke from microvascular problems. For example, eye disease (see Chapter 17), clinically known as retinopathy, is a microvascular complication. Blindness is a serious problem, but you won't die from it.

People with Type 1 diabetes (see Chapter 1) are more vulnerable to microvascular complications, but a good portion of people with Type 2 diabetes suffer from them, too. Microvascular complications are known as the sugar-related complications. The small blood vessel damage is caused by high blood sugar levels over long periods of time. The Diabetes Control and Complications Trial, referred to throughout this book and discussed in detail in Chapter 13, showed that by keeping blood sugar levels as normal as possible, *as often as possible,* through frequent self-testing, microvascular complications can be prevented.

UNDERSTANDING DIABETIC NEUROPATHY

When your blood sugar levels are too high for too long, you can develop a condition known as diabetic neuropathy or nerve disease. Somehow, the cells that make up your nerves are altered in response to high blood sugar. Different groups of nerves are affected by high blood sugar; keeping your blood sugar levels as normal as possible is the best way to prevent many of the following problems. Drugs that help to prevent chemical changes in your nerve cells can also be used to treat nerve damage.

Types of Neuropathy

Polyneuropathy is a disease that affects the nerves in your feet and legs. The symptoms are burning, tingling and numbness in the legs and feet. This is what can lead to amputations in extreme cases. Chapter 20 is devoted solely to foot problems and amputations.

Autonomic neuropathy is a disease that affects the nerves you don't notice: the nerves that control your digestive tract (see gastrointestinal tract section below), bladder, bowel, blood pressure, sweat glands, overall balance and sexual functioning (see genitals section on page 253). Treatment varies depending on what's affected, but drugs can control individual parts of the body, such as the digestive tract.

Proximal motor neuropathy is a disease that affects the nerves that control your muscles. It can lead to weakness, burning sensations in the joints (hands, thighs and ankles are the most common). These problems can be individually treated with physiotherapy and/or specific medication. When the nerves that control the muscles in the eyes (see Chapter 17) are affected, you may experience problems with your vision, such as double vision. Finally, nerve damage can affect the spine, causing pain and loss of sensation to the back, buttocks and legs.

NERVE DAMAGE HEAD TO TOE

Below is an overview of the body parts most commonly affected by diabetic neuropathy, listed in order from head to toe. Keep in mind that this list is not exhaustive as there are hundreds of nerve-related problems that can occur. These are the "majors" that affect people with Type 2 diabetes.

Eyes

For details on all eye and vision problems caused by diabetes, see Chapter 17.

Gastrointestinal Tract (G.I. Tract)

When high blood sugar levels affect your nerve cells, the nerves that control your entire gastrointestinal tract may be affected as well. In fact, 30 to 50 percent of people with diabetes suffer from dysmotility, a condition in which the muscles in the digestive tract become uncoordinated, causing bloating, abdominal pain and reflux (heartburn).

What is your G.I. tract?

Imagine that your digestive tract is one long subway tunnel with different stops. If you were to look at the G.I. "subway map," the first stop is your mouth. The next stop is your pharynx, and the third stop is your esophagus. The esophagus is a major "connecting stop." This is where the train stops for a while before switching tracks and moving on to the more active parts of your gut: the stomach, which connects to your duodenum, which connects to your small intestine, which connects to the last stop on the line, your large intestine.

Swallowing your food triggers all the muscles in your digestive tract to begin contracting in wavelike motions known as peristalsis. The act of swallowing is voluntary, but once the food is down the throat, the rest of the movement through the digestive tract is involuntary, or beyond our control. Our nervous system takes over. The food goes down the throat into the pharynx and into the esophagus. The esophagus connects your throat to your stomach.

In order for your food to get from the esophagus to the stomach, it must go through a crucial tunnel known as the lower esophageal sphincter (LES). When you swallow your food, the LES relaxes to allow your food to pass from the esophagus into the stomach. This is necessary in order to prevent your digested food from backing up into the esophagus.

The stomach is an accordionlike bag of muscle and other tissue near the centre of the abdomen just below the rib cage. The bag expands to accommodate food and shrinks when it is empty. The stomach itself is a holding tank for your food until it can pass through the gastrointestinal tract.

In the same way that the larger coffee grinds stay in the filter, the larger solid particles of food go from the stomach into the duodenum for further digestion, while the mushy, nicely "worked over" food remnants from the stomach will quickly pass from the duodenum into the small intestine (a.k.a. midgut or small bowel). The small intestine is usually called just that, but technically, it can be categorized as the duodenum, jejunum and ileum. For simplicity, most refer to it as "the small intestine."

A series of various tubes along your G.I. tract empty food particles from one into the next. This process depends on continuous movement, known as *motility*, which is controlled by nerves, hormones and muscles. In fact, if you're experiencing problems with other parts of your body, the motility can be slowed down (you'll be constipated and bloated) or speeded up (you'll have diarrhea).

By the time your food gets into the small intestine, your food is now mushed up by the digestive secretions of your stomach, pancreas and biliary tract. All this mush stays in the small intestine for a relatively long period of time, and all the usable nutrients are absorbed through the intestinal walls. These nutrients include digested molecules of food, water and minerals from the diet. The waste products are sent to the large intestine (a.k.a. colon or large bowel), where they sit around for about a day or two before they are expelled in the form of stools.

Diabetic nerve disease affects the G.I. tract north of the colon—that is, everything between the esophagus and small intestine. A number of things can go wrong north of the colon because hundreds of nerves and secretions (hormones, enzymes and chemicals that help to break down your food into usable nutrients) go to work for us whenever we eat. If even one hormone or enzyme is "off" in your system, there will be consequences. There are upper G.I. disorders and lower G.I. disorders. The upper G.I. disorders, which can be caused by diabetic nerve disease, can include heartburn/reflux, a symptom of a larger problem of dysmotility (see below), also known as gastroesophageal reflux disease (GERD). Diabetic nerve disease can also cause problems south of the colon, where muscles controlling the bowel become uncoordinated, causing them to open, leak stool and allow bacteria to grow abnormally in the colon, resulting in bacterial-related diarrhea. This can be controlled with antibiotics.

Understanding dysmotility

Dysmotility means "things not moving very well." Food travels from your esophagus into your stomach, which slowly releases it into the small intestine. There can be problems on any or all "floors" of this elevator. Things can get stuck between the esophagus and stomach, causing symptoms of heartburn and reflux (see further on). In this case, the lower esophageal sphincter relaxes when it should be taut, allowing food to come back up. Or things can get stuck between the stomach and small intestine, which causes symptoms of bloating, early fullness and gas. So when things aren't moving very well, you can have a lot of discomfort. This is known as a motility disorder.

Dysmotility, with all of its varying symptoms, is typically a very chronic condition. Symptoms keep coming back, and by the time dysmotility is finally diagnosed, most people have had these symptoms for a long time. The only way you can stop symptoms from recurring is by changing certain lifestyle habits (losing weight, quitting smoking and staying in control of blood sugar levels may improve your condition) or taking a motility drug as a "maintenance" drug. If your dysmotility goes on for a long time, it could also lead to inflammation of the esophageal lining, a condition known as esophagitis. This can lead to the narrowing of the esophagus. (When your esophagus is inflamed, it narrows, just the way your shoes are suddenly too tight when your feet expand.)

Understanding heartburn/reflux

As described above, your food must pass from your esophagus into your stomach through the lower esophageal sphincter, which opens and closes through a variety of involuntary muscular contractions. If you have diabetic nerve disease, the sphincter may not shut completely after dumping your ingested food particles into the stomach. So what happens? The food, now bathed in your stomach acid, can actually come back up the sphincter, causing a burning sensation in your chest, and even a spreading pain throughout your neck and arms, which may even be mistaken for a heart attack. You can also experience nausea, belching and regurgitation of that half-digested food. When it comes back up the sphincter, it doesn't taste as good as it did going down. Thanks to the acid and enzymes it's been exposed to, the food will taste sour and bitter in your throat. The problem will be aggravated when you bend forward or lie down. In fact, you may even find that after an experience like this, you wake up with a sore throat. This problem is clinically called *acid reflux*, and in lay terms it is known as heartburn or acid indigestion. For the remainder of this book, the term "heartburn/reflux" will be used.

Heartburn/reflux usually lasts about two hours. Most people find that standing up relieves the burning; that's because gravity helps. You could also take an antacid to clear acid out of the esophagus. Not everyone will experience the same degree of heartburn. Heartburn/reflux can be mild, moderate or severe. It all depends on why it's occurring, how often it occurs, when it occurs and how much food backup you have. But for the most part, chronic heartburn/reflux is the first sign of a more serious, underlying health problem such as dysmotility or GERD.

A number of atypical, unusual or "odd" symptoms can suggest you have heartburn/reflux, too. They include

- morning hoarseness,
- drooling,
- coughing spells,
- waking up with a sore throat, or
- asthmalike symptoms (or the worsening of asthma symptoms if you are asthmatic). In these cases, you may be having heartburn/reflux at night, which is obstructing your breathing passages, causing all the strange symptoms from coughing to asthma.

Managing diabetes-related dysmotility

If you suffer dysmotility, there are a number of drugs that can help. A common drug is known as a prokinetic drug, which will improve motility and get things moving again. These agents tell your brain to send the right messages to the muscles that control the G.I. tract. Those muscles include the lower esophageal sphincter, which will stop relaxing when it should be contracting. In essence, a prokinetic drug helps your food get from the esophagus into the stomach, and then from the stomach into the small intestine. It does this by improving LES pressure and peristalsis, which gets rid of the acid in the esophagus and improves gastric emptying. Once that happens, you'll notice that all those symptoms, caused by food sitting around in your stomach too long, will disappear. Other drugs, known as H2 receptor antagonists or proton pump inhibitors, can help suppress or control stomach acid.

Skin

High blood sugar levels, combined with poor circulation, puts the skin—on your whole body—at risk for infections ranging from yeast to open wound-related infections. You may form scar tissue or develop strange yellow pimples (a sign of high fat levels in the blood), boils or a range of localized infections. Yeast infections, which typically plague women who experience them in the form of vaginal yeast infections (see "Genitals"), can develop not just in the vagina, but in the mouth (called thrush), under the arms or wherever there are warm, fatty folds. And all skin, whether on the feet or elsewhere, can become dry and cracked, requiring a daily regimen of cleaning, moisturizing and protecting.

Kidneys

Diabetic kidney disease is very serious and requires a separate chapter. For details, please see Chapter 19.

Gallbladder

The gallbladder stores bile for the liver. But you don't really need the gallbladder since the liver is large enough to store as much bile as you'd ever want or need anyway. Nevertheless, we do come equipped with this extra storage space. Bile isn't a very reliable product to store because it can form into little stones inside the gallbladder, known as gallstones (or calculi). When your gallbladder isn't emptying properly, a process controlled by nerves and one that can be impaired with diabetic nerve disease, you can form gallstones. Symptoms occur when the stones become large enough to obstruct the bile ducts. And when this happens, you are said to have *gallbladder disease.*

The symptoms of a gallbladder attack are quite severe; you'll feel sudden, intense pain in the upper abdominal region (which may shoot into your back), often after a fatty meal, but it may not be related to meals. Vomiting frequently brings relief, although nausea is not a symptom. The pain may then subside over several minutes or hours. Many people mistake gallstone symptoms for heartburn or a heart attack.

The obstruction can become infected or even gangrenous, which is a dire emergency (you don't want gangrene inside your abdominal cavity!). Usually gallbladder disease presents itself as a series of gallbladder "attacks" in which you'll feel the pain after a meal and, if there's infection, may even experience a fever. The attacks will become progressively worse until you decide to have the darned thing removed! As a rule, any abdominal pain accompanied by a fever means there is some sort of serious infection going on in there, which is an emergency, warranting emergency medical attention.

Because of other factors, such as taking estrogen (many women take some form of estrogen product), gallbladder problems are much more common in women than men (one in five women after age 50 versus one in 20 men), and are also common in women who are on hormone replacement therapy after menopause. Estrogen-containing oral contraceptives are also associated with gallstones.

Since the late 1980s, gastroenterologists have been able to widen the ducts with endoscopy to allow the gallstones to pass, avoiding major surgery in people who are not up to it or who do not want it. Removal of the gallbladder is called a *cholecystectomy*, one of the most common surgical procedures performed. Over half a million North Americans have their gallbladders removed annually for a variety of reasons, not all of which are related to diabetes.

Bladder

Nerves that control the bladder can be affected, which causes you to lose your sense of bladder urge and your ability to force a bladder contraction (that is, to urinate). Ultimately this can lead to incontinence as urine will start to leak out. Women, in particular, can also suffer from repeated urinary tract infections caused by insufficient emptying of the bladder, resulting in bacteria overgrowth. Learning to go to the bathroom on a schedule (every four hours or so), instead of waiting for the urge, is one solution. Drugs can also increase the force of bladder contraction if your problem involves the inability to force bladder contraction.

Genitals

Fifty percent of men with diabetes and 30 percent of women with diabetes suffer from sexual dysfunction.

Men

Microvascular complications can lead to impotence, or erectile dysfunction (ED, the new, politically correct term for impotence), because the small blood vessels responsible for causing an erection can be damaged, or the nerves controlling sexual response could be damaged. As well, macrovascular disease can affect the flow of blood to the penis.

In the first case, when nerves to the penis are damaged, blood flow is limited, preventing erection. Roughly 60 percent of all men with diabetes (Type 1 or 2) over age 50 suffer from erectile dysfunction (ED), which means that about 33 percent of all ED is caused by diabetes.

To be considered impotent, you have to be unable to achieve or sustain an erection long enough to have intercourse—for a period of at least six months. In other words, we're not talking about one of those movie scenes where a frustrated couple lies in bed and the woman turns to the man and says, "It happens," and the man replies, "Not to me." Premature ejaculation is also not considered to be ED, although it can happen when you have ED. When a physical problem is at work, signs come on gradually. Over time, you'll notice that your penis becomes less rigid, until you are unable to obtain or sustain an erection completely.

Just because you have diabetes doesn't mean your impotence is caused by it. Therefore, to diagnose physical impotence, doctors will tell you to place a paper band around your penis before you go to sleep. Since all healthy men have erections during their sleep, if you wake up with a broken band, it means your impotence is not physical but psychological. If the band is intact upon waking, your problem is physical (although not necessarily related to diabetes—it could be hormonal).

Once it's established that you have a physical disorder, your doctor can rule out nerve damage rather than blood vessel damage by checking out both. To check nerve damage, a test involving painless electrical current can measure your penis's response.

To check blood vessel damage, a device similar to testing blood pressure in your arm can be used on your penis, or a drug that bypasses your nerves can be injected into your penis to see if you can have an erection. If you can't, blood vessel damage is indeed the problem, and it's most likely a macrovascular one. Ultrasound and a tracer dye can confirm impotence caused by macrovascular disease. This procedure allows the doctor to actually see whether the blood is flowing freely through the vessels into the penis.

Another physical cause of impotence is blood pressure-lowering medication, while smoking and alcohol are considered aggravating factors.

One of the most popular treatments for ED is Viagra (sildenafil citrate). It is a pill that you take about an hour prior to potential sexual contact. You will get an erection only if you are aroused. Viagra should begin to take effect in about 30 minutes and lasts up to four hours. Viagra works by increasing blood flow to the penis, and it works in about four out of five men who take it, regardless of how long they have had ED, what caused it or how old they are. But men over 65 and men who have cardiovascular problems, kidney problems or liver problems should consult their physicians about the safety of Viagra. If you are on medications for the treatment of HIV, you should also consult your physician about the safety of Viagra. In some cases, depending on the severity of your other health problems, your doctor may okay it, but the makers of Viagra caution against it. Furthermore, if you take any drugs containing nitroglycerine or nitrates, you must not take this drug as it can lead to a heart attack or stroke (see Chapter 15). Nitrates are found in many prescription medications that are used to treat angina (chest pain due to heart disease). If you cannot take Viagra or if it doesn't work, there are older remedies such as the following:

- **Drug injections:** Various drugs can be injected into the penis prior to intercourse; they will increase blood flow and produce an erection for at least

30 minutes. Prolonged erection is a side effect, however. (In Europe, certain "patch" medications, intended for heart disease, are being used by *healthy* men to prolong their normal erections!)

- **Vacuum devices:** A vacuum device is used to enlarge the penis, then a tension band is placed around the penis to maintain the erection for intercourse. Bruising can occur if the rubber band is on longer than 20 minutes.
- **Penile implants:** Either an inflatable or semirigid rod is placed inside the penis to enable you to have an erection whenever you want.
- **Blood vessel surgery:** Blood vessels that are blocking blood flow to the penis can be corrected through surgery.
- **Yohimbine:** This is a sexual stimulant that increases nerve sensitivity in the penis; if nerve damage has occurred, you may want to ask your urologist about the benefits of this drug.

Women

Nerve damage can also affect arousal for women. Special nerve fibres and blood vessels connect to the clitoris, vaginal wall and vulva, which are necessary for achieving orgasm and lubrication. If you have sustained nerve damage, you may notice a loss of sensation in your genital area, which can be a frustrating experience. Estrogen therapy and lubricants may help, as well as trying different positions to increase arousal.

Vaginal dryness has a domino effect: The dryness itself can increase your vulnerability to yeast infections. Dry vaginas can be torn during intercourse, and the resultant wounds can become vulnerable to yeast infection. High blood sugar levels also increase the amount of sugar in the vaginal walls, which can also cause yeast infections.

Sexual dysfunction in women is also related to nerve damage to the bladder (see above). When the bladder is not emptied sufficiently, it leads to bacterial bladder infections, which makes sex uncomfortable. Since Type 2 diabetes often coincides with menopause, many women will notice a compromised libido anyway due to natural estrogen loss, which can be aggravated by nerve damage. Or vice versa. Antibiotics prescribed to women for the purposes of clearing up the bladder infection can predispose them to yeast infections, too, a classic side effect that all women can experience when they take antibiotics for any reason. Yeast infections are caused by a yeast known as *candida albicans,* a one-cell fungus that belongs to the plant kingdom. Under normal circumstances, candida is always in your vagina, mouth and digestive tract. It is "friendly" fungus. For a variety of reasons, candida will overgrow and reproduce too much of itself, changing from a harmless one-cell fungus into long branches of yeast cells, called mycelia. This is known as *candidiasis*.

Generally, any changes to your vagina's normal acidic environment can make you vulnerable to candidiasis. The list of factors that affect your vaginal environment is quite long. High blood sugar levels increase the amount of sugar stored in the vaginal cell walls, and yeast *love* sugar. In fact, women who suffer from chronic yeast infections are encouraged to be screened for diabetes since they are so common in women with diabetes.

Anything that interferes with the immune system will make yeast thrive, too. Antibiotics, for example, not only kill the harmful bacteria, but often the friendly bacteria that are always in the vagina and which are necessary to fend off infection.

Severe itching and a curdlike or cottage-cheesy discharge are classic symptoms of candidiasis. The discharge, interestingly, may also smell like baking bread, fermenting yeast or even brewing beer. So if the discharge *is* foul-smelling or fishy, you can rule out yeast. The discharge may also be thinner and mucus-like, but it is always white. Other symptoms are swelling, redness and irritation of the outer and inner vaginal lips, painful sex and painful urination due to an irritation of the urethra.

When yeast is in the throat, it is called *thrush* and usually occurs in immune-deficient women (they may be HIV-positive or undergoing cancer treatments). Thrush is unsettling because the mouth and throat are coated with a milky-white goop. It can also be present in newborns, when yeast-infected mothers give birth. Thrush is treated orally with nystatin drops. Finally, since yeast is present in the intestines, HIV-positive women can develop severe, life-threatening esophageal yeast infections.

Vaginal yeast infections are so common that over-the-counter antifungal agents in creams, suppositories or pill form are available at all drugstores. A doctor will confirm yeast by taking a culture swab.

Plain yogurt, also an antifungal, is the best way to fend off yeast. Simply eat a small container of any kind of yogurt daily; so long as it has active bacterial culture, any brand is fine. Alternatively, you can take *lactobacillus acidophilus*, which is generally available in capsule form at any drugstore. If you find that you have thrush, *citrus seed extract* (Citricidal) and *tea-tree oil* can be used as a gargle.

Following an "antiyeast" diet may also be helpful. Certain foods interfere with the vagina's acidity, something you need to prevent yeast. The diet entails avoiding the following: sugar, honey, maple syrup, molasses and any foods that contain them; alcoholic beverages; vinegars and foods containing vinegar such as pickled foods, salad dressings, mustard, ketchup and mayonnaise; mouldy nuts, such as peanuts, pistachios and cashews; soy sauce, miso and other fermented products; dairy food with the exception of butter, buttermilk and yogurt; coffee, black tea and sweetened pop; dried fruits; processed foods.

Try to incorporate more of the following foods to compensate: whole grains such as rice, millet, barley, buckwheat, etc.; breads, crackers, muffins that are yeast-free and preferably wheat-free; raw or cooked fresh vegetables; fish, chicken and lean meats (organically fed and hormone- and antibiotic-free); nuts and seeds that are not mouldy; fruit in moderation (limiting sweeter fruits).

There are some other ways to avoid yeast infections:

1. **Don't wear tight clothing around your vagina:** Tight pants, panties and nylon pantyhose prevent your vagina from breathing and make it warmer and moister for yeast. Wear looser pants that allow your vagina to breathe, switch to knee highs or old-fashioned stockings, or wear pantyhose only for special occasions. And go "bottomless" to bed to let air into your vagina.

2. **Wear only 100 percent cotton clothing and/or natural fibres around your vagina:** Synthetic underwear and polyester pants are not good ideas. All cotton underwear, denim, wool or rayon pants that are loose fitting are fine.

3. **Avoid vaginal deodorants or sprays:** These products are unnecessary and disturb the vagina's natural environment, which is fully designed to "self-clean."

4. **Don't douche unless it's for purely medicinal purposes:** Douching can push harmful bacteria up higher into the vagina, disturb the vagina's natural ecosystem or interfere with a pregnancy. Always a bad idea!

5. **Watch your toilet habits:** Always wipe from front to back with toilet paper. When you do it the other way around, you can introduce fecal material and germs into your vagina. After a looser bowel movement, wet the toilet paper and clean your rectal area thoroughly so that fecal material doesn't stay on your underwear and wind up in your vagina. If you're in a less hygienic bathroom that doesn't have running water near the toilet, spit on your toilet paper and clean the rectal area. (It's better than nothing.)

6. **Don't insert anything into a dry vagina:** Whether it's a penis or a tampon, make sure your vagina is well lubricated before insertion.

7. **Avoid wearing tampons.**

8. **Avoid long car trips on vinyl seats:** New research indicates that vinyl seats increase a woman's risk of developing a yeast infection because the vinyl traps moisture and doesn't allow the crotch area to breathe.

The next chapter focuses on one of the most notorious microvascular (small blood vessel) complications: diabetes eye disease.

Chapter 17

DIABETES EYE DISEASE

● ● ● ● ● ● ● ● ● ●

Diabetes is the leading cause of new blindness in adults. Seventy-eight percent of people with Type 2 diabetes experience diabetes eye disease, clinically known as diabetic retinopathy. Microvascular complications (see Chapter 16) damage the small blood vessels in the eyes. High blood pressure, associated with macro-vascular complications (see Chapter 2), also damages the blood vessels in the eyes.

While 98 percent of people with Type 1 diabetes will experience eye disease within 15 years of being diagnosed, in Type 2 diabetes eye disease is often diagnosed *before* the diabetes; in other words, many people don't realize they have diabetes until their eye doctors ask them if they have been screened for diabetes. In fact, 20 percent of people with Type 2 diabetes already have diabetes eye disease before their diabetes is diagnosed. The longer you've had diabetes, the more at risk you are for diabetes eye disease. Because people are living longer with diabetes, it is now considered the most common cause of blindness under age 65, and the most common cause of new blindness in North America. Right now, about 400 Canadians go blind each year as a result of diabetes eye disease.

Eighty percent of all eye disease is known as non-proliferative eye disease, meaning "no new blood vessel growth" eye disease. This is also called background diabetic eye disease. In this case, the blood vessels in the retina (the part of your eyeball that faces your brain, as opposed to your face) start to deteriorate, bleed or hemorrhage (known as microaneurysms) and leak water and protein into the centre of the retina, called the macula; this condition is known as macular edema and causes vision loss, which sometimes is only temporary. However, without treatment, more permanent vision loss will occur. Although non-proliferative eye disease rarely leads to total blindness, as many as 20 percent of those with non-proliferative eye disease can become legally blind within five years.

Proliferative eye disease means "new blood vessel growth" eye disease. In this case, your retina says, "Since all my blood vessels are being damaged, I'm just going to grow *new* blood vessels!" This process is known as neovascularization. The problem is that these new blood vessels are deformed, or abnormal, which makes the problem worse, not better. These deformed blood vessels look a bit like Swiss cheese; they're full of holes and have a bad habit of suddenly bleeding, causing severe damage without warning. They can also lead to scar tissue in the retina, retinal detachments and glaucoma, greatly increasing the risk of legal blindness.

Diabetes can also cause cataracts, a clouding of the lens inside the eye that blurs vision.

This chapter will cover signs of eye disease and failing vision, laser treatment to slow vision loss, visual aids and coping with low vision or blindness. But first, the best step is *prevention*.

PREVENTING DIABETES EYE DISEASE

The adage "Early detection is your best protection" is perhaps no truer when it comes to diabetes eye disease! *It's crucial to have frequent eye exams.* The average person has an eye exam every five years. And if you're walking around with undiagnosed Type 2 diabetes, you can also be walking around with early signs of diabetes eye disease. So, as soon as you're diagnosed with Type 2 diabetes, get to an eye specialist for a complete exam and make it a yearly "gig" from now on.

During an eye exam, an ophthalmologist will dilate your pupil with eye drops, then use a special instrument to check for

- tiny red dots (signs of bleeding),
- a thick or "milky" retina, with or without yellow clumps or spots (signs of macular edema),
- a "bathtub ring" on the retina—a ring shape that surrounds a leakage site on the retina (also a sign of macular edema), or
- "cottonwool spots" on the retina—small fluffy white patches in the retina (signs of new blood vessel growth, or more advanced eye disease).

Today, it's estimated that if everyone with impaired glucose tolerance (see Chapter 1) went for an eye exam once a year, blindness from diabetes eye disease would drop from 8 percent in this group to 1 percent.

Stop Smoking

Since smoking also damages blood vessels, and diabetes eye disease is a blood vessel disease, smoking will certainly aggravate the problem. Quitting smoking may help to reduce eye complications. See Chapter 2 for more details on smoking cessation.

Avoid Eye Infections

High blood sugar can predispose you to frequent bacterial infections, including conjunctivitis (pink-eye). Eye infections can also affect your vision. To prevent eye infections, make sure you wash your hands before you touch your eyes, especially before you handle contact lenses.

Stay in Control

The Diabetes Complication and Control Trial showed that Type 1 patients, who suffer most from diabetes eye disease, were able to delay the onset of eye damage by staying in tight blood sugar control (see Chapter 2). Also, by controlling your blood pressure and cholesterol (see Chapter 7), you can help to reduce the effects of swelling in the central part of the retina.

SIGNS OF EYE DISEASE

Seventy-eight percent of people with Type 2 diabetes will experience eye changes as a result of diabetes eye disease, and one-fifth will actually show signs of eye disease when they are first diagnosed. In the early stages of diabetes eye disease, there are no symptoms. That's why you need to have a thorough eye exam every six months. As the eye damage progresses, you may notice blurred vision. The blurred vision is due to changes in the shape of the lens of the eye. During an eye exam, your ophthalmologist may notice yellow spots on your retina, signs that scar tissue has formed on the retina from bleeding. If the disease progresses to the point where new blood vessels have formed, vision problems may be quite severe as a result of spontaneous bleeding or detachment of the retina.

Vision can fail in two areas: central vision and peripheral vision. Central vision is identifying an object in focus. Peripheral vision is seeing out of the corner of your eye. When we lose our central vision, we lose the ability to focus on fine detail: print, television images, details of faces. When we lose our peripheral vision, we develop "tunnel vision" (a common sign of glaucoma, for example). This restricts us from seeing obstructions, causing us to bump into corners of chairs and doors and trip on many objects. Diabetes eye disease affects both central and peripheral vision.

Vision loss is often very gradual. It may not be something you notice suddenly. Signs of failing vision are important clues that you may have diabetes eye disease that is progressing. The following are classic signs of failing or deteriorating vision:

- You sit closer and closer to the television.
- You're squinting in order to see.
- You need a stronger prescription for your glasses or contacts.
- You have difficulty reading the newspaper.
- You're bothered by bright lights.
- You're more accident-prone, bumping into chairs or doors; tripping over curbs and steps; and knocking things over all the time.
- You can't see well in the dark or at night; night driving is difficult.

If you have signs of failing vision, any of the following eye specialists can help:

- **An ophthalmologist:** This is a medical doctor who specializes in eye conditions. Ophthalmologists can be referred by your family doctor or an optometrist. Ophthalmologists perform eye surgery, prescribe glasses or contacts and recommend visual aids.
- **An optometrist:** This is not a doctor, but a professional who is trained to correct vision problems with refractions, visual exercises and visual aids. Optometrists can diagnose and recognize eye disease and can refer you to an ophthalmologist.
- **An optician:** This is the specialist who makes lenses for glasses and who is frequently on hand at optical stores to answer questions. He or she may be your first point of contact in finding help, particularly if you think you just need stronger glasses or contacts. Opticians often recognize more serious problems with the eyes and can recommend (but not *formally* refer you to) an ophthalmologist.

Much of the time, these specialists help you see better with what you've got. They can help you get around and complete daily tasks with visual aids (see the section in this chapter), enlarging images, assisting with lighting and improving colour contrasts.

CAN YOU TREAT DIABETES EYE DISEASE?

Not completely. A procedure known as laser photocoagulation can burn and seal off the damaged blood vessels, which stops them from bleeding or leaking. In the earlier stages of eye disease, this procedure can restore your vision within about six months. In most cases, however, laser surgery only slows down vision loss, rather than restoring vision. In other words, without the treatment, your vision will get worse; with the treatment, it will stay the same.

If new blood vessels have already formed, a series of laser treatments are done to purposely scar the retina. Since a scarred retina needs less oxygen, blood vessels stop re-forming, reducing the risk of further damage.

In more serious cases, surgery known as a vitrectomy is performed. In this procedure, blood and scar tissue on the retina is surgically removed.

After-Effects of Laser Treatment

While you're healing from laser surgery, you may notice blurred vision that lasts anywhere from a few weeks to a few months. You may also notice that it takes longer for your eyes to adapt to very bright or very dark lighting (called night vision). This may or may not improve and is a common side effect of all laser eye surgery, even in people who are having it done to improve astigmatism. Finally, you may notice "floaters," which are evidence that there is bleeding inside the eye.

ALL ABOUT VISUAL AIDS

If your vision is deteriorating, a range of visual aids are available that can make living and working far easier than it was for many of our parents and grand-parents who suffered from partial or complete vision loss. This is, in part, due to a range of technologies that can enhance images through magnification, lighting and colour contrast. A number of tactile products exist as well using the Braille alphabet.

Visual aids are used by people with partial sight, also known as low vision, reduced vision or impaired vision. Some people still refer to low vision as "legally blind" or partial blindness. These terms are slowly falling out of favour because of myths surrounding what blindness means in most cases (see further on). Of the Canadians who identify themselves as visually impaired, fewer than 20 percent are totally blind—without any usable vision. When you hear that "diabetes causes blindness," it is not untrue, but it usually refers to a scenario in which you are visually impaired with *some usable vision left*, which makes you a candidate for visual aids (a.k.a. low-vision aids).

Making Things Larger

One of the most common visual aids involves products that can magnify an image, known as magnification devices. These devices can extend the image over a large enough area of the retina for it to be detected by the healthy cells at the edges, or periphery. Magnification devices typically magnify as much as 22 times the normal size. Even as I write these words now, my computer can magnify my screen so that the words I'm typing are 500 percent larger than they actually are. Magnification aids commonly used can be telescopes, which make distant objects appear closer; binoculars, which many people can use for watching television, movies or plays; monoculars, which can help you read distance objects such as street names, house numbers or bus numbers; or pocket magnifiers, illuminated magnifiers or stand-mounted magnifiers, which are frequently used for a wide assortment of tasks, from working to crafts and leisure activities.

Some people need different visual aids for different tasks. Typically one aid will be used for fine detail tasks, such as reading; another one for watching television; and another one for outdoor use.

You can also buy many items with large print, including large-print books, telephones and clocks.

High-tech magnification devices

Magnification devices can be low tech (as in magnifying reading glasses) or high tech (as in software or hardware). People with diabetes have a wide variety of income levels. If you can afford it, here is a sample of some of the higher-tech magnification products you can find. Typically, high-technology products work with existing hardware you may already own, such as desktop or laptop computers, palm devices and so on. They may be sold as software that works with your equipment, or sold as an "interface," a smaller piece of hardware you connect to something like a computer, which can transform data, manipulate data and so on.

Many computer companies offer a range of adaptive products. For example, Xerox makes a product called the Reading Edge, which is a transportable reading machine that offers magnification, scanning, speech synthesizer (if you can't read it, you can hear the data), optical character recognition, allowing you to dictate letters that come out in print, and so on. Another product, called the Reading AdvantEdge, is a software program that can make your home computer do all of these things (except perhaps to scan).

Large-print computer access products are another kind of high-tech aid that allow you to select a preferred font for the computer's display of characters; change the foreground or background colours of the screen; and display large print as full-screen mode. Almost any word-processing software has some capacity to magnify, but these products, such as MAGic, can magnify the screen image from 2 through 20 times the normal size. A range of other options to optimize visual image are offered with these various large-print packages.

Closed-circuit television (CCTV) can also help with magnification. This is a system that is similar to a video camcorder device. Anything you place in front of the camera will be broadcast on your TV screen so you can see it more closely: Books, recipes, prescriptions, photographs and so on can all be enhanced with CCTV systems. One product called Magni-Cam, for example, is a hand-held electronic magnifier that connects to any television set. The camera weighs only 198 g (7 oz.) and doesn't require any focusing.

There are literally hundreds of high-tech visual aids available. The best way to find them is through the Internet, by going to your favourite software/hardware manufacturer's Web site and searching for "adaptive products," "products for the visually impaired" or "visual aids." You can also find a wealth of information on high-tech products by visiting the Web site of the Canadian Institute for the Blind (CNIB): www.cnib.ca.

Making Things Brighter

Products that improve lighting are also visual aids. Direct light sources can dramatically improve the ability of people with low vision to complete tasks by reducing glare, improving background light and so forth. Low-tech solutions involve

- a direct light source focused on the task, not on the person,
- increasing the light bulb wattage on lamps,

- using high-intensity lights that reduce glare but increase light,
- retrofitting the home with adjustable indirect track lighting for flexibility,
- installing fluorescent lighting under kitchen cabinets and near the sink and stove,
- keeping a flashlight by the stove,
- equipping the home with night lights to ease the transition from darkness to light,
- getting a few floor lamps or other non-glare light sources near the TV,
- installing dimmer switches or three-way light bulbs,
- sitting with your back to the window to reduce glare (especially in public places),
- wearing a hat with a visor for light sensitivity outdoors, and
- getting ultraviolet-inhibitor sunglasses for outdoor glare (ask your optician).

Making Things Stand Out

You can make objects stand out by using colour coding, another type of visual aid. The general rule is to contrast the background with the foreground; smoother textures tend to make colours appear light, while uneven surfaces tend to make colours appear darker.

In the home, for example, using colour contrast can make it easier to find things or identify objects. You can buy markers that are brightly coloured and that dry into a hard plastic. (e.g., Hi-marks). They can be used to mark appliances, such as the stove, washer or dryer. Nail polish or coloured tape can be used on keys or mailboxes. Brightly coloured elastic bands can be used as markers for jars or tins. You can even use coloured magnets for metal surfaces (such as coloured alphabet letters). In the kitchen, dark pots against a white stove (or the reverse) can help. Otherwise, you can put coloured tape near the end of the pot handles. When you eat, colour contrast between placemats or tablecloth and dishes makes it easier to distinguish between them than using table coverings with glossy finishes or patterns. Electrical outlets should also contrast with the surrounding walls; just buy coloured wall plates for your outlets.

A little redecorating using colour can work wonders: Colour-contrasting paint can be used around door frames or to paint cupboards.

Colour contrasting can be used to separate your clothes (by colour or texture). For the bathroom, you can use coloured toothpaste that will contrast with white bristles on the toothbrush; a colour-contrasted bath mat will help, as well as using a coloured soap in the shower or bath. Using different colours for towels and washcloths can help you tell which you're using. For more information on implementing a colour-coding system, contact the CNIB.

Making Things Touchy-Feely

Tactile products are "touchy-feely." Such products are either designed with Braille lettering (the raised dots system invented by Louis Braille back in the 19th century and still used today). Essentially, Braille is another way to read and write printed information. It is equivalent, in every way, to print. You can read or write words, numbers, music notations and any other symbols that appear in print. It works by arranging combinations of the six dots of the Braille "cell." Braille is read by touch and is therefore a tactile language. Most people use the first finger on one or both hands to read it. Braille can be used for any language, mathematics, scientific equations and computer notations. The only people who can't use Braille are those who suffer from numbness in their fingers or hands, but most people with diabetes-related numbness will feel it in their legs or feet (see Chapter 16), not their fingers.

You can get hundreds of Braille-adapted products, including glucose meters, pill organizers, thermometers and so on. Braille is actually all around us in modern architecture, but the sighted population doesn't always notice. (For example, most elevators are equipped with Braille lettering on the buttons.) There are also Braille computers with Braille keyboards and a refreshable Braille screen. (Braille computers are very expensive, however, with each Braille cell retailing at roughly $55.)

In short, the availability of tactile products is not the problem; everything you could possibly need in life either comes in Braille lettering or can probably be specially ordered (check with the CNIB).

Braille as a second language

The problem with tactile products has more to do with people's reluctance to learn Braille. Most people equate learning Braille with being totally blind, which is truly unfortunate. Braille is just as useful for people who have partial sight, and in many situations knowing it can make life a little easier. It's like knowing a second language to enhance your communications skills. For example, learning Spanish comes in handy in all kinds of situations, from being able to communicate and make friendships with Spanish-speaking people to ordering food in a

Mexican restaurant. It's the same thing with Braille: *It comes in handy* and can enhance, rather than detract from, your life.

People who lose their hearing are similarly reluctant to learn sign language (a.k.a. signing), but in numerous situations, signing would make a hearing-impaired person's life easier.

When you know a different language, it allows you access to a new community of people, too, which is very important when you feel isolated or alone. You already know that when you can talk to someone else who has diabetes, you immediately "connect" with one another because you share a common struggle. It's the same thing with vision loss; meeting someone else who is coping with vision loss helps you feel less alone and allows you to talk to someone who knows what you're going through. Imagine Braille as a bridge to new friends and a new community. It can also keep you employed as it enables you to make notes on documents, read a spreadsheet, take minutes at a meeting, file materials, read label diskettes and so on.

Braille also lessens your dependency on voice synthesizers (for reading or writing), audiotape recordings, magnifiers and other print enhancers. These are great visual aids, but are not convenient in all circumstances. At home, you can also use Braille to label CDs, clothing, spices, cans, etc. You can also play games—cards, Scrabble, backgammon, chess and so on.

For more information on Braille or Braille products, contact the CNIB at 1-800-268-8818.

Making Things Talk

An obvious visual aid is a product that talks. Before the popularity of voice synthesizers, audio-taped books were about the only talking product available. Today, voice synthesizers can be used with almost any information product, including small things such as thermometers. With scanners, you can scan printed material into a voice-synthesized computer that can tell you what something says, including labels or fine print. One danger is an overreliance on voice-synthesized products, however.

COPING WITH LOW VISION OR BLINDNESS

The hardest part of losing some or all of your vision is coping with it. This has a lot to do with misconceptions about what "blindness" means, which is defined as total loss of sight. That said, more than 80 percent of people who are considered blind can usually make out the outlines of objects, identify the sources of light, ascertain the direction of light, distinguish light from dark, etc.

Registered Blind

There are degrees of blindness that go from low or impaired vision to profound vision loss. All these definitions can be classified as "Registered Blind," a category that allows you to be eligible for income tax and other government benefits. You are considered Registered Blind when you have visual acuity in your better eye, after correction, of 20/200 or less. That means that you can see at 20 feet what someone with perfect vision can see at 200 feet. (Visual acuity refers to the sharpness and clarity of "near vision"—close-up objects.) You can also be Registered Blind if your visual field (a.k.a. peripheral vision) results in a narrowing of your central vision to 20 degrees or less (you may be able to read, but walking around is hazardous because you can't see what's around you).

So that means that most people who are Registered Blind see *something*. A lot of people who appear sighted in public and who seem to get around just fine with some visual aids are Registered Blind.

Rehabilitation Services

You have access to a range of rehabilitation services through the CNIB (you can request a CNIB rehabilitation teacher) and other organizations, which can help you improve your mobility with daily living—cooking, banking, grooming and getting around town.

Trained individuals (volunteers or professionals) are on hand through these organizations to take you out and get you used to walking around and travelling by yourself, with perhaps the aid of a cane. These individuals can also help you find the right visual aids (see previous section) to enhance your usable vision; they can also help you find mobility aids, guide dogs and canes.

The white cane is often perceived as an announcement to the world that you are visually impaired, *but that's not necessarily a bad thing.* One of the cane's chief purposes is to get people to be considerate and *move out of your way* when you are trying to get around. It also gives permission for people to approach you to offer their assistance. For example, as a Toronto subway passenger, I have never witnessed a caned individual attempt to get on and off a train without being deluged with offers of assistance. All kinds of people, from a myriad of age groups and backgrounds, offer to help. The offers of assistance also help to reinforce a sense of community for the sighted subway travellers; it's good to see people get involved and offer unsolicited help!

An identification cane is a collapsible white cane that primarily identifies you as visually impaired, but it can also be used for depth perception on stairs or curbs. There is also the white support cane, which says, "I have vision loss, *and* I have trouble walking." This cane is designed to support your weight. Finally, a long cane is like your "whiskers"—it is a probe that senses things in front of you. It is mostly used in the home or in unfamiliar surroundings. Before you use it, the CNIB encourages a training session with an orientation and mobility instructor.

A Word About Denial

Coping with vision loss often involves overcoming denial that you are losing your sight. This is a normal reaction, but it can also foster behaviours that are not helpful in the long run. It can lead to a lesser quality of life because those in denial often refuse help with visual aids or the CNIB. Some people may also become overly dependent on others, which can foster a range of unhealthy relationships with friends or family members. You may rely on family members to cook, clean, shop for you and so on. Vision loss does *not* have to mean loss of mobility, and with the right visual aids and training, you can do lots of things on your own and regain your independence.

Distinguishing Your Medications

People with perfect vision can make all kinds of mistakes when it comes to medications; they can confuse pills, misread labels and so forth. Keeping track of your medications is especially challenging if you're visually impaired. The following tips from the CNIB may help. You're also encouraged to contact the CNIB and arrange for a CNIB rehabilitation teacher to work with you on designing a system for keeping track of all your medications. In the meantime, try some or all of the following:

- Get a pill organizer with different sections. (These come with Braille lettering, too.)
- Arrange your medications alphabetically on the shelf.
- Get some large-print labels, colour labels or Braille labels to identify them.
- Put personal markings on the lids, and keep your personal marked lid for refills.
- Try to use different-sized or shaped bottles for your medications.

- Use elastic bands to indicate the number of doses per bottle you need to take. (A bottle with two bands around it means you take it twice a day, and so on.) Remove a band as you take your dose and replace it the next day.

Staying Physically Active

As you know from Chapter 8, staying physically active is an important way to manage your diabetes and help to stabilize blood sugar. Visual impairment does not mean you need to be inactive. Swimming, golfing, skiing, curling, tandem bicycling and walking are just a few of the many activities you can enjoy with a few adaptations. For example, you can utilize a sighted guide to help you with some of these activities. You can incorporate brightly coloured guide wires in swimming pools; you can find a sighted partner for tandem cycling (it may be a sighted friend who needs to get active too and could use a partner). You can find beeping balls for ball sports or tactile markers for bowling. The range of visual aids or adaptations is endless, and you're encouraged to contact the CNIB to discuss how to use adaptations to accommodate your activities.

Coping with Blind Ignorance

The most disabling part of vision loss is the ignorance you encounter from the general public. You may want to pass on the following tips to friends and family members (who, in turn, can tell a few more people), which can make life a little easier for everyone.

- When speaking to someone with vision loss, face them and speak clearly in a moderate tone. Don't shout. Vision loss does not mean the person is hearing impaired, too.
- Anyone can act as a sighted guide. Just offer your arm and say, "My name is X. Here's my arm if you need some assistance." Then allow the person to take it. Never just grab someone's arm without permission. When acting as a sighted guide, walk at a normal pace. You can hesitate slightly before stepping up or down.
- Don't pat a guiding dog, please. And speak to the person, not the dog!
- If you're giving directions, use phrases such as "on your left" or "right behind you" instead of "over there" or "over here."
- At social gatherings, describe who is in a large group; don't just leave someone alone in the middle of the room with no sense of who's in it.

- Identify yourself when you approach a visually impaired guest so she or he knows who's talking.
- When dining with a visually impaired person, describe what's on the table to elicit a mental image of the food and help enhance appetite.
- Describe what's on the plate clockwise to make it easier.
- Assist with cutting meat if it's requested.
- Use extra large napkins if possible.

Hopefully this chapter has helped to alleviate some of your fears about maintaining independence with vision loss. As you can see, vision loss is certainly not the end of the world, but it *is* a preventable problem. By staying in control of your diabetes and keeping your blood sugar levels as normal as possible as much as possible, you may be able to avoid severe vision loss and the eye problems that so many people with diabetes develop. But did you know that the same strategy can help you avoid losing your teeth? Gum disease and tooth decay are other diabetes complications that are a growing problem mainly because of a lack of awareness about the relationship between diabetes and tooth decay. The next chapter will benefit anyone, whether he or she has diabetes or not. Losing your teeth can be a very uncomfortable experience (as anyone with dentures will tell you) that you ought to avoid if you can.

Chapter 18

BRUSHING UP ON TOOTH DECAY

● ● ● ● ● ● ● ● ● ● ●

High blood sugar levels get into your saliva and feed the bacteria in your mouth. The bacteria, in turn, break down the starches and sugars to form acids that eventually break down your tooth enamel. This is how cavities are formed.

Moreover, damage to the small blood vessels in your gums can lead to periodontal problems, while blood sugar levels naturally rise when you're fighting a gum infection (known as a periodontal infection), such as an abscess. Preventing dental problems means the usual regimen (see "Combatting Gum Disease"). You're also advised to have your teeth cleaned and examined at least every six months or more depending on your periodontal health, and to avoid sugary foods (which you should be doing anyway). Unfortunately, this is just not enough information for most people with diabetes, especially if they already have gum disease.

GUM DISEASE AND HEART DISEASE

Here is some news you don't want, but must have: Gum disease increases your risk of heart disease. The link has been known for years, but very few people are aware of it. It's believed that inflamed gums can produce inflammatory by-products that affect the cardiovascular system. Also, the bacteria that spread in gum disease can produce damage to blood platelets, causing clots. Since people with Type 2 diabetes are already at high risk for heart disease and stroke (see

Chapter 15), this means that Type 2 diabetes, combined with gum disease, puts you at extreme risk for heart disease. Treating or preventing gum disease can have a positive effect on your cardiovascular health! For more information about heart disease and stroke, see Chapter 15.

DIABETES-RELATED GUM DISEASE

Gum disease, also called periodontitis, is often not noticeable until it's serious. It's caused by bacteria that are normally in the mouth, which can vary in aggressiveness. The bacteria settle around and under the gum line (where the gums and teeth meet); this is called plaque. Brushing and flossing can remove the plaque, preventing it from hardening into tartar (also called calculus). Bacterial infections can develop from tartar. At this stage, it's called gingivitis, but as the bacterial infection worsens, you're looking at full-blown gum disease or periodontitis.

Healthy gums go around the tooth the way a cuff goes around your wrist. When the gums fit more loosely, the bacteria get high up, alongside the tooth, near the bone, where no toothbrush or floss can go (but a periodontist can with special cleaning instruments). The bacteria can cause an inflammatory reaction that erodes the bone supporting the teeth, making them loose. Eventually, you may have to have your teeth pulled and wear dentures.

Roughly 90 percent of all Canadians have gum disease at some point in their lives. Because people with diabetes have more frequent infections and are slower to heal due to inefficient white blood cells, this can also affect the gums. Second, any kind of infection, such as a urinary tract infection, or even a cold or a flu, will increase blood sugar levels. So when the gums become infected, it can have serious consequences for your overall health. Damage to small vessels (a.k.a. microvascular complication) can also affect the support tissues in the gums.

Two things are going on with diabetes-related gum disease: High blood sugar can make you vulnerable to gum disease, and gum disease can increase your blood sugar levels even more because it is an active infection. (Of course, the same can be said for any infection, but many of us don't think of gum disease as an active infection.)

The Smoking Gum

If you've read other chapters in this book, you know what a bad combination smoking and diabetes is. Unfortunately, smoking can predispose you to gum disease, making your already high risk from diabetes higher still. More smokers than non-smokers have gum disease; at least half of all cases of gum disease are directly linked to smoking, and some studies show that as much as 75 percent of gum disease is smoking-related.

If you quit smoking, you can reduce the likelihood of developing gum disease; the longer you've not smoked, the greater the chances you will not suffer gum disease.

Smokers have the highest risk of gum disease, ex-smokers have the next highest and non-smokers have the lowest risk. But diabetes is another significant risk factor, which means if you smoke and have diabetes, you're at highest risk of developing serious gum disease. See Chapter 2 for information on smoking cessation. Quitting smoking will make it easier for you to treat your gum disease, too.

COMBATTING GUM DISEASE

The strategy is to try to prevent gum disease, if possible, by employing all of those boring "dentist" rules (see "Doing the Right Thing the Right Way") that have been drilled into you since you can remember: brushing after eating, flossing, rubber-tip massage, fluoride rinses, etc., and, most of all, frequent checkups. Going for regular cleaning by your dentist or dental hygienist to remove built-up tartar is considered a "first-line" prevention strategy; however, it is what you do at home that can really make the difference. Ask your dentist or hygienist to show you how to brush and floss properly; it's amazing how many of us were taught the wrong way by our parents or dentists of yesteryear, and these poor habits contribute to dental problems. We also should not be using hard brushes, but soft only.

If you have diabetes, consider going for routine dental cleanings every three months instead of every six months, too. Extra cleaning can really help to reduce plaque, which is the building block of gum disease.

Doing the Right Thing the Right Way

Whether you want to prevent gum disease or are being treated for gum disease, brushing and flossing are "doing the right thing," but many of us are doing the right thing *the wrong way*! The first thing most people do when their gums start to bleed from brushing or flossing is stop. This is the worst response. Keep at it; the bleeding should stop after a few days as you strengthen the gums.

Sometimes people use the wrong brushes. Use soft bristles; hard bristles can damage the gums, and you can "brush off" gum tissue, which can lead to recession and root exposure.

Next, people buy the wrong floss and then assume that flossing doesn't "work" for them. If you're finding that your floss is shredding or breaking, get another brand. If your teeth are very close together, finer, unwaxed floss is better. If shredding is a problem, a thicker, waxed floss is better.

I'm all for recycling, but *please* don't recycle your floss. Use a clean piece for each tooth. Take a long piece of floss and inch your way to the end with each tooth. If the plaque you remove is foul smelling, by the way, that is a sign you have bad breath. You can recheck for the smell when you floss next; if the smell improves, so has your breath, and you can rest assured that it was a plaque problem and not a chronic, unsolvable problem.

Brushing your teeth for five seconds is better than nothing, but the Canadian Dental Association recommends you need to brush every 24 hours at least, for about three minutes. Again, use soft instead of hard brushes. With soft brushes, you can also massage your gums and loosen plaque that is high up. Ask your dentist to show you how to do this and for a sample of a special brush you can use for hard-to-reach places; it can brush behind your front teeth, for example, an area often missed, or behind your side teeth.

Many years ago, the manufacturers of Close Up toothpaste used the line "How's your love life?" to sell their toothpaste. Well, they were onto something. *Did you know that gum disease can be transmitted by kissing?* If your lover has gum disease, chances are he or she has aggressive bacteria that can be transferred to your mouth, too. For more information about gum disease transmissibility, it's worth visiting the Web site www.periotrans.com.

A Gum-Smart Diet

A gum-smart diet can start with the right chewing gum! If you don't have the opportunity to brush after eating, chew some "dental gum," a new product that has exploded onto the shelves "in the toothpaste section," as one commercial tells us. Dozens of chewing gum brands have introduced dental gums. These gums may have tartar-fighting or whitening agents, are sugar free and so on. When you chew a sugar-free gum after eating, you get the saliva activated, which can wash away bacteria that form plaque.

All that stuff you tell your kids about sugar and cavities still applies! Use the same rules for yourself. Avoid sticky sweets and sugary snacks—something you need to do anyway if you're managing diabetes and planning meals (see Chapter 6). Ask your dietitian about "gum-smart" snacks (e.g., nuts, seeds, raw fruits and vegetables).

If you plan to eat something sweet, have it with a meal so your saliva can wash it down. After meals, if you can't brush, rinse your mouth with water and chew some sugar-free or dental gum.

SIGNS OF GUM DISEASE

Any of the following are signs that you already have gum disease:

- **Bleeding gums:** This is often the first sign of gum disease. You may notice bleeding when you brush your teeth or floss. If your gums are bleeding, it's always a sign of gum disease, but you can also have gum disease and not have bleeding gums.
- **Receding gums:** This occurs when the gum is not covering as much tooth as it should, sometimes exposing the roots.
- **New spaces between teeth:** This is called migration and refers to two teeth that used to "touch" but that no longer do.
- **Chronic bad breath (a.k.a. halitosis):** Bad breath can be caused by poor digestion, or by insufficient cleaning and a buildup of plaque. And, of course, there are many foods that cause bad breath. But if bad breath persists after proper cleanings and a good oral hygiene routine (including brushing the tongue), gum disease is probably the reason, where pus and bleeding are contributing to the bad breath problem.
- **Red gums:** Healthy gums should be the colour of salmon or coral, not blood. If you breathe through your mouth, red gums are more common, too.
- **Loose teeth.**
- **Less tapered gum "coverage" around the teeth:** The gum should meet the tooth at a knife-edge margin. If this margin is rolled and swollen, it's a sign of gum disease.
- **Shiny gums:** Gums should have some "stippling" to them (little dots) so they don't shine; shiny red gums are not a good thing.

When you notice any of these signs of gum disease, see your dentist. Your dentist will look for a host of things you can't see yourself, such as root cavities, pockets in the gums, tooth decay under the gum line and so on.

WHAT TO DO IF YOU HAVE GUM DISEASE

See a Gum Specialist

If gum disease has progressed beyond the early-stage gingivitis, you'll be referred to a periodontist. This is a dentist who has done a three-year "residency" of sorts in treating gum problems and gum disease. Periodontists can restore gum tissue or regenerate it. At your first visit, the periodontist will use a special probe that can measure gaps between the gums and teeth, as well as look for exposed roots, which need special care, too. Gaps between the gum and teeth are called pockets and normally shouldn't be deeper than 1–3 mm. Pockets deeper than this can be a sign of serious gum disease.

Periodontists may also do special cleanings called root planing, where the gum tissues are usually anaesthetized, and the roots of the teeth (these may be exposed or still covered by gums) are cleaned. The goal is to get rid of as much plaque and tartar as possible to prevent bacterial infections from developing or progressing once they have developed. Root planing may also involve using antibiotics to help kill off the bacteria high inside the gums. Gum surgery involves restoring the gumline to a more readily cleanable state by reducing the pockets and removing the diseased state.

If you have gum disease, it must be treated. Doing so will lower your blood sugar levels and can improve your overall health and ability to control your diabetes. If gum disease has progressed to the point where your teeth are loose, or keep becoming infected (forming root infections, abscesses and so on), dentures may be the next step. Compared to losing your eyesight (see Chapter 17) or a kidney (see Chapter 19) or a foot (see Chapter 20), dentures are certainly not the end of the world. But each set of dentures comes with its own set of problems. For more information on dentures, contact the Canadian Dental Association. If you still have your teeth, the information in this chapter can help you keep them.

The road to complications doesn't stop at the mouth. It keeps on going. What you put in your mouth can help prevent kidney failure if you're showing signs of diabetes-related kidney disease, discussed next.

Chapter 19

KEEPING YOUR KIDNEYS

● ● ● ● ● ● ● ● ● ●

Diabetic kidney disease, also known as diabetic nephropathy, is what happens when macrovascular complications *and* microvascular complications converge. The high blood pressure that is caused by macrovascular complications, combined with the small blood vessel damage caused by microvascular complications, together can cause kidney failure—something you *can* die from unless you have dialysis (filtering out the body's waste products through a machine) or a kidney transplant. About 15 percent of people with Type 2 diabetes will develop kidney disease, which often goes by the term "renal disease" or "nephropathy." When your kidneys have failed and you require dialysis, this is known as end-stage renal disease (ESRD); diabetes is considered to be the leading cause of kidney disease, responsible for roughly 45 percent of all cases of end-stage renal disease. Put another way, roughly 45 percent of all dialysis patients have diabetes. Certain population groups, such as Aboriginal Canadians (in the United States Aboriginal groups include American Indians, Native Hawaiians, and Alaskan Natives) and people of African or Hispanic descent, are more at risk for kidney failure than Caucasians. The good news is that the risk of developing chronic kidney disease increases with the length of time you've had diabetes, so by getting your diabetes under control early in the game, you may be able to prevent kidney disease or kidney failure.

WHAT DO YOUR KIDNEYS DO ALL DAY?

Kidneys are the public servants of the body; they're busy little bees! If they go on strike, you lose your water service, garbage pickup and a few other services you don't even appreciate.

Kidneys regulate your body's water levels; when you have too much water, your kidneys remove it by dumping it into a large storage tank, your bladder. The excess water stays there until you're ready to "pee it out." If you don't have enough water in your body (or if you're dehydrated), your kidneys will retain the water for you to keep you balanced.

Kidneys also act as your body's sewage filtration plant. They filter out all the garbage and waste that your body doesn't need and dump it into the bladder; this waste is then excreted into your urine. The two waste products your kidneys regularly dump are *urea* (the waste product of protein) and *creatinine* (waste products produced by the muscles). In people with high blood sugar levels, excess sugar will get sent to the kidneys, and the kidneys will dump it into the bladder, too, causing sugar to appear in the urine.

Kidneys also balance calcium and phosphate in the body, needed to build bones. Kidneys operate two little side businesses on top of all this. They make hormones. One hormone, called renin, helps to regulate blood pressure. Another hormone, called erythropoietin, helps bone marrow make red blood cells.

WHAT AFFECTS YOUR KIDNEYS

The Macro Thing

When you suffer from cardiovascular disease, you probably have high blood pressure. High blood pressure damages blood vessels in the kidneys, which interferes with their job performance. As a result, they won't be as efficient at removing waste or excess water from your body. And if you are experiencing poor circulation, which can also cause water retention, the problem is further aggravated.

Poor circulation may cause your kidneys to secrete too much renin, which is normally designed to regulate blood pressure, but in this case increases it. All the extra fluid and the high blood pressure place a heavy burden on your heart— and your kidneys. If this situation isn't brought under control, you'd likely suffer from a heart attack before kidney failure, but kidney failure is inevitable.

The Micro Thing

When high blood sugar levels affect the small blood vessels, that includes the small blood vessels in the kidney's filters (called the nephrons), hence the term "diabetic nephropathy." In the early stages of nephropathy, good, usable protein is secreted in the urine. That's a sign that the kidneys were unable to distribute usable protein to the body's tissues. (Normally, they would excrete only the waste product of protein—urea—into the urine.)

Another microvascular problem affects the kidneys: nerve damage. The nerves you use to control your bladder can be affected, causing a sort of sewage backup in your body. The first place that sewage hits is your kidneys. Old urine floating around your kidneys isn't a healthy thing. The kidneys can become damaged as a result, aggravating all the conditions discussed so far in this section.

The Infection Thing

There's a third problem at work here. If you recall, frequent urination is a sign of high blood sugar. That's because your kidneys help to rid the body of too much sugar by dumping it into the bladder. Well, guess what? You're not the only one who likes sugar; bacteria, such as *E. coli* (the "hamburger bacteria"), like it, too. In fact, they thrive on it. So all that sugary urine sitting around in your bladder and passing through your ureters and urethra can cause this bacteria to overgrow, resulting in a urinary tract infection (UTI) such as cystitis (inflammation of the bladder lining). The longer your urethra, the more protection you have from UTIs. Men have long urethras; women have very short urethras, however, and at the best of times are prone to these infections—especially after a lot of sexual activity, explaining the term "honeymoon cystitis." Sexual intercourse can introduce even more bacteria (from the vagina or rectum) into a woman's urethra due to the close space the vagina and urethra share. Women who wipe from back to front after a bowel movement can also introduce fecal matter into the urethra, causing a UTI.

Any bacterial infection in your bladder area can travel back up to your kidneys, causing infection, inflammation and a big general mess, aggravating all the other problems!

The Smoking Thing

In the same way that smoking contributes to eye problems (see Chapter 17), it can also aggravate kidney problems. Smoking causes small vessel damage throughout your body.

SIGNS OF DIABETIC KIDNEY DISEASE

Obviously, there are a lot of different problems going on when it comes to diabetes and kidney disease. If you have any of the following early warning signs of kidney disease, see your doctor as soon as possible:

- Bad taste in the mouth (sign of toxins building up; see also Chapter 18 on tooth decay)
- Blood or pus in the urine (a sign of a kidney infection)
- Burning or difficulty urinating (a sign of a urinary tract infection)
- Fever, chills or vomiting (a sign of *any* infection)
- Foamy urine (a sign of kidney infection)
- Foul-smelling or cloudy urine (a sign of a urinary tract infection)
- Frequent urination (a sign of high blood sugar and/or urinary tract infection)
- High blood pressure (see Chapter 2)
- Itching
- Leg swelling or leg cramps (a sign of fluid retention)
- Less need for insulin or oral diabetes medications
- Morning sickness, nausea and vomiting
- Pain in the lower abdomen (a sign of a urinary tract infection)
- Protein in the urine (a sign of microvascular problems)
- Puffiness around eyes, swelling of hands and feet (sign of edema, or fluid retention)
- Weakness (a sign of anemia)

In the early stages of kidney disease, there are often no symptoms at all. Many of the symptoms above are signs that your kidney function has deteriorated to the point where toxins and wastes have built up, causing, for example, nausea and vomiting, fluid retention, even chronic hiccups. Heart failure (not to be confused with a heart attack, discussed in Chapter 15) and fluid in the lungs are characteristic of very late stages of kidney failure.

When you experience any of these symptoms, it's crucial to have a blood test that looks for creatinine levels. Again, creatinine is a waste product removed from the blood by healthy kidneys. A creatinine blood test greater than 1.2 for women and 1.4 for men is a sign of kidney disease. Another test that looks for blood urea nitrogen (BUN) is also important; when the BUN "rises," so to speak, it's a sign of kidney disease, too. Other more sensitive tests that detect the level of kidney function include creatinine clearance, glomerular filtration rate (GFR) and urine albumin.

TREATING KIDNEY DISEASE

If you have high blood pressure, getting it under control through diet, exercise or blood pressure-lowering medication will help to save your kidneys. If you have high blood sugar, treating any UTI as quickly as possible with antibiotics is the best way to avert kidney infection, while drugs known as ACE inhibitors can help to control small blood vessel damage caused by microvascular complications. In general, slowing the progression of kidney disease can be done by

- controlling high blood pressure (see Chapter 2)
- controlling blood sugar levels (see Chapter 4)
- adopting a kidney-smart diet (see below)
- avoiding medications that may damage the kidneys (sit down with your pharmacist or doctor and try to find substitutes for medications that can affect the kidneys; there are many substitutes for commonly prescribed medications)
- treating urinary tract infections (see Chapter 16 on neuropathy)
- exercise and weight loss (see Chapter 10 on obesity and Chapter 8 on active living)

The Kidney-Smart Diet

To prolong the life of your kidneys when you experience signs of kidney disease or are in the early stages and perhaps have been alerted through blood test results, you can adjust your diet to cut down on the work your kidneys normally do as well as meet nutritional needs, such as increasing iron intake, which may be lower due to anemia. Diet can even control the buildup of food wastes and reduce fatigue, nausea, itching and a bad taste in the mouth that can occur when toxins build up in the body. And, of course, diet will help to control high blood sugar. When you think about a kidney-smart diet, remember "3PS," a term I've coined to remember protein, potassium, phosphorus and sodium. The diet involves *cutting down on 3PS*. A dietitian or nutritionist can help you make the cuts necessary to save your kidneys, but keep you as healthy as possible.

Protein

Protein is a good thing normally; it builds, repairs and maintains your body tissues, and also helps you fight infections or heal wounds. But as protein breaks down in the body, it forms urea, which is a waste product. The kidney normally flushes out urea. When it can't, urea builds up in the blood, so cutting down on protein is necessary. You need to eat enough for health, however. Meat, fish, poultry, eggs, tofu and dairy products are high in protein.

Potassium

Your nerves and muscles normally rely on the mineral potassium to work well. But without the filtering process of your kidneys, too much can build up in your blood, which can affect your heart. Normally your kidneys get rid of potassium excess, so most of us never think about it. But when your kidneys aren't functioning well, we can cut down on potassium-rich foods, such as potatoes, squash, bananas, oranges, tomatoes, dried peas and beans.

Phosphorus (a.k.a. phosphate)

Your bones normally rely on the mineral phosphorus to stay healthy and strong. When phosphorus levels rise, usually the kidneys just filter out excess phosphorus and we feel fine. But when the kidneys aren't working well, phosphorus levels rise until we get itchy skin or painful joints. Limiting foods with phosphorus will help reduce toxic levels of this mineral. These foods include anything with protein (see "Protein"), seeds, nuts, dried peas, beans and processed bran cereals. You'll need some phosphorus-containing foods for health. When you ingest them, you can also take a phosphate binder, a medication that binds with the phosphorus in your intestine so it can pass in your stool. Ask your doctor about prescribing the binder.

Sodium

As discussed in the high blood pressure section in an earlier chapter, sodium affects your body fluids and blood pressure. Reducing sodium means cutting down on salt and packaged or canned products with sodium (canned soups are notorious). Start reading labels and stop salting your foods. Avoid foods with a high sodium content. Processed foods, such as deli meats, fast foods, salty snacks and anything with salty seasonings, are high in sodium. There are many herbs you can use instead; lemon and vinegar are terrific substitutes, too.

A word about fluids

Kidneys produce urine, which eliminates many of our wastes. When kidneys are not functioning well, not as much urine is produced, and this can cause fluid retention—swelling in hands, legs, feet and so on. Limiting your fluid intake may help, but it isn't necessary in all cases. Fluids include water, soup, juice, milk, popsicles and gelatin; you and your doctor should discuss how to limit your fluid intake.

FROM KIDNEY DISEASE TO KIDNEY FAILURE

Kidney failure is also known as chronic renal insufficiency (CRI); this term means your kidneys are operating at 50 percent or less than normal capacity. By this point, your kidneys are working with "half the staff" and are not able to remove the bodily wastes as efficiently. Again, you may not notice symptoms of kidney failure at all; the disease progresses slowly, and as the kidneys continue to fail and more waste products build up, you'll begin to feel sick. Because your kidneys stop making enough of the crucial hormone erythropoietin (EPO), you can suffer from low iron levels or anemia, as well as weakness. When the kidneys are functioning at less than 10 percent of their capacity, you'll need to consider dialysis or even a kidney transplant, if possible. By this point, you've progressed to end-stage renal disease.

When You Need Dialysis

Dialysis comes from the root word dissolution, which means to "set free." It is a life-saving treatment that replaces many of your kidney's functions, such as removing waste, salt and extra water to prevent them from building up in the body; it keeps levels of potassium, sodium and bicarbonate in check, and helps to control your blood pressure. Dialysis has been available since the mid-1940s and began to be used as a regular treatment for people with kidney failure in the 1960s. Dialysis allows people with kidney failure to live a long time, often as long as someone with functioning kidneys. In Canada, the cost of dialysis is covered by the provinces. In the United States, many people simply die because they don't have health insurance coverage for dialysis and can't afford it. (Yay Canada!) However, the need for dialysis in Canada is putting a strain on our resources. While there are dialysis units across Canada, you need to plan your treatments several months in advance due to limited staff and space. This may mean you have to travel great distances and pay for many expenses yourself: accommodation, travel costs and so on. Your local Kidney Foundation office has information about the nearest dialysis units in your area and can give you some advice about making suitable arrangements for accommodations. Dialysis can be done at home, but it requires supervision with a trained health care professional. You still need to be "retrofitted" for home dialysis, get the equipment, make arrangements and so on.

There are two types of dialysis: hemodialysis ("hemo" means blood) and peritoneal dialysis ("peritoneal" means abdominal).

Hemodialysis

Hemodialysis involves cleaning your blood through an artificial kidney machine (a.k.a. dialyzer). The blood flows into the machine and goes back into your body nice and clean, free of waste products and excess buildup from chemicals and fluid.

You are connected to the artificial kidney through a blood vessel in your arm or leg. If there are problems finding a healthy blood vessel, a "bridge" can be created through a graft or catheter (a narrow plastic tube). The connection process can be uncomfortable, depending on how it's done.

The length of time a hemodialysis treatment lasts depends on the functioning capacity of your kidneys, how much waste has built up, how much fluid builds up between treatments, your overall size and the type of artificial kidney used. Typical treatments last about four hours and are required three times per week. Only a small amount of your blood can be handled by the machine so it takes a while. The blood has to circulate many times before it is clean. Hemodialysis can be done in a hospital, in an out-patient care centre or at home.

Peritoneal dialysis

Peritoneal dialysis filters the blood from within the body. This treatment can involve using a machine (known as continuous cycling peritoneal dialysis—CCPD), or a catheter and bag, similar to an ostomy or ileostomy (known as continuous ambulatory peritoneal dialysis—CAPD), available since 1976. CAPD does *not* mean you have dialysis in an ambulance; it means that you can remain *ambulatory*—able to walk around.

CCPD is usually done at home; in this case the catheter is connected to a special machine called a "cycler."

If you opt for CAPD, you do this procedure yourself, which is required about four or five times a day. The usual procedure is to put a bag of dialysate (about 2 L/2 quarts) through your catheter and into your peritoneal cavity. The dialysate stays there for about four or five hours before it is drained back into your catheter bag. When the bag is full, toss it and exchange it for a new bag of dialysate and new catheter bag. This allows you to carry on with your normal activities without planning your life around a dialysis machine.

Lifestyle adjustments for dialysis

Dialysis treatments, unlike some other treatments such as chemotherapy, do not leave you feeling sick or weak afterwards; they leave you feeling healthier. But during the procedure, you may feel muscle cramps, nausea or dizziness because the waste products are removed more abruptly than they are when kidneys are functioning. Low blood pressure can also occur, causing dizziness, headaches and even vomiting. As you have more treatments, these side effects should pass.

Dialysis also means you have to stay on your 3PS diet (see above), cutting down on protein, potassium, phosphorus and sodium.

You can travel while on dialysis; you just have to contact a dialysis centre in your place of destination (or closest dialysis centre to your place of destination) and make arrangements for a treatment. If you're using CAPD, don't worry about it. Just pack your equipment and luggage and go.

You can also continue to work if you're on dialysis; you just need to arrange your work schedule around your dialysis treatments. Physical jobs involving heavy lifting, digging and so on do not mix well with kidney failure. You can't do hard labour when you're on dialysis.

Stopping dialysis

Dialysis is a medical treatment that keeps you alive. As discussed in an early chapter about stroke (Chapter 15), when someone has no quality of life, life-saving medical interventions can be withdrawn. This decision is legal and is not in any way the same thing as euthanasia, which means you use medical intervention to stop a life. In the film *Whose Life Is It Anyway?* Richard Dreyfus plays a quadriplegic who is dependent on dialysis (as most people with spinal cord injury are). Because he cannot move on his own, he feels his life does not have quality or value, and he asks for withdrawal of all medical treatment, including dialysis.

Stopping dialysis may be a decision you make yourself, or it may be a decision your "surrogate" makes (this is the person, such as a spouse or child, you appoint to make decisions on your behalf when you're not conscious or are incapacitated).

There may be other health problems behind this choice; you may be experiencing failing health as a result of stroke or cancer, for example. In these cases, you may decide to stop your dialysis treatment.

You may also decide that being on dialysis is not allowing you the quality of life you want; if this is the case, you may be a candidate for a kidney transplant (see further on), but that may involve dialysis until a donor comes forward. Depending on your age, level of mobility and other circumstances in your life, you may decide to refuse dialysis treatment and die a natural death of kidney failure. These are all choices that are yours to make and no one else's.

You may also decide to state the conditions under which dialysis should be stopped, such as in the event of a coma or stroke that leaves you with no quality of life (see Chapter 15). This is called an advanced directive. In the same way that you can stipulate in an advanced directive (a.k.a. living will) that you do not want to be resuscitated if you die of a heart attack, you can stipulate that dialysis be stopped in such an event.

Palliative Care for Kidney Failure

If your kidneys fail and you do not choose dialysis, and you are not a candidate for a kidney transplant, you can die a peaceful death from kidney failure and be made comfortable with palliative care. As the toxins build up in your body, fluid will fill your lungs and can cause shortness of breath. The fluid can be removed manually or through diuretics, which will make you comfortable. You can also be pain-free through medications, but usually kidney failure is not painful; the discomfort comes from breathing difficulties as fluids build up in the lungs. Dying from kidney failure is more like drowning and "slipping away" rather than experiencing agony and pain.

WHEN YOU WANT A KIDNEY TRANSPLANT

The good news is that you can get a new kidney when the one you have stops working. Kidney transplants are an option for people with kidney failure. That's because we have two kidneys, but can live with only one. As long as people are healthy, they can give away a kidney to someone who needs it. (In fact, kidney donation is so doable, medical ethicists are worried that some people are selling their kidneys as a way to make money, creating a scenario where the rich buy kidneys from the poor!)

Living Donors

In the film *Steel Magnolias* (which I mentioned earlier), Sally Fields plays mother to Julia Roberts, whose character has Type 1 diabetes. When Julia Roberts's kidneys fail, Sally Fields donates one kidney to her. The general rule is this: If you've got a donor, you've got a new kidney! The person donating the kidney is called a living donor. Kidney donation is similar to bone marrow donation, in that the blood type and tissues should match as closely as possible to avoid the kidney being rejected as foreign by your body. Relatives are always good bets, but you can use anybody's kidney if the match is there. With a living donor, success rates are greater than 90 percent in the first year.

Transplant Waiting Lists

If you don't know anyone willing to give you a kidney, you have to wait for a kidney from someone who has filled out a donor card on a driver's licence. Many people die each day in car accidents and other types of accidents, but unless they specify that they *want* to donate their organs, they cannot be a donor. People who donate organs after they die are called cadaver donors, which is a terrible term. I prefer the term "posthumous donor." The success rates with posthumous donors are not as high as those with living donors, but it's still about 80 percent successful for the first year.

Without a living donor, you have to be on a transplant waiting list, and the wait can be long when you factor in the blood and tissue matching. When you don't have a donor, transplant patients receive kidneys according to need, rather than "first come, first serve." But your overall health is also weighed. For example, if your kidneys are failing because you're in terrible health as a result of out-of-control diabetes and a host of other complications, a new kidney may not fare very well in your body and may eventually fail, too. Someone in better health may get a kidney faster than you because they have a greater chance of being a successful recipient.

Generally, to be considered for a transplant from either a live or posthumous donor, you must be healthy enough to have the surgery and be free from infection or other diseases, such as cancer. You must also be willing to take antirejection drugs, which can have side effects.

Preparing for a Transplant

Obviously you don't just bring your sister to a hospital and say, "Give me her kidney." Preparing for a transplant is rather involved. First, you will need to meet with a transplant surgeon or a team of transplant specialists to find out whether the risks of the transplant surgery and antirejection medications outweigh the inconveniences of dialysis. In other words, is a new kidney going to give you a better quality of life than the one you have now? In many cases, the answer is *yes*, but in a significant number of cases, the answer is *no* because of health complications.

In most transplant units, you're provided with some names of recipients you can talk to about the process. You then have to prepare for major surgery, which can be planned in advance if you have a living donor. Numerous tests and workups determine your fitness for undergoing a transplant surgery. In a nutshell, if you're a good candidate for a kidney transplant and you can find a donor, you may have a better quality of life than you do on dialysis, provided the rejection drugs used for the transplant don't cause worse side effects.

Complications run head to toe and unfortunately do not bypass the kidneys, as you can see. If you are successful in either saving your kidneys by preventing kidney disease or kidney failure, or finding success through treatments such as transplant or dialysis, don't put on your dancing shoes until you read the next chapter. You can be a "walking complication" and not even know it.

Chapter 20

FOOT NOTES

● ● ● ● ● ● ● ● ● ● ●

Foot complications related to diabetes were dramatized in the mid-1980s film *Nothing in Common,* in which Jackie Gleason plays the ne'er-do-well diabetic father, and Tom Hanks plays the son who cannot accept him. In a heartbreaking scene, Tom Hanks is shocked to discover how ill his father really is when he finally sees his feet. They are swollen, purple and badly infected. Ultimately, the story ends with the father and son coming to terms as Gleason must undergo surgical amputation.

I share this example with you because many of us are used to ignoring and abusing our feet. We wear uncomfortable shoes, we pick at our calluses and blisters, we don't wear socks with our shoes, and so on. You can't do this any more. Your feet are the targets of both macrovascular (large blood vessel) complications and microvascular (small blood vessel) complications. In the first case, peripheral vascular disease affects blood circulation to your feet. In the second place, the nerve cells to your feet, which control sensation, can be altered through microvascular complications. Nerve damage can also affect your feet's muscles and tendons, causing weakness and changes to your foot's shape.

WHAT CAN HAPPEN TO YOUR FEET

The combination of poor circulation and numbness in your feet means that you can sustain an injury to your feet and not know it. For example, you might step on a piece of glass or badly stub your toe and not realize it. If an open wound becomes infected, and you have poor circulation, the wound will not heal properly, and infection could spread to the bone or gangrene could develop. In this situation, amputation may be the only treatment. Or, without sensation or proper circulation in them, your feet could be far more vulnerable to frostbite or exposure than they would be otherwise. Diabetes can also cause your feet to thicken as a result of poor circulation. In this case the skin on the foot becomes very thin and blood vessels are visible through the skin, which has a shiny appearance and looks red. Thinner skin can be more easily pierced and infected.

As if this weren't enough for your feet, they can also be damaged from bone loss: osteoporosis of the feet! Diabetes can cause your body to take more calcium from bones. Because there are 26 bones in your foot alone, bone loss in the foot can weaken it, and it can break more easily or become deformed with bigger arches and a claw-like toe. All of this can cause calluses that can get infected, leading to gangrene and amputation, too.

Diabetes accounts for approximately half of all non-emergency amputations, but all experts agree that doing a foot self-exam every day (see below) can prevent most foot complications from becoming severe. Those most at risk for foot problems are people who still smoke (smoking aggravates *all* diabetic complications) or who are overweight (overweight people with diabetes have a 5 to 15 percent risk of undergoing amputation during their lifetime). In Winnipeg, which has a high Aboriginal Canadian population, 60 percent of all amputations are related to diabetes complications; 80 percent of those amputations could have been prevented with proper foot care.

Signs of Foot Problems

The most common symptoms of foot complications are burning, tingling or pain in your feet or legs. These are all signs of nerve damage. Numbness is another symptom that could mean nerve damage or circulation problems. If you do experience pain from nerve damage, it usually gets worse with time (as new nerves and blood vessels grow), and many people find that it's worse at night. Bed linens can actually increase discomfort. Some people notice foot symptoms only after exercising or a short walk. But many people don't notice immediate symptoms until they've lost feeling in their feet.

Other symptoms people notice are frequent infections (caused by blood vessel damage), hair loss on the toes or lower legs, or shiny skin on the lower legs and feet. Foot deformity or open wounds on the feet are also signs.

When you knock your socks off

When you take off your socks at the end of the day, get in the habit of doing a foot self-exam. This is the only way you can do damage control on your feet. You're looking for signs of infection or potential infection triggers. If you can avoid infection at all costs, you will be able to keep your feet. Look for the following signs:

- Reddened, discoloured or swollen areas (blue, bright red or white areas mean that circulation is cut off)
- Pus
- Temperature changes in the feet or "hot spots"
- Corns, calluses and warts (potential infections could be hiding under calluses; do not remove these yourself—see a podiatrist)
- Toenails that are too long (your toenail could cut you if it's too long)
- Redness where your shoes or socks are rubbing due to a poor fit (When your sock is scrunched inside your shoe, the folds could actually rub against the skin and cause a blister.)
- Toenail fungus (under the nail)
- Fungus between the toes (this is athlete's foot, common if you've been walking around barefoot in a public place)
- Breaks in the skin (especially between your toes), or cracks, such as in calluses on the heels; this opens the door for bacteria

If you find an infection, wash your feet carefully with soap and water; *don't use alcohol.* Then see your doctor or a podiatrist (a foot specialist) as soon as possible. If your foot is irritated but not yet infected (redness, for example, from poor-fitting shoes but no blister yet), simply avoid the irritant—the shoes—and it should clear up. If not, see your doctor. If you're overweight and have trouble inspecting your feet, get somebody else to check them for the signs listed above. In addition to doing a self-exam, see your doctor to have the circulation and reflexes in your feet checked four times a year.

Foot Steps

By following these "foot steps," you can prevent diabetes foot complications:

- Walk a little bit every day; this is a good way to improve blood flow and get a little exercise!
- Don't walk around barefoot; wear proper-fitting, clean cotton socks with your shoes daily, and get in the habit of wearing slippers around the house and shoes at the beach. If you're swimming, wear some sort of shoe (plastic "jellies" or canvas running shoes). This doesn't mean you have to look like

the geek who wears white sports socks with Greek sandals; there are lots of options. If it's cold out, wear woollen socks.

- Before you put on your shoes, shake them out in case something such as your (grand)child's Lego piece, a piece of dry cat food or a pebble is in there.
- Trim your toenails straight across to avoid ingrown nails. Don't pick off your nails. Use only a nail clipper, and be sure not to cut into the corners of the nails. Use a nail file or emery board to smooth or round rough edges.
- No more "bathroom surgery" on your feet, which may include puncturing blisters with needles or tweezers, shaving your calluses and the hundreds of crazy things people do to their feet (but never disclose to their spouses).
- When you're sitting down, feet should be flat on the floor. Sitting cross-legged or in crossed-legged variations can cut off your circulation—and frequently does in people without diabetes.
- Wear comfortable, proper-fitting footwear. See the box on page 295 for tips about shoe shopping.
- Avoid heat. Extreme heat, such as heating pads, very hot water and even hot sun can cause swelling or burn your feet.
- Don't wear clothing that restricts blood flow to your legs and feet, including girdles, garters, tight pantyhose or socks that cut off the circulation.
- If you're overweight, lose some weight; this will put less pressure on your feet.

The Foot Self-Exam (FSE)

Ever heard of a breast self-exam? Well, this is a foot self-exam you can do, which I've compiled from different sources. Do this each day and you can prevent serious foot complications.

1. Look for redness. Redness is a sign of irritation or pending breaks in the skin.
2. Look for breaks in the skin, which include blisters or cracks, especially between the toes. They can become infected.
3. Look for calluses, which can turn into sores or blisters.
4. Look for changes in foot shape, such as deformity.
5. Look for signs of swelling, which could also mean fluid retention related to kidney disease (see previous chapter).
6. Wash your feet and lower legs every day in lukewarm water with mild soap. Dry them really well, especially between the toes.
7. Baby your feet. When the skin seems too moist, use baby powder or a foot powder your doctor or pharmacist recommends (especially between the toes).

When your feet are too dry, moisturize them with a lotion recommended by your doctor or pharmacist. The reason is simple: Breaks in the skin happen if feet are too moist (such as between the toes) or too dry (such as cracking). Use a foot-buffing pad on your calluses after bathing.

HOW TO SHOE SHOP FOR HEALTH

To save your feet, you may not be able to save on your next pair of shoes. These are new shoe-shopping rules:

▶ Shoe shop at the time of day when your feet are most swollen (such as afternoons). That way, you'll purchase a shoe that fits you in "bad times" as well as good times.

▶ Don't even think about high heels or any type of shoe that is not comfortable or that doesn't fit properly. Say goodbye to thongs. That strip between your toe can cause too much irritation.

▶ Buy leather; avoid shoes with the terms "man-made upper" or "man-made materials" on the label; this means the shoes are made of synthetic materials and your foot will not breathe. Cotton or canvas shoes are fine, as long as the insole is cotton, too. Synthetic materials on the very bottom of the shoe are fine as long as the upper — the part of the shoe that touches your foot — is leather, cotton, canvas or something breathable.

▶ Remember that leather does, indeed, stretch. When that happens, the shoe could become loose and cause blisters. On the other hand, if the shoe is too tight and the salesperson tells you the shoe will stretch, forget it. The shoe will destroy you in the first few hours of wear, which sort of "defeets" the purpose.

▶ If you lose all sensation and cannot "feel" whether the shoe is fitting, make sure you have a shoe salesperson fit you.

▶ Avoid shoes that have been on display. A variety of people try these shoes on; you never know what bacteria and fungi these previously tried-on shoes harbour.

WHEN YOU HAVE AN OPEN WOUND

Open wounds on the feet are also called "foot ulcers" and affect between 80,000 and 200,000 Canadians with diabetes; about 20 percent of diabetes-related foot ulcers don't heal, leading to amputation to prevent gangrene. Any tear in the skin can lead to an open wound that becomes infected. Blisters, cracks in the feet from dryness and stepping on something sharp (see above) are the most common causes of open wounds.

Healing Open Wounds

The first order of business is removing the source of irritation that caused the sore, such as bad shoes or poor hygiene (see "Foot Steps" above). In many cases antibiotics can heal the wounds, as well as dressing the wound well (cleaning it, using proper bandages and so on). Keeping pressure off the feet can also help to heal them. Often healing a foot ulcer requires home care; you may need to have a nurse or home health care worker come into your home and dress your wounds. When wounds are open and not healing well, an odour can develop that is very unpleasant. Waiting for your daily dressing while you heal your foot sore can be pretty isolating and depressing for many people. One experience with this is often enough for you to take prevention steps seriously (see above).

When wounds don't heal

Not all open wounds heal. To heal cuts, sores or any open wound, your body normally manufactures macrophages, special white blood cells that fight infection, as well as special repair cells, called fibroblasts. These "ambulance cells" need oxygen to live. If you have poor circulation, it's akin to an ambulance not making it to an accident scene in time because it gets caught in a long traffic jam.

When wounds don't heal, gangrene infections can set in. Until recently, amputating the infected limb was the only way to deal with gangrene. But a new therapy is available at several hospitals throughout Canada called hyperbaric oxygen therapy (HBO). The procedure involves placing you in an oxygen chamber or tank and feeding you triple the amount of oxygen you'd find in the normal atmosphere. To heal gangrene on the feet, you'd need about 30 treatments (several per day for a week or so). The result is that your tissues become saturated with oxygen, enabling the body to heal itself. In one research trial, 89 percent of diabetics with foot gangrene were healed, compared to 1 percent of the control group. This treatment sounds expensive, but it's much cheaper than surgery, which is why HBO is catching on.

Not everybody is an HBO candidate, and not everybody in Canada has access to this therapy. But if you're being considered for surgical amputation, you should definitely ask about HBO first.

There are also two new wound-healing products on the market. One is "replaceable skin" called Dermagraft, which is made of skin cells that are grown in a lab. Dermagraft is applied once a week to the wound and actually replenishes the skin. Another product, Regranex, contains natural growth factors in our skin cells and comes in a gel applied once a day to jump-start healing. These products don't always work, but are a good option for wounds that won't heal.

WHEN YOU REQUIRE AN AMPUTATION

Many people are amputees, including former Quebec premier Lucien Bouchard. When you require an amputation to stop a gangrene infection, there are a few ways you can maximize your health prior to surgery; they'll also help you heal after surgery.

Quit smoking. (See Chapter 2 for more details on smoking-cessation programs.) Smoking restricts your blood vessels, as I've said many times in this book. You need your blood vessels to be as healthy as possible prior to surgery and after.

The next step is to review with your surgeon the risks of general anaesthetic over what's called "continuous epidural anaesthetic," which has lower risks. Discuss whether the continuous epidural anaesthetic can be continued for a few days after the procedure to decrease phantom sensations and pain.

Ask whether your nerves will be anaesthetized, too; they should be injected with a long-acting local anaesthetic before they're severed during the procedure. Find an amputee support group on-line. There are quite a few. It's important to be in touch with others who have been through this procedure. It lessens your isolation and fears. You can reach out across the border, too. For example, the Amputee Coalition of America networks with thousands of amputees across the United States. They can be reached at 800-355-8772.

Getting an Artificial Limb

Artificial limbs are also called prosthetic limbs, or simply a prosthesis. In Canada, some of the costs for the prosthesis are covered by the province (usually about 70 percent of the costs are covered). If you have private health insurance on top of that, through your job, for example, it will cover the rest of the costs. You can also look into non-profit agencies for help.

Doctors do not have prosthetic limbs you can purchase. You have to go to a special artisan of sorts, known as an orthotist or prosthetist, a person who is trained in making artificial limbs and understands amputees' needs. The orthotist or prosthetist must have a doctor's prescription before they make the limb. Some prosthetic companies have catalogues, allowing you to order direct, and sometimes bypassing the prescription, but it's best to be fitted for a limb in person and to work directly with a prosthetist. Ordering from the Internet or a catalogue is akin to ordering a breast implant from a catalogue: You should be fitted. Amputees recommend shopping around for an orthotist or prosthetist; the limb prices vary wildly from manufacturer to manufacturer and prosthetist to prosthetist.

Most prosthetists are willing to work with you and answer the many questions you may have about how the limb is made, durability, ranges of motions and so on.

ASKING THE RIGHT QUESTIONS WHEN SHOPPING FOR ARTIFICIAL LIMBS

1. What is the alignment of the limb? Refers to the position of prosthetic socket in relation to foot and knee.

2. Is this assistive or adaptive equipment? Refers to devices that assist in performance or mobility, including ramps and bars, changes in furniture heights, environmental control units and specially designed devices.

3. Will you prepare a check socket, or test socket? This is a trial socket, which is often transparent, made to evaluate comfort and fit prior to the final prosthesis design.

4. What is a control cable? This is a steel cable used to move and lock mechanical joints and to operate body-powered prostheses.

5. What material will you use for the cosmetic cover? This refers to the material from which the surface of the limb is made, giving it a more natural appearance. Materials used could be plastic, foam, rubber laminate or stocking. An endoskeletal limb is one in which the prosthesis consists of a lightweight plastic or metal tube encased in a foam cover.

An exoskeletal limb is a prosthesis made of plastic over wood or rigid foam.

6. Will it be made with energy-storing feet? This refers to prosthetic feet with plastic springs or carbon fibres designed to help move the prosthesis forward.

7. Will it be designed with knee components? This refers to devices designed to create a safe, smooth walking pattern.

8. Will it have a single axis? This refers to a free-swinging knee with a small amount of friction.

9. Will it have stance control? This refers to a friction device with an adjustable brake mechanism to add stability.

10. Will this limb be polycentric? This refers to a multiple-axis joint, which is particularly useful with a very long residual limb.

11. Will it have manual locking? This refers to a device that locks the knee in complete extension to prevent buckling and falls.

12. Will it have pneumatic or hydraulic controls? This provides controlled changes in the speed of walking.

13. Will it be a myoelectric prosthesis? This means it has electrodes mounted within the socket to receive signals from muscle contraction to control a motor in the terminal device, wrist rotator or elbow.

14. Will it have nudge control? This is a mechanical switch that operates one or more joints of the prosthesis.

15. Will I see a preparatory prosthesis before the "definitive" prosthesis? "Definitive" means the final product, which meets accepted clinical standards for comfort, fit, alignment, function, appearance and durability. A preparatory prosthesis refers to a short-term prosthesis, generally without cosmetic finishing, which is provided in the early phase of fitting to expedite prosthetic wear and use; it also aids in the evaluation of amputee adjustment and component selection.

16. How is the socket constructed? This refers to a portion of the prosthesis that fits around the residual limb or stump and to which prosthetic components are attached. A "hard socket" is a prosthetic socket made of rigid materials; a "soft socket" refers to the inner socket liner of foam, rubber, leather or other material for cushioning the residual limb.

17. What materials will be designed to protect my residual limb (or "stump")? Ask about things such as a stockinette (a tubular open-ended cotton or nylon material); a stump sock (a wool or cotton sock worn over a residual limb to provide a cushion between the skin and socket interface); and a stump shrinker (an elastic wrap or compression sock worn on a residual limb to reduce swelling and shape the limb).

Source: Questions above compiled from material retrieved in July 2001 from the Amputee Web Site www.amputee-online.com.

Some Surprising Sexual Issues

When I was researching this section, it became apparent that new amputees are unprepared for a surprising and sometimes disturbing issue—encountering someone with a "stump fetish." This is a type of sexual fetish that can be very disturbing for people who have just undergone amputation. A person with such a fetish is called an acrotomophile. On the amputee Web sites, they are also called "devotees," a somewhat kinder label. Acrotomophiles tend to pose as "fellow amputees" in chat rooms on the Internet, inviting e-mail exchanges and so on. The e-mails can then develop into very solicitous and unpleasant sexual invitations that can really disturb you. Some acrotomophiles are open and honest about their fetish, and if you don't mind, that's fine. But many are covert about their fetishes and can be very manipulative. You may also be approached in public if you are on crutches or in a wheelchair.

Encounters with acrotomophiles are more likely if you're sexually active and single. Women are harassed more than men, and because of gender roles, they may fall prey to an acrotomophile unwittingly. Stay alert, and look this subject up on the Internet. The information on "devotees" is abundant.

HOW TO COMBAT HARASSING E-MAIL

1. *Do not* respond to any of the e-mails. If you have any filtering capabilities on your e-mail program, use them. Eudora Pro (for Mac and Windows) has extensive filtering capabilities, which might be worth the small investment; you will never see the e-mails once the software is configured correctly.

2. Contact the postmaster@domain.xxx. If the Internet service provider is aboveboard, the company is obligated to notify their client that a complaint has been received. If the deviant behaviour continues, the harasser will have his or her Internet account or privileges revoked.

3. If you get no satisfaction or results with the Internet service provider, contact your own service provider with the domain name of the harasser and copies of the offending e-mail. The ISP can track down where the e-mail has been routed from and locate the source of the e-mail. (AOL and similar on-line services that can change user addresses easily are often the source of unwanted e-mail.)

4. You can also perform your own research with any major Web search engine. Simply perform a Web search under a domain name such as "portal.ca." You should be able to find where that ISP is located from a Web search.

5. Contact the authorities in that city or town. Contacting the police or university campus security may not result in a conviction, but it may result in a visit to the offending person's front door, which can have an interesting way of changing one's behaviour. If the harasser is sending mail from a company address, contact the person's superior or postmaster.

Source: Reprinted with permission from the Amputee Web Site www.amputee-online.com.

APPENDIX I
A BRIEF HISTORY OF DIABETES

● ● ● ● ● ● ● ● ● ● ●

1552 B.C.: Earliest known record of diabetes mentioned on Third-Dynasty Egyptian papyrus by physician Hesy-Ra; mentions polyuria (frequent urination) as a symptom.

First Century A.D.: Diabetes described by Arateus as "the melting down of flesh and limbs into urine."

A.D. 164: Greek physician Galen of Pergamum mistakenly diagnoses diabetes as an ailment of the kidneys.

Up to 11th Century: Diabetes commonly diagnosed by "water tasters," who drank the urine of people suspected of having diabetes; the urine of people with diabetes was thought to be sweet-tasting. *Mellitus*, the Latin word for honey (referring to its sweetness) is added to the term *diabetes* as a result.

1500s: Swiss-born alchemist and physician Paracelsus identifies diabetes as a serious general disorder.

Early 1800s: First chemical tests developed to indicate and measure the presence of sugar in urine.

1800s: French researcher Claude Bernard studies the workings of the pancreas and the glycogen metabolism of the liver.

1800s: Czech researcher I.V. Pavlov discovers the links between the nervous system and gastric secretion, making an important contribution to science's knowledge of the physiology of the digestive system.

Late 1800s: Italian diabetes specialist Catoni isolates his patients under lock and key in order to get them to follow their diets.

Late 1850s: French physician Priorry advises diabetes patients to eat extra-large quantities of sugar as a treatment.

1870s: French physician Bouchardat notices the disappearance of glycosuria in his diabetes patients during the rationing of food in Paris while under siege by Germany during the Franco-Prussian War; formulates idea of individualized diets for his diabetes patients.

1869: Paul Langerhans, a German medical student, announces in a dissertation that the pancreas contains two systems of cells. One set secretes normal pancreatic juice; the function of the other was unknown. Several years later, these cells are identified as the islets of Langerhans.

1889: Oskar Minkowski and Joseph von Mering at the University of Strasbourg, Austria, first remove the pancreas from a dog to determine the effect of an absent pancreas on digestion. They proved that without its pancreas a dog becomes severely diabetic. They also showed through experiments with duct ligation (surgically tying off different parts of tissue) that the pancreas indeed has two secretions: the *external* (which fed directly into the bloodstream and regulated carbohydrate metabolism) and a mysterious *internal* secretion, which appeared to be the "missing secretion" in diabetics. This connection between diabetes and the pancreas resulted in a series of early experiments using pancreatic extracts to treat animals and humans. But unfortunately, these experiments didn't work and even served to challenge the entire hypothesis of this internal secretion.

November 14, 1891: Frederick Banting born near Alliston, Ontario. His parents, devout Methodists, try to pressure their son into joining the ministry; however, Banting enrols in medical school at the University of Toronto in 1912 instead.

February 28, 1899: Charles Best born in West Pembroke, Maine.

1900–1915: "Fad" diabetes diets include the "oat-cure" (in which the majority of the diet was made up of oatmeal), the milk diet, the rice cure, "potato therapy," and even the use of opium.

1906: German scientist Georg Zuelzer makes some interesting progress on June 21, 1906. He injects pancreatic extract under the skin of a comatose 50-year-old diabetic. The man is momentarily revived, reinforcing the connection between pancreatic extract (a.k.a. pancreatic secretion) and diabetes. Zuelzer obtains funding from the Schering drug company to produce a viable extract for therapy. By 1907, he produces what appears to be a workable pancreatic extract, but the Schering company decides that the results of his work don't justify their costs and pulls funding. This was a shame, considering that Zuelzer's formula was the first pancreatic extract to suppress *glycosuria* (sugary urine). Unfortunately, Zuelzer's extract also causes many toxic side effects—what we know today as insulin shock. What should have been a major breakthrough in research is viewed by pancreatic researchers as a setback. Caution rules, and the risks of these "toxic side effects" interferes with many pancreatic extract experiments.

1910–1920: Frederick Madison Allen and Elliot P. Joslin emerge as the two leading diabetes specialists in the United States. Joslin believes diabetes to be "the best of the chronic diseases" because it is "clean, seldom unsightly, not contagious, often painless and susceptible to treatment."

1913: After three years of diabetes study, Frederick Allen publishes *Studies Concerning Glycosuria and Diabetes*, a book that is significant for the revolution in diabetes therapy that developed from it. J.J.R. Macleod, a professor of medicine at the University of Toronto, publishes a book called *Diabetes: Its Pathological Physiology*. Library records show that Frederick Banting borrowed Macleod's book for his research in 1920.

1919: Frederick Allen publishes *Total Dietary Regulation in the Treatment of Diabetes*, citing exhaustive case records of 76 of the 100 diabetes patients he observed, and becomes the director of diabetes research at the Rockefeller Institute.

1919–1920: Frederick Allen establishes the first treatment clinic in the United States, the Physiatric Institute in New Jersey, to treat patients with diabetes, high blood pressure and Bright's disease; wealthy and desperate patients flock to it.

July 1, 1920: Dr. Banting opens his first office in London, Ontario; he receives his first patient on July 29; total earnings for his first month of work are $4.

October 30, 1920: Dr. Banting conceives of the idea of insulin after reading

Moses Barron's "The Relation of the Islets of Langerhans to Diabetes with Special Reference to Cases of Pancreatic Lithiasis" in the November issue of *Surgery, Gynecology and Obstetrics*. In fact, Banting's notebook from that night is fully preserved at the Academy of Medicine in Toronto. In it he writes, "Diabetus. Ligate pancreatic ducts of dogs. Keep dogs alive till acini degenerate leaving Islets. Try to isolate the internal secretion of these to relieve glycosurea."

November 1920: Banting approaches Dr. J.J.R. Macleod with his idea. In that meeting, Macleod apparently brings Banting up to date on a variety of research attempts in the area of pancreatic extract. Macleod concedes that no one thought about the fact that the digestive agents of the pancreas may be responsible for destroying the secretion made by the islets of Langerhans. Banting proposes to Macleod that by using duct-ligated pancreases to make an extract, which would destroy the digestive secretions, they could find a treatment for diabetes. (Macleod was apparently irritated by Banting's clear lack of knowledge in the area of diabetes. Nevertheless, it is a damned good idea! Macleod, it would appear, was sorry the idea never occurred to him.) For the next year, with the assistance of Charles H. Best, J.B. Collip and J.J.R. Macleod, Dr. Banting continues his research using a variety of different extracts on de-pancreatized dogs.

December 30, 1921: Dr. Banting presents a paper entitled "The Beneficial Influences of Certain Pancreatic Extracts on Pancreatic Diabetes," summarizing his work to this point at a session of the American Physiological Society at Yale University. Among the attendees are Frederick Allen and Elliot Joslin. Little praise or congratulation is received.

January 23, 1922: One of Banting's insulin extracts is first tested on a human being, a 14-year-old boy named Leonard Thompson, in Toronto; treatment considered a success by the end of the following February.

May 21, 1922: James Havens becomes the first American successfully treated with insulin.

May 30, 1922: Pharmaceutical manufacturer Eli Lilly and Company and the University of Toronto collaborate on the mass production of insulin in North America.

October 25, 1923: Dr. Banting and Dr. Macleod awarded the Nobel Prize for Medicine; Banting shares his award with Best; Macleod then shares his award with Collip. (History would not remember Macleod's nor Collip's role in the discovery of insulin. While Banting, Best, Collip and Macleod would privately acknowledge they were a team, they could never admit it to each other. For Banting's obituary tribute, Collip wrote that his own contribution to insulin was trivial compared to Banting's. Banting apparently admitted in his later years that he and Best wouldn't have "achieved a damned thing" without Collip.*)

1934: Dr. Banting is knighted and becomes Sir Frederick Banting.

February 21, 1941: Sir Frederick Banting is killed in an airplane crash over Newfoundland while en route to England.

1971: 50th anniversary of the discovery of insulin celebrated worldwide.

1996: 75th anniversary of the discovery of insulin celebrated.**

* In 1978, Banting's first biographer, Lloyd Stevenson, published an article that contained Macleod's personal account of the insulin discovery. Although Macleod had died in 1935, the University of Toronto did not want to reopen old wounds and for many years prevented the publication of that account. Macleod's account was bitter. He left the University of Toronto in 1928 and returned to Scotland as Regius Professor at the University of Aberdeen; it is believed that he moved away from Toronto because he couldn't stand living in the shadow of Banting's idea.

Charles Best replaced Macleod as professor of physiology at the University of Toronto when he was just 29 years old. He went on to enjoy a long, distinguished career and many awards and honours until he died in 1978. Best continued Macleod's work on the properties of insulin and received delayed credit for insulin's discovery after Banting's death in 1941. The Best Institute was erected next door to the Banting Institute in 1953.

J.B. Collip attempted to invent another version of insulin he called *gluclokinin*, and then abandoned it. He is also known for pioneering work on parathyroid hormone. Collip received his M.D. and eventually became Chair of Biochemistry at McGill University. He became a world-renowned endocrinologist in Canada, and in 1947 was made Dean of Medicine at the very university that triggered Banting's idea: the University of Western Ontario. Collip enjoyed a great career and died in 1965 at the age of 72.

** New evidence challenges whether Canadians have the right to claim complete ownership of the insulin discovery at all. Romanian scientist Nicolas Paulesco, who was concentrating on measuring the impact of *his* pancreatic extract (called "pancreine") on blood sugar, likely would have been the discoverer of insulin had we Canadians not beaten him to human testing. In 1971, on the 50th anniversary of the discovery of insulin, a campaign was launched by Bucharest medical students to honour Paulesco's work and give him due credit.

SOURCES

Bliss, Michael. "Rewriting Medical History," *Journal of History of Medicine and Allied Sciences, Inc.*, 1993, Vol. 48: 253–74.

_____. *Banting: A Biography.* Toronto: McClelland & Stewart, 1984.

_____.*The Discovery of Insulin.* Toronto: McClelland & Stewart, 1982.

Canadian Diabetes Association. *Diabetes Timeline*. Toronto: The Canadian Diabetes Association, 1997.

Williams, Michael J. "J.J.R. Macleod: The Co-discoverer of Insulin." *Proceedings of the Royal College of Physicians of Edinburgh*, July 1993, Vol. 23, No. 3.

APPENDIX 2
WHERE TO GO FOR MORE INFORMATION

● ● ● ● ● ● ● ● ● ●

Note: This list was compiled from dozens of sources. Because of the nature of many health and non-profit organizations, some of the addresses and phone numbers below may have changed since this list was compiled. For Web site addresses, please see Appendix 3.

DIABETES ORGANIZATIONS

Canadian Diabetes Association
National Office
15 Toronto St., Suite 800
Toronto, Ont.
M5C 2E3
ph. 416-363-3373
fax 416-363-3393

Alberta/NWT Division
Suite 1010, Royal Bank Building
10117 Jasper Ave., N.W.
Edmonton, Alta.

T5J 1W8
ph. (403) 423-1232/1-800-563-0032
fax (403) 423-3322

British Columbia/Yukon Division
1091 West 8th Ave.
Vancouver, B.C.
V6H 2V3
ph. (604) 732-1331/1-800-665-6526
fax (604) 732-8444

Manitoba Division
102-310 Broadway
Winnipeg, Man.
R3C 0S6
ph. (204) 925-3800/1-800-782-0175
fax (204) 949-0266

New Brunswick Division
165 Regent St., Suite 3
Fredericton, N.B.
E3B 7B4
ph. (506) 452-9009/1-800-884-4232
fax (506) 455-4728

Newfoundland and Labrador Division
354 Water St., Suite 217
St. John's, Nfld.
A1C 1C4
ph. (709) 754-0953
fax (709) 754-0734

Nova Scotia Division
6080 Young St., Suite 101
Halifax, N.S.
ph. (902) 453-4232
fax (902) 453-4440

Prince Edward Island Division
P.O. Box 133
Charlottetown, PEI
C1A 7K2
ph. (902) 894-3005
fax (902) 368-1928

Association Diabete Quebec
(Quebec CDA Affiliate)
5635 Sherbrooke Ave. East
Montreal, Que.
H1N 1A2
ph. (514) 259-3422
fax (514) 259-9286

Saskatchewan Division
104-2301 Avenue C.N.
Saskatoon, Sask.
S7L 5Z5
ph. (306) 933-4446/1-800-996-4446
fax (306) 244-2012

Juvenile Diabetes Foundation Canada
89 Granton Dr.
Richmond Hill, Ont.
L4B 2N5
ph. (905) 889-4171/1-800-668-0274
fax (905) 889-4209

DIABETES EDUCATION HOSPITALS

Note: This list is not exhaustive; it is intended as a "starting point" for English-speaking Canadians looking for specific hospitals across the country that provide diabetes education.

Alberta
Mista Hia Regional Health Authority
Grande Prairie Health Unit
10320-99 St.
Grande Prairie, Alta. T8V 6J4
ph. (403) 532-4441
fax (403) 532-1550

University of Alberta Hospitals
2F2 Metabolic Center
Brenda Cook, RD
8440-112 St.
Edmonton, Alta. T6G 2B7
ph. (403) 492-6696
fax (403) 492-8291

Clinical Nutrition Services
Foothills Hospital
1403-29th St. NW
Calgary, Alta. T2N 2T9
ph. (403) 670-1522
fax (403) 670-1848

British Columbia
University of Northern British Columbia
Department of Community Health
3333 University Way
Prince George, B.C. V2N 4Z9
ph. (250) 960-5671
fax (250) 960-5743

S. Okanagan Diabetes Education Program
S. Okanagan Health Unit
740 Carmi Ave.
Penticton, B.C. V2A 8P9
ph. (250) 770-3492
fax (250) 770-3470

Diabetes Education Program
1305 Summit Ave.
Prince Rupert, B.C. V8J 2A6
ph. (250) 624-0294
fax (250) 627-1244

Manitoba
Manitoba Health
(Teaching text for Type 2 diabetes
and Aboriginal population)
303-800 Portage Ave.
Winnipeg, Man. R3G 0N4
ph. (204) 945-6735
fax (204) 948-2040

Maritimes
Nova Scotia Diabetes Center
Queen Elizabeth II Health Science Center
Gerrard Hall, 5303 Morris St., 2nd Floor
Halifax, N.S. B3J 1B6
ph. (902) 496-3722
fax (902) 496-3726

Ontario
Diabetes Education Centre
Doctors Hospital
340 College St., Suite 560
Toronto, Ont. M5T 3A9
ph. 416-963-5288
fax 416-923-1370

Mount Sinai Hospital
600 University Ave.
Toronto, Ont. M5G 1X5
ph. 416-586-4800
fax 416-586-8785

Tri-Hospital Diabetes Education Centre (TRIDEC)
[All Toronto hospital patients referred here]
Women's College Hospital
60 Grosvenor St.
Toronto, Ont. M5S 1B6
ph. 416-323-6170
fax 416-323-6085

Diabetes Care and Research Center
Chedoke McMaster Hospitals
McMaster Division, 1200 Main St. West
Hamilton, Ont. L8S 4J9
ph. (905) 521-2100 Ext. 6818
fax (905) 521-2653

Education Department
Hamilton Civic Hospitals
General Division
Robert Panchyson, BScN
237 Barton St. East
Hamilton, Ont. L8L 2X2
ph. (905) 527-4322 Ext. 6245

Hamilton Civic Hospitals
(Patient Teaching)
711 Concession St.
Hamilton, Ont. L8V 1C3
ph. (905) 527-4322 Ext. 2024, Paging 2110
fax (905) 575-2641

Diabetes Education Centre
Kitchener-Waterloo Health Centre
Grand River Hospital
835 King St. West
Kitchener, Ont. N2G 1G3
ph. (519) 749-4300
fax (519) 749-4317

Sioux Lookout Diabetes Program
Box 163, 73 King St.
Sioux Lookout, Ont.
P8T 1A3
ph. (807) 737-4422
fax (897) 737-2603
E-mail: slktdiab@sioux-lookout.lakeheadu.ca

Lawrence Commanda Diabetes
Education & Resource Centre
Ken Goulais, Resource Clerk
24 Semo Rd.
Garden Village, R.R. #1, Sturgeon Falls, Ont.
P0H 2G0
ph. (705) 753-3355
fax (705) 753-4116

Porcupine Health Unit
Teresa Taillefer
Bag 2012
Timmins, Ont. P4N 8B2
ph. (705) 267-1181
fax (705) 264-3989

Quebec
SMBD Jewish General Hospital
Diabetes Clinic
Pav. E104
3755 Cote St. Catherine Rd.
Montreal, Que. H3T 1E2
ph. (514) 340-8222, Loc. 5787
fax (514) 340-7529

Saskatchewan
Royal University Hospital
103 Hospital Dr.
Saskatoon, Sask. S7N 0W0
ph. (306) 655-2615
fax (306) 655-1044

DIETITIANS

Dietitians of Canada
480 University Ave., Suite 601
Toronto, Ont.
M5G 1V2
phone: 416-596-0857
fax: 416-596-0603
www.dietitians.ca

FOOD/NUTRITION

Canadian Organic Growers Inc.
National Branch
Box 6408, Station J
Ottawa, Ont.
K2A 3Y6

National Institute of Nutrition
302-265 Carling Ave.
Ottawa, Ont.
K1S 2E1
ph. (613) 235-3355
fax (613) 235-7032

HEART AND STROKE

Heart and Stroke Foundation of Canada
222 Queen Street, Suite 1402
Ottawa, Ont. K1P 5V9
ph. (613) 569-4361
fax (613) 569-3278
www.na.heartandstroke.ca

KIDNEY

The Kidney Foundation of Canada
National Branch
5165 Sherbrooke Ave. West, Suite 300
Montreal, Que.
H4A 1T6
ph. 1-800-361-7494

MEDIC ALERT

MedicAlert Foundation
250 Ferrand Dr., Suite 301
Postal Station Don Mills, Box 9800
Toronto, Ont.
M3C 2T9
ph. 1-800-668-1507
Local Toronto: 416-696-0267

PODIATRISTS

Canadian Podiatric Medical Association
2 Sheppard Ave. East, Suite 900
Willowdale, Ont.
M2N 5Y7
ph. 416-927-9111/1-888-220-3338
fax 416-733-2491

VISUALLY IMPAIRED/BLIND REHABILITATION

Canadian National Institute for the Blind
National Office
320 McLeod St.
Ottawa, Ont.
K2P 1A3
ph. (613) 563-4021
fax (613) 563-1898

OUTSIDE OF CANADA

Belgium
International Diabetes Federation (IDF)
40 Rue Washington
1050, Brussels, Belgium
32-3/647-4414
www.idf.org

United States
American Association of Diabetes Educators
444 N. Michigan Ave., Suite 1240
Chicago, Ill., 60611
ph. (312) 644-2233
www.aadenet.org

The American Diabetes Association
ADA National Service Center
1660 Duke St.
Alexandria, Va., 22314
ph. (703) 549-1500
www.diabetes.org

International Diabetic Athletes Association
1647-B West Bethany Home Road
Phoenix, Ariz., 85015
ph. (602) 433-2113

TOLL-FREE HOTLINES

American Dietetic Association and National Center for Nutrition and Dietetics
(NCND) Consumer Nutrition Hot Line (1-800-366-1655)

The Becel Heart Health
Information Bureau
ph. 1-800-563-5574
fax 1-800-442-3235

LifeScan TELELIBRARY
1-800-847-SCAN (7226)

LifeScan Customer Care Line
1-800-663-5521
Lilly/BMC Diabetes Care
ph. 1-800-361-2070
fax (514) 668-7009

McNeil Consumers
ph. 1-800-561-0070

Monoject Diabetes Care Products
Sherwood Medical Industries Canada Inc.
ph. 1-800-661-1903

Novo Nordisk Canada Inc.
ph. 1-800-465-4334/(905) 629-4222
fax (905) 629-2596

Pharma Plus Pharma Answers Phone Line
(24 hour access to a pharmacist)
ph. 1-800-511-INFO

APPENDIX 3
LINKS FROM
sarahealth.com

● ● ● ● ● ● ● ● ●

For more information about disease prevention and wellness, visit me on-line at www.sarahealth.com, where you will find over 300 links—including these—related to your good health and wellness.

- Abbott Laboratories: www.abbott.com
- About.com (Diabetes):
  http://diabetes.about.com.health/diabetes/mbody.htm
- American Diabetes Association: www.diabetes.org
- American Association of Clinical Endocrinologists: www.aace.com
- Amputation Prevention Global Resource Center: prevention, causes, signs and symptoms, treatment. www.diabetesresource.com
- Bayer Corp: www.glucometer.com/product.htm
- Blindness and Diabetes Resource and Support: includes back issues of the "Voice of the Diabetic" from the National Federation of the Blind. www.prevent-blindness.org
- Canadian Diabetes Association: www.diabetes.ca
- Canadian National Institute for the Blind: www.cnib.ca
- Canadian Organic Growers Association: www.cog.ca

- Chronimed Inc: www.chronimed.com
- Diabetes.com (Diabetes and Sexual Intimacy): award-winning site with health library, products and prescriptions, newsroom. www.diabetes.com/site
- Diabetic Gourmet Magazine: free newsletter, daily tidbits, menus and forum. http://gourmetconnection.com/diabetic
- Diabetes mall: targets both a general audience and medical professionals. Information about research, prevention and education. With support group. www.diabetesnet.com/index.html
- Diabetes monitor: great source of patient information, research, statistics and education. Registry of links. www.diabetesmonitor.com
- Diabetes Type II Resource and Discussion Page: information specific to those with Type II Diabetes. http://home.ptd.net/~hwagner/2r.htm
- Diabetes Type 2—from the American Medical Association; symptoms, screening, diagnosis, complications, etc. www.ama-assn.org/insight/spe_con/diabetes.htm
- HealthNet-Diabetes: treatment, patient education, advice. www.healthnet.com
- The Islet Foundation: foundation dedicated to finding a cure for insulin-dependent diabetes. Interesting resources and information on the future of diabetes. www.islet.org
- The Kidney Foundation of Canada: www.kidney.ca
- Life Scan Inc: U.S.— www.lifescan.com / Canada — www.lifescan-can.com
- LXN Corp: www.lxncorp.com
- Managing your Diabetes: official site of Eli Lilly & Co. Lots of great information about diabetes products. http://diabetes.lilly.com
- Medic Alert: site of the trademarked Medic Alert emblem. www.medicalert.org
- Medic Alert: www.medicalert.ca
- National Diabetes Fact Sheet (from the U.S. Center for Disease Control and Prevention): www.cdc.gov/diabetes
- National Diabetes Information Clearinghouse (and diabetes database): www.niddk.nih.gov/NDIC/NDIC.html
- National Institute of Diabetes and Digestive Kidney Disease: www.niddk.nih.gov

- NutraSweet: facts about this artificial sugar substitute. www.alaskanet:/80/~tne
- Olestra: information about this synthetic fat product now available in the U.S. www.diabetesmonitor.com/olestra.htm
- Polymer Tech Systems Inc: www.diabetes-testing.com
- QuestStar Medical Inc: www.queststarmedical.com
- Recipe of the Day: features a new healthy recipe every day, Monday through Thursday. From the ADA. www.diabetes.org/ada/rcptoday.html
- The Roche Group (Accu-Check): www.roche.com

GLOSSARY

● ● ● ● ● ● ● ● ● ●

Note: Some definitions below also appear in The Diabetes Dictionary, *found at the Web site of The Canadian Diabetes Association at www.diabetes.ca.*

Adrenaline: a hormone your body secretes that creates "fight-or-flight" symptoms of increased heart rate, sweating, nervousness, dizziness and so on.

Aerobic activity: any activity that causes the heart to pump harder and faster, causing you to breathe faster, which increases the level of oxygen in the bloodstream.

Alpha-glucosidase inhibitors (a.k.a. acarbose or Prandase): drugs that delay the breakdown of sugar in your meal.

Andrologist: a doctor who specializes in male reproductive problems.

Antioxidants: vitamins A, C, E and beta carotene, found in coloured (i.e., non-green) fruits and vegetables. Antioxidants prevent the oxidation of cell membranes, which can lead to cancer; they are the "cancer-fighting GIs."

Autoimmune disease: a disease in which a person's own antibodies destroy body tissues, such as the beta cells in the pancreas, which is what occurs in Type 1 diabetes.

Betaglucan: a phytochemical found in legumes, oats and other grains that is believed to help prevent diabetes by delaying gastric emptying and by slowing down glucose absorption in the small intestine.

Biguanides (Metformin): a type of oral hypoglycemic agent.

Binge-eating disorder: refers to compulsive overeating, or bingeing without purging.

Bulimia nervosa: bingeing followed by purging in the form of self-induced vomiting, laxative or diuretic abuse, or abusing other medications to induce weight loss.

Carbohydrates: the building blocks of most foods, which provide energy to the body to fuel the central nervous system; they help the body use vitamins, minerals, amino acids and other nutrients.

Certified Diabetes Educator (CDE): a healthcare provider who has taken a diabetes educator certification course; teaches diabetes patients about diet and management.

Cholesterol: a whitish, waxy fat made in vast quantities by the liver. (See also HDL; LDL)

Community Health Representative (CHR): someone from the community who works with you and your family, as well as with other health care professionals, to educate you about various health issues, including diabetes.

Complex carbohydrates: more sophisticated foods that have larger molecules in them, such as grain foods and foods high in fibre.

Creatinine: waste products produced by the muscles and released by the kidneys.

Cystitis: urinary tract infection (UTI) resulting in an inflammation of the bladder lining.

Dextrose tablets: tablets that contain pure dextrose to boost the blood sugar level quickly in case of hypoglycemia.

Diabetes: a condition in which the body either cannot produce insulin or cannot effectively use the insulin it produces.

Diabetic ketoacidosis (DKA): an emergency that can lead to death; signs of DKA include frequent urination, excessive thirst, excessive hunger and a fruity smell to your breath.

Diabetic neuropathy: diabetic nerve disease; occurs when the cells that make up nerves are altered in response to high blood sugar.

Diabetic retinopathy: diabetes eye disease, characterized by damage to the back of the eye or retina, and other problems.

Diastolic pressure: one of the readings in a blood pressure measurement; the pressure occurring when the heart rests between contractions.

Dysmotility: occurs when the muscles in the digestive tract become uncoordinated, causing bloating, abdominal pain and reflux (heartburn).

Edema: the swelling or puffiness caused by fluid collecting in the tissues. Also known as "water retention."

End-stage renal disease: a term used to describe advanced stage kidney failure.

Erythroepoetin: a hormone produced by the kidneys that helps bone marrow to make red blood cells.

Fasting blood glucose readings: what your blood sugar levels are before you've eaten (normally between 3.5 and 7 mmol/L).

Fatty acids: crucial nutrients for cells, which also regulate hormone production.

Fibre: part of a plant that cannot be digested; can lower cholesterol levels or improve regularity; also causes a slower rise in glucose levels, which lowers the body's insulin requirements.

Fructose: a monosaccharide or single sugar that combines with glucose to form sucrose and is one and a half times sweeter than sucrose.

Functional foods: foods that have significant levels of biologically active disease-preventing or health-promoting properties.

Gastroenterologist: a doctor who is a G.I. (gastrointestinal) specialist.

Gerontologist: a doctor who specializes in diseases of the elderly.

Gestational diabetes mellitis (GDM): develops during pregnancy due to a deficiency of insulin during pregnancy (between the 24th and 28th week) that disappears following delivery. Women who have had gestational diabetes are at a high risk of developing Type 2 diabetes later in life.

Gestational hypertension: high blood pressure during pregnancy.

Glucagon: a hormone produced by the pancreas that stimulates the liver to produce large amounts of glucose. It is given by injection for hypoglycemia and generally restores blood sugar within five to ten minutes.

Glucose: a monosaccharide or single sugar that combines with fructose to form sucrose; can also combine with glucose to form maltose, and with galactose to form lactose; slightly less sweet than sucrose.

Glycogen: the main carbohydrate storage material, which is stored in the liver and muscles for use when energy is required.

Glycosuria: sugary urine, sometimes a symptom of very high blood sugar.

Glycosylated hemoglobin levels: detailed blood sugar test that checks for glycosylated hemoglobin (glucose attached to the protein in red blood cells), known as glycohemoglobin or HbA_{1c} levels; this test can determine how well blood sugar has been controlled over a period of two to three months.

Guar gum: a high source of fibre made from the seeds of the Indian cluster bean. When you mix guar with water, it turns into a gummy gel, which when ingested slows down the digestive system, similar to acarbose.

HDL: high-density lipoproteins, known as the "good" cholesterol.

High-fructose corn syrup (HFCS): a liquid mixture of about equal parts glucose and fructose from cornstarch, which has the same sweetness as sucrose.

Human insulin: a biosynthetic product that has the advantage of eliminating the allergic reactions that occur with the use of animal insulins and more closely matching insulin produced by the pancreas.

Hydrogenation: process that converts liquid fat to semisolid fat by adding hydrogen.

Hyperglycemia: high blood sugar, a condition in which blood sugar levels are too high; defined by a fasting blood sugar level of over 7.0 mmol/L.

Hyperinsulinemia: a condition in which the pancreas produces too much insulin; a condition caused by insulin resistance, or by injecting too much insulin.

Hypertension (a.k.a. high blood pressure): the tension or force exerted on the artery walls; a condition that damages the small blood vessels as well as the larger arteries.

Hypertensive drug: a drug designed to lower blood pressure.

Hypoglycemia: low blood sugar; defined by a blood sugar level less than 3.5 mmol/L any time.

Impotence: the inability to obtain or sustain an erection long enough to have intercourse; also called erectile dysfunction (ED).

Insulin lispro: an insulin analogue that is very short-acting (also called immediate-acting).

Insulin resistance: occurs when the pancreas is making insulin but the cells are not responding to it.

Insulin: a hormone made by the islets of Langerhans, a small island of cells afloat in the pancreas; it regulates blood sugar levels.

Intensive insulin therapy: a treatment program involving close monitoring of blood sugar levels combined with taking short-, intermediate- or long-acting insulin prior to meals.

Islets of Langerhans: one of two cell systems located inside the pancreas, which secretes insulin.

Isokinetic exercise: an activity such as wrestling or weightlifting that is short but intense.

Ketones (a.k.a. ketone bodies): a poisonous by-product the body produces when there is not enough glucose in the cells, and the body burns fat as an alternative fuel; this situation can occur when blood sugar levels are 14 mmol/L at any one time.

Lancet: tiny needle used to prick the finger for a blood sample.

Laser photocoagulation: a procedure that can burn and seal off damaged blood vessels, stopping them from bleeding or leaking; this can restore vision in the earlier stages of diabetes eye disease.

LDL: low-density lipoproteins, known as the "bad" cholesterol.

Leptin: a hormone currently being used as an experimental treatment for obesity (a leptin deficiency is thought to cause weight gain); also being tested as a preventive drug for Type 2 diabetes.

Macrosomia: a condition that occurs in gestational diabetes, when high blood sugar levels cross the placenta and feed the fetus too much glucose, causing it to grow too large for its gestational age; technically defined by a birth weight greater than 4,000 g; babies with macrosomia are usually not able to fit through the birth canal because their shoulders get stuck (known as shoulder dystocia).

Macrovascular complication: a "large blood vessel complication," one that is body-wide, or systemic, such as cardiovascular problems.

Mellitus: Latin for "honey"; added to the term "diabetes" because in the past, diabetes was diagnosed through sweet-tasting urine.

Microvascular complication: a problem with the smaller blood vessels (a.k.a. capillaries) that connect to various body parts, such as eyes.

mmol: millimole, a unit of measurement that counts molecular volume per litre.

Modifiable risk factor: a risk factor that can be changed by alterations in lifestyle or diet.

Monosodium glutamate (MSG): the sodium salt of glutamic acid; an amino acid that occurs naturally in protein-containing foods such as meat, fish, milk and many vegetables.

Nephrologist: a kidney specialist.

Neurologist: a nerve and brain specialist.

Non-nutritive sweeteners: sugar substitutes or artificial sweeteners, such as saccharin and sucralose, that do not have any calories and will not affect blood sugar levels.

Nutritive sweeteners: sweeteners such as table sugar, molasses and honey, which have calories or contain natural sugar.

Obesity: a condition in which you weigh more than 20 percent of your ideal weight for your age and height.

Omega-3 fatty acids: acids naturally present in fish that swim in cold waters; crucial for brain tissue, are all polyunsaturated, and not only lower cholesterol levels, but are said to protect against heart disease.

Ophthalmologist: an eye specialist.

Oral glucose tolerance test: Standard method of diagnosing impaired glucose tolerance (IGT) or diabetes; blood sugar is tested every 30 minutes for two hours following a period of fasting.

Oral hypoglycemic agents (OHAs): drugs that help the pancreas release more insulin.

Orlistat: an antiobesity drug now available in Canada; goes by the brand name Xenical.

Pancreas: a bird beak-shaped gland situated behind the stomach.

Peripheral vascular disease (PVD): occurs when the blood flow to the limbs (arms, legs and feet) is restricted, causing cramping, pains or numbness.

Phytochemicals: "plant chemicals" (*phyto* is Greek for "plant"); disease-fighting or protective chemicals found in plant foods such as tomatoes, oats, soya, oranges and broccoli.

Polydipsia: excessive thirst.

Polyphagia: excessive hunger.

Polyuria: excessive urination.

Postprandial: postmeal or after a meal, as in postprandial blood sugar levels.

Premixed insulin: insulin produced when both short-acting insulin and inter-mediate-acting insulin are mixed together.

Primary care doctor: the doctor you see for a cold, flu or an annual physical; the doctor who refers you to specialists; general and family practitioners (GPs and FPs) or internists are common primary care doctors.

Renin: a hormone produced by the kidneys that helps to regulate blood pressure.

Risk marker: a risk factor that cannot be changed, such as age or genes.

Saturated fat: a solid fat at room temperature (from animal sources) that stimulates the body to produce LDL, or "bad" cholesterol.

Secondary diabetes: occurs when diabetes surfaces as a side effect of a particular drug, surgical procedure or other condition, such as cancer or trauma.

Soluble fibre: fibre that is water-soluble, or dissolves in water; forms a gel in the body that traps fats and lowers cholesterol.

Stroke: occurs when a blood clot travels to the brain and stops the flow of blood and oxygen carried to the nerve cells in that area, at which point cells may die or vital body functions controlled by the brain may be temporarily or permanently damaged.

Sucrose: A diasaccharide or double sugar made of equal parts glucose and fructose; known as table or white sugar; found naturally in sugar cane and sugar beets.

Sugar alcohols: nutritive sweeteners that are half as sweet as sugar; found naturally in fruits or manufactured from carbohydrates (i.e., Sorbitol).

Sulfonylureas: an oral hypoglycemic agent that helps the pancreas release more insulin.

Systolic pressure: one of the readings in a blood pressure measurement; the pressure occurring during the heart's contraction.

Thiazoladinediones (troglitazone or Rezulin): an agent that makes the cells more sensitive to insulin.

Traditional healer: a vital health care professional within the Aboriginal population.

Trans-fatty acids (a.k.a. hydrogenated oils): harmful, artificial fats that not only raise the level of "bad" cholesterol (LDL) in the bloodstream, but lower the amount of "good" cholesterol (HDL) that's already there; produced through the process of hydrogenation.

Triglycerides: a combination of saturated, monounsaturated and polyunsaturated fatty acids and glycerol.

Type 1 diabetes: insulin-dependent diabetes mellitus (IDDM), a disease usually diagnosed before age 30, in which the pancreas stops producing insulin; Type 1 diabetes, also known as juvenile diabetes, requires daily insulin injections for life.

Type 2 diabetes: "non-insulin-dependent diabetes mellitus" (NIDDM), also called "late-onset" or "mature-onset" diabetes because it's usually diagnosed after age 45; the body is either not producing enough insulin or the insulin it does produce cannot be used efficiently.

Unsaturated fat: known as "good fat" because it doesn't cause the body to produce "bad" cholesterol and increases the levels of "good" cholesterol; partially solid or liquid at room temperature.

Urea: the waste product of protein released by the kidneys.

BIBLIOGRAPHY

● ● ● ● ● ● ● ● ● ●

"Acarbose (Prandase)." *New Drugs/Drug News,* Ontario College of Pharmacists Drug Information Service Newsletter, Vol. 14, No. 2 (March/April 1996).

The Accu-Chek Advantage System. Patient information. Eli Lilly of Canada Inc., distributed 1997.

"Actos (pioglitazone) Product Monograph." Takeda America Research and Development Center, July 1999, retrieved March 2000 from www.actos.com.

"The Ad Hoc Technical Committee Working Group on Development of Management Principles and Guidelines for Subsistence Catches of Whales by Indigenous (Aboriginal) Peoples." *International Whaling Commission and Aboriginal/Subsistence Whaling: April 1979 to July 1981.* Special Issue 4, International Whaling Commission, Cambridge, England. "Advocacy in Action." *Diabetes Dialogue,* Vol. 43, No. 3 (Fall 1996).

"The Agony of De-Feet."*Equilibrium,* Issue 1 (1996): 12–14.

"AHA Stroke Connection." Patient information retrieved on-line July 2001 from the American Heart Association www.americanheart.org.

Alcohol and Diabetes—Do They Mix? Booklet. Canadian Diabetes Association, distributed 1996.

All About Insulin. Booklet. Novo Nordisk Canada Inc., distributed 1996.

All About Insulin: Novolin Care. Patient information manual from Novo Nordisk Canada Inc.

Allard, Johane P. Excerpts from "International Conference on Antioxidant Vitamins and Beta-Carotene in Disease Prevention: A Canadian Perspective," 1996.

Allsop, Karen F., and Janette Brand Miller. "Honey Revisited: A Reappraisal of Honey in Preindustrial Diets." *British Journal of Nutrition,* Vol. 75 (1996): 513–520.

American Board for Certification in Orthotics and Prosthetics Inc. Retrieved on-line July 2001 from the Amputee Web Site www.amputee-online.com.

American Diabetes Association. "An Introduction to Oral Medications for Diabetes." Posted to Diabetes.com, January 1999.

_____. "Standards of Medical Care for Patients with Diabetes Mellitus." *Diabetes Care,* Vol. 21, Supp. 1, Clinical Practice Recommendations, 1998.

_____. "The United Kingdom Prospective Diabetes Study (UKPDS) for Type 2 Diabetes: What You Need to Know About the Results of a Long-Term Study." Posted to www.diabetes.org, January 1999.

_____. On-line information. Document ID: ADA035, 1995.

Amputation Prevention Global Resource Center. *Prevent Foot Ulcers and Amputations.* Booklet. Retrieved from www.diabetesrousource.com, July 2001.

Anderson, Pauline. "Researchers Predict 'Beginning of the End' of Diabetes." *The Medical Post* (August 22, 1995).

"Antibiotics in Animals: An Interview with Stephen Sundlof, D.V.M., Ph.D." International Food Information Council, 1100 Connecticut Avenue N.W., Suite 430, Washington D.C. 20036, 1997.

The Antioxidant Connection: Visiting Speakers Discuss Immunity, Diabetes. Published by the Vitamin Information Program of Hoffman-La Roche Ltd., September 1995.

Antonucci, T., et al. "Impaired Glucose Tolerance Is Normalized by Treatment with the Thiazoladinedione." *Diabetes Care,* Vol. 20, Issue 2 (February 1997): 188–193.

Appavoo, Donna, Rayanne Waboose, and Stuart Harris. ACPM Dialogue, "Sioux Lookout Diabetes Program." *Diabetes Dialogue,* Vol. 41 No. 3 (Fall 1994): 19–20.

Armstrong, David G., Lawrence A. Lavery and Lawrence B. Harkless. "Treatment-Based Classification System for Assessment and Care of Diabetic Feet." *Journal of the American Podiatric Medical Association,* Vol. 87, No. 7 (July 1996): 303–308.

Augustine, Freda. "Helping My People." *Diabetes Dialogue,* Vol. 41, No. 3 (Fall 1994): 42–43.

Avandia (rosiglitazone). Product Monograph. Smith-Kline Beecham, 2000.

Badley, Wendy. "Across the Country." *Diabetes Dialogue,* Vol. 41, No. 3 (Fall 1994): 32.

Balancing Your Blood Sugar: A Guide for People with Diabetes. Patient information. Canadian Diabetes Association, distributed 1997.

Barnie, Annette. "'At Risk' in Northern Ontario: Looking for Answers in the Sioux Lookout Zone." *Diabetes Dialogue*, Fall Vol. 41, No. 3 (1994): 18–20.

Barwise, Kim, and Danielle Sota. "Two Views." *Diabetes Dialogue*, Vol. 43, No. 3 (Fall 1996): 42–43.

"Bayer Launches Major International Research Project into Prevention of Diabetes." Media Release, March 5, 1997.

Bell, S.J., and R.A. Forse. "Nutritional Management of Hypoglycemia." *Diabetes Education*, Vol. 25, No. 1 (Jan.–Feb. 1999): 41–47.

Bequaert Holmes, Helen, and Laura M. Purdy, eds. *Feminist Perspectives in Medical Ethics.* Bloomington: Indiana University Press, 1992.

Berndl, Leslie. "Understanding Fat." *Diabetes Dialogue*, Vol. 42, No. 1 (Spring 1995): 17–20.

Best, Henry. "Charles Herbert Best: 1899–1978." *Diabetes Dialogue*, Vol. 43, No. 4 (Winter 1996): 20–21.

The Better Health & Medical Network Collective Work & Database. Transmitted to the Internet: 8/18/97.

Beyers, Joanne. "How Sweet It Is!" *Diabetes Dialogue*, Vol. 42, No. 1 (Spring 1995): 6–8.

Biermann, June, and Barbara Toohey. *The Diabetic's Book.* New York: Perigee Books, 1992.

"A Bill of Health for the IUD: Where Do We Go from Here?" *Advances in Contraception* 10 (1994): 121–131.

Bliss, Michael. "Rewriting Medical History." *Journal of History of Medicine and Allied Sciences, Inc.* Vol. 48 (1993): 253–274.

_____. *Banting: A Biography.* Toronto: McClelland & Stewart, 1984.

_____. *The Discovery of Insulin.* Toronto: McClelland & Stewart, 1982.

Blood Glucose Monitoring: Guidelines to a Healthier You. Patient information from Bayer Inc. Healthcare Division, distributed 1997.

"Blood Pressure: Check It Out." *Countdown USA: Countdown to a Healthy Heart*, Allegheny General Hospital and Voluntary Hospitals of America, Inc., 1990.

Blood Sugar Testing Diary. Patient information. Becton Dickinson Consumer Products, 1996.

Boctor, M.A., et al. "Gestational Diabetes Debate: Controversies in Screening and Management." *Canadian Diabetes*, Vol. 10, No. 2 (June 1997): 5–7.

Bonen, Arent. "Fueling Your Tank." *Diabetes Dialogue*, Vol. 42, No. 4 (Winter 1995): 13–16.

Bril, Vera. "Diabetic Neuropathy—Can It Be Treated?" *Diabetes Dialogue*, Vol. 41, No. 4 (Winter 1994): 8–9.

British Columbia Women's Community Consultation Report. *The Challenges Ahead for Women's Health.* Vancouver: B.C. Women's Hospital and Health Centre Society, Vancouver, 1995.

Britt, Beverley. "Pesticides and Alternatives." Excerpted from the Canadian Organic Growers Toronto Chapter's Spring Conference, 1–4, 1991.

Brubaker, Patricia L. "Glucagon-like peptide-1." *Diabetes Dialogue*, Vol. 41, No. 4 (Winter 1994): 17–18.

Bureau of Human Prescription Drugs, Drugs Directorate, Health Protection Branch, Health Canada. *Drugs Directorate Guidelines, Directions for Use of Estrogen-Progestin Combination Oral Contraceptives.* Ottawa: Bureau of Human Prescription Drugs, 1994.

Burkman, Ronald T. Jr. "Noncontraceptive Effects of Hormonal Contraceptives: Bone Mass, Sexually Transmitted Disease and Pelvic Inflammatory Disease, Cardiovascular Disease, Menstrual Function, and Future Fertility." *American Journal of Obstetrics and Gynecology*, Vol. 170, No. 5, Part 2 (1994).

"Buying Your Prosthesis." Retrieved on-line July 2001 from the Amputee Web Site www.amputee-online.com.

Canadian Diabetes Association. "Guidelines for the Nutritional Management of Diabetes Mellitus in the New Millennium." A position statement. Reprinted from *Canadian Journal Diabetes Care*, Vol. 23, No. 3 (2000): 56–69.

_____. "Health ... the Smoke-Free Way." *Equilibrium*, Issue 1 (1996): 1-4.

Canadian Institute of Child Health. "Aboriginal Children." In *The Health of Canada's Children: A CICH Profile*, 2nd ed., 131–148. Ottawa: The Institute, 1994.

Canadian Medical Association Journal and the Canadian Diabetes Association. "1998 Clinical Practice Guidelines for the Management of Diabetes in Canada." Supplement to *CMAJ*, Vol. 159, No. 8, Suppl. (1998): s1–s27.

Canadian Pharmacists Association. *Compendium of Pharmaceuticals and Specialties*, 35th ed. Toronto: Webcom Ltd., 2000.

_____. *Compendium of Pharmaceuticals and Specialties*, 36th ed. Toronto: Webcom, Ltd., 2001.

Canadian Task Force on the Periodic Health Examination. *The Canadian Guide to Clinical Preventive Health Care.* Ottawa: Health Canada, 1994.

"Canons of Ethical Conduct for Prosthetists." March 1997, Committee on Professional Discipline. Retrieved on-line from The Amputee Web Site www.amputee-online.com, July 2001.

"Carbohydrate Counting: A New Way to Plan Meals." American Diabetes Association. Posted to: Diabetes.com, January 1999.

Cattral, Mark. "Pancreas Transplantation." *Diabetes Dialogue*, Vol. 43, No. 4 (Winter 1996): 6–8.

Chabun, Roxanne, and Debbie Stiles. "Bar None." *Diabetes Dialogue*, Vol. 43, No. 3 (Fall 1996): 18–21.

Chaddock, Brenda. "Activity Is Key to Diabetes Health." *Canadian Pharmacy Journal* (March 1997): 45.

_____. "Blood-Glucose Testing: Keep Up with the Trend." *Canadian Pharmacy Journal* (September 1996): 17.

_____. "Doing the Things That Make a Difference." *Canadian Pharmacy Journal* (July/August 1996): 19.

_____. "The Right Way to Read a Label." *Canadian Pharmacy Journal* (May 1996): 26.

_____. "Foul Weather Fitness: The Hardest Part Is Getting Started." *Canadian Pharmacy Journal* (March 1996): 42.

_____. "The Magic of Exercise." *Canadian Pharmacy Journal* (September 1995): 45.

The Challenge: Newsletter of the International Diabetic Athletes Association Vol. XI, No. I (Spring 1997): 1–2.

"Choosing Your Sweetener." Product information. PROSWEET Canada, 1997.

Christrup, Janet. "Nuts About Nuts: The Joys of Growing Nut Trees." *Cognition* (July 1991): 20–22.

Clarke, Bill. "Action Figures." *Diabetes Dialogue*, Vol. 43, No. 3 (Fall 1996): 14–16.

Clarke, Peter V. "Hemoglobin A1c Test Helps Long-Term Diabetes Management." *Monitor*, Vol. 1, No. 1 Medisense Canada Inc. 1996: 1–3.

Cleave, Barbara. "Viewpoint." *Diabetes Dialogue*, Vol. 44, No. 2 (Summer 1997): 2.

"CMA's Submission to the Royal Commission on Aboriginal Peoples." In *Canadian Medical Association Bridging the Gap: Promoting Health and Healing for Aboriginal Peoples in Canada*, 9–17. Ottawa: The Association, 1994.

"Complications: The Long-Term Picture." *Equilibrium*, Issue 1 (1996): 8–10. Canadian Diabetes Association.

"Cooked Food Byproducts May Be Hazardous to Diabetics." *The Medical Post* (July 2, 1996): 55.

"Corn and the Environment—Historical Perspectives." Ontario Corn Producers Association (OCPA) Corn and Environment Index Homepage, 1997.

Cox, Bruce Alan, ed. *Native People, Native Lands: Canadian Indians, Inuit and Metis.* Ottawa: Carleton University Press, 1988.

Creighton, Donald. *The Forked Road: Canada 1939–1957.* Toronto: McClelland & Stewart.

Cronier, Claire. "Sweetest Choices." *Diabetes Dialogue*, Vol. 44, No. 1 (Spring 1997): 26–27.

Cunningham, John J. "Vitamins, Minerals and Diabetes." Excerpted from Canadian Diabetes Association Conference, 1995.

"Dental Care." Retrieved on-line July 2001 from the Canadian Dental Association www.cda-adc.ca.

Deutsch, Nancy. "Vitamin C Stores Critical for Diabetics." *Family Practice*, 11 (November 1996): 24.

Dextrolog: For Recording Blood and Urine Glucose Test Results. Booklet. Bayer Inc. Healthcare Division, distributed 1997.

Diabetes and Kidney Disease. Patient information. The Kidney Foundation of Canada, 1995.

"Diabetes and Kidney Disease." Retrieved on-line July 2001 from the Kidney Foundation of Canada www.kidney.ca.

Diabetes and Non-Prescription Drugs: Guidelines to a Healthier You. Patient information. Bayer Inc. Healthcare Division, distributed 1997.

"Diabetes and the Eye." Retrieved on-line July 2001 from the Blindness and Visual Impairment Centre, Canadian National Institute for the Blind www.cnib.ca.

Diabetes Education. Patient information. Canadian Diabetes Association, distributed 1997.

"Diabetes Implants Tested." *Los Angeles Daily News* (Jan. 23, 1997).

"Diabetes Raises Dementia Risk." Reuters (Feb. 13, 1997).

Diabetes. Patient information. Pharma Plus, distributed 1997.

"Diabetes: An Undetected Time-Bomb." *CARP News* (April 1996): 12.

"Diabetes: Facts and Figures." *News from the VIP*, No. 2 (Fall 1995): 1. Vitamin Information Program, Fine Chemicals Division of Hoffman-La Roche Ltd.

"Diabetes: What Is It?" *Equilibrium*, Canadian Diabetes Association, Issue 1 (1996): 1–4.

Dickens, B.M. "The Doctrine of Informed Consent." In *Justice Beyond Orwell*, edited by R.S. Abella and M.L. Rothman, 243–63. Montreal: Yvon Blais, 1985.

_____. "Health Care Practitioners and HIV: Rights, Duties and Liabilities." In *HIV Law, Ethics and Human Rights – Text and Materials*, Jaysuriya (ed.), 66–98. New Delhi: UNDP Regional Project on HIV and Development, 1995.

"Diets Slow Reaction Times." Reuters (April 8, 1997).

"Discovery of Insulin Marked Turning Point in Human History." *The Globe and Mail* (November 1, 1996).

"Double Trouble." *Countdown USA: Countdown to a Healthy Heart*. Allegheny General Hospital and Voluntary Hospitals of America, Inc., 1990.

Doyle, Patricia. "Insulin—The Facts." Canadian Diabetes Association, 1995.

Drum, David, and Terry Zierenberg. *The Type 2 Diabetes Sourcebook*. Los Angeles: Lowell House, 1998.

Dutcher, Lisa. "A Wholistic Approach to Diabetes Management." *Diabetes Dialogue*, Vol. 41, No. 3 (Fall 1994): 42.

Emanuel, Ezekiel J., and Linda L. Emanuel. "Four Models of the Physician-Patient Relationship." *Journal of the American Medical Association*, Vol. 267, No. 16 (1992): 2221–2226.

Engel, June. "Eating Fibre." *Diabetes Dialogue*, Vol. 44, No. 1 (Spring 1997): 16–18.

_____. "Beyond Vitamins: Phytochemicals to Help Fight Disease." *Health News*, Vol. 14 (June 1996): 1.

Etchells, E., et al. "Disclosure." *Canadian Medical Association Journal*, Vol. 155 (1996): 387–91.

_____. "Voluntariness." *Canadian Medical Association Journal*, Vol. 155 (1996): 1083–1086.

Etchells, E., Gilbert Sharpe, et al. "Consent." *Canadian Medical Association Journal* Vol. 155 (1996): 177–180.

Exercise: Guidelines to a Healthier You. Patient information. Bayer Inc. Healthcare Division, distributed 1997.

The Expert Committee on the Diagnosis and Classification of Diabetes Mellitus. *Report of the Expert Committee on the Diagnosis and Classification of Diabetes Mellitus*, American Diabetes Association, January 1, 1998.

Farquhar, Andrew. "Exercising Essentials." *Diabetes Dialogue*, Vol. 43, No. 3 (Fall 1996): 6–8.

"The Fat Trap." *Countdown USA: Countdown to a Healthy Heart*. Allegheny General Hospital and Voluntary Hospitals of America, Inc., 1990.

"FDA Approves Drug to Reduce Insulin Needs for Some Diabetics." The Associated Press (Jan. 30, 1997).

"Feeding Your Child for a Lifetime." Reuters (April 10, 1997).

Feig, Denice S. "The Fourth International Workshop Conference on Gestational Diabetes Mellitus." *Canadian Diabetes*, Vol. 10, No. 2 (June 1997): 2.

Findlay, Deborah, and Leslie Miller. "Medical Power and Women's Bodies." In B.S. Bolaria and R. Bolaria, eds., *Women, Medicine and Health*. Halifax: Fernwood, 1994.

"First New Insulin in 14 Years Approved for Use in Canada." Media Release. Eli Lilly of Canada Inc./ Boehringer Mannheim Canada, October 9, 1996.

"Flick Your Risk: By Tossing Out Those Cigarettes, You Can Slash Your Chances of Heart Disease." *Countdown USA: Countdown to a Healthy Heart*, Allegheny General Hospital and Voluntary Hospitals of America, Inc., 1990.

"Folic Acid Surveys Say Consumer Awareness Is Low." *News from the VIP*, No. 2 (Fall 1995): 1–2. Vitamin Information Program, Fine Chemicals Division of Hoffman-La Roche Ltd.

"Following the Patient with Chronic Disease." *Patient Care Canada*, Vol. 7, No. 5 (May 1996): 22–38.

"Following the Patient With Stable Chronic Disease: Type II Diabetes Mellitus." *Patient Care Canada*, Vol. 7, No. 5 (May 1996): 22–41.

Food and Drug Administration, Press Release, "Rezulin to Be Withdrawn from the Market" (March 21, 2000).

———. "Nutrient Claims Guide for Individual Foods." Special Report, Focus on Food Labeling. FDA Publication no. 95-2289.

Food and Exercise: Guidelines to a Healthier You. Patient information. Bayer Inc. Healthcare Division, distributed 1997.

"Foot Care and Ulcer Prevention for People with Diabetes: Is Amputation the Only Answer?" Retrieved on-line July 2001 from the University of Manitoba (www.umanitoba.ca) Diabetes Research & Treatment Centre.

Fox, Mary Lou. "Zeesbakadapenewin: Words of an Elder Grandmother About the Sugar Disease." *Diabetes Dialogue*, Vol. 41, No. 3 (Fall 1994): 22–24.

Foxman, Stuart. Adapted from "Human vs. Beef/Pork Insulin." *The Report of the Ad Hoc Committee on Beef-Pork Insulins* by Nahla Aris-Jilwan, et al. Canadian Diabetes Association, June 6, 1996.

Fraser, Elizabeth, and Bill Clarke. "Loafing Around." *Diabetes Dialogue*, Vol. 44, No. 1 (Spring 1997): 32–33.

Gabrys, Jennifer. "Ask the Professionals." *Diabetes Dialogue*, Vol. 43, No. 4 (Winter 1996): 60–61.

Gauthier, Serge G., and Patricia H. Coleman, Reviewers. "Nutrition and Aging." *The Lederle Letter*, Vol. 2, No. 2 (April 1993), Lederle Consumer Health Products Department.

Gerth Mulvad, Gerth, and Henning Sloth Pedersen Mulvad. "Orsoq—Eat Meat and Blubber from Sea Mammals and Avoid Cardiovascular Disease." *Inuit Whaling*, published by Inuit Circumpolar Conference, Special Issue (June 1992).

"Get Off the Diet Rollercoaster." *Countdown USA: Countdown to a Healthy Heart*, Allegheny General Hospital and Voluntary Hospitals of America, Inc., 1990.

Get the Best Out of Life. Patient information. Canadian Diabetes Association, distributed 1997.

Getting to the Roots of a Vegetarian Diet. Baltimore: Vegetarian Resource Group, 1997. "Glory Enough for All: The Discovery of Insulin." Film. Gemstone Productions Ltd. and Primedia Productions, Ltd., 1988.

Gordon, Dennis. "Acarbose: When It Works/When It Doesn't." *Diabetes Forecast* (February 1997): 25–28.

Graham, Joan. "Impotence—The Complication No One Wants to Talk About." Canadian Diabetes Association, 1995.

Graham, Peg. "Rising Expectations." *Diabetes Dialogue*, Vol. 44, No. 2 (Summer 1997): 32–33.

Gregson, Ian. "An Amputee's Perspective." Retrieved on-line July 2001 from the Amputee Web Site www.amputee-online.com.

"Grieving Necessary to Accept Diabetes." *Diabetes Dialogue*, Vol. 41, No. 3 (Fall 1994): 35–36.

"Guidelines for the Nutritional Management of Diabetes in Pregnancy." A position statement by the Canadian Diabetes Association, Vol. 15, No. 3 (September 1991).

Guillebaud, J. *Contraception: Your Questions Answered.* New York: Churchill-Livingston, 1993.

"The Gum Disease Project." Retrieved July 2001 from www.periodiabetes.com.

Guthrie, Diana, and Richard A. Guthrie. *The Diabetes Sourcebook.* Los Angeles: Lowell House, 1996.

Halvorson, Mary, Francine Kaufman and Neal Kaufman. "A Snack Bar Containing Uncooked Cornstarch to Diminish Hypoglycaemia." American Diabetes Association 56th Scientific Sessions, 1996.

Harrison, Pam. "Rethinking Obesity." *Family Practice* (March 11, 1996): 24.

Hatcher, Robert A., et al. *Contraceptive Technology,* 16th rev. ed. New York: Irvington Publishers, 1994.

"Health and Healing: Inroads of Chronic Disease." *Final Report on Royal Commission on Aboriginal Peoples*, Vol. 3, Ch. 3. Posted to the Internet at www.libraxus.com.

Health Record for People with Diabetes. Patient information booklet. The Canadian Diabetes Association/Lifescan Canada, Ltd., McNeil Consumer Products Company, 1996.

Health Record for People with Diabetes. Patient Information. Canadian Diabetes Association, distributed 1997.

"Heart and Stroke Foundation's Annual Report Card." Retrieved on-line July 2001 from the Heart and Stroke Foundation of Canada www.na.heartandstroke.ca.

Heart and Stroke Foundation of Canada. *The Canadian Family Guide to Stroke: Prevention, Treatment, Recovery.* Toronto: Random House, 1996.

"Heart Attack No Stranger to Canadians." Retrieved on-line July 2001 from the Heart and Stroke Foundation of Canada www.na.heartandstroke.ca.

"Heart Attack Picture in Canada Receives Mixed Grade." (February 7, 2001) Retrieved on-line from the Heart and Stroke Foundation of Canada www.na.heartandstroke.ca.

"Heart Attack Survival in Canada." Retrieved on-line July 2001 from the Heart and Stroke Foundation of Canada www.na.heartandstroke.ca.

Heart Disease and Stroke. Patient information. The Heart and Stroke Foundation of Ontario, distributed 1997.

"The Heart Healthy Kitchen." *Countdown USA: Countdown to a Healthy Heart.* Allegheny General Hospital and Voluntary Hospitals of America, Inc., 1990.

Helwick, Caroline. "Apnea, Diabetes Linked." *The Medical Post* (May 28, 1996): 24.

"Hemodialysis." Retrieved on-line July 2001 from the Kidney Foundation of Canada www.kidney.ca.

High Blood Pressure and Your Kidneys. Patient information. The Kidney Foundation of Canada, 1995.

"High-Carbohydrate Diet Not for Everyone." Reuters (April 16, 1997).

The History of Contraception Museum, Ortho-McNeil Inc., distributed 1993.

Ho, Marian. "Learning Your ABCs, Part Two." *Diabetes Dialogue*, Vol. 43, No. 3 (Fall 1996): 38–40.

Hommel, Cynthia Abbott. "The SUGAR Group." *Diabetes Dialogue*, Vol. 41, No. 3 (Fall 1994): 21–23.

"Hostility and Heart Risk." Reuters Health Summary (April 22, 1997).

Houlden, Robyn. "Health Beliefs in Two Ontario First Nations Populations." *Diabetes Dialogue*, Vol. 41, No. 4 (Winter 1994): 24–25.

"How Adults Are Learning to Manage Diabetes with Their Lifestyle." *The Globe and Mail* (November 1, 1996).

How Do I Choose a Healthy Diet? Patient information. The Heart and Stroke Foundation of Ontario, distributed 1997.

How to Choose Your New Blood Glucose Meter. Patient information. LifeScan Canada Inc., distributed 1997.

How to Cope with a Brief Illness: A Guide for the Person Taking Insulin. Patient information. The Canadian Diabetes Association, March 1996.

How to Take Insulin. Patient information. Monoject Diabetes Care Products, distributed 1997.

Hunt, John A. "Fueling Up." *Diabetes Dialogue*, Vol. 41, No. 4 (Winter 1994): 20–21.

Hunter, J.E., and T.H. Applewhite. "Reassessment of Trans Fatty Acid Availability in the U.S. Diet." *American Journal of Clinical Nutrition*, 54 (1991): 363–369.

Hurley, Jane, and Stephen Schmidt. "Going with the Grain." *Nutrition Action* (October 1994): 10–11.

IFIC Review: Intense Sweeteners: Effects on Appetite and Weight Management. International Food Information Council, 1100 Connecticut Avenue N.W., Suite 430, Washington D.C. 20036, November 1995.

IFIC Review: Uses and Nutritional Impact of Fat Reduction Ingredients. International Food Information Council 1100 Connecticut Avenue N.W., Suite 430, Washington D.C. 20036, October 1995.

"The Importance of Braille Literacy." Retrieved on-line July 2001 from the Blindness and Visual Impairment Centre, Canadian National Institute for the Blind www.cnib.ca.

"Improving Treatment Outcomes in NIDDM: The Questions and Controversies." *The Diabetes Report*, Issue 1, Vol. 2 (1996): 1–2.

"Increased Awareness of Stroke Symptoms Could Dramatically Reduce Stroke Disability—New NIH Public Education Campaign Says Bystanders Can Play Key Role." (May 8, 2001) Retrieved on-line from the American Heart Association www.americanheart.org.

"Insulin and Type 2 Diabetes."*Equilibrium*, Issue 1 (1996): 29–30.

Insulin Management Information. Patient information from Eli Lilly and Co., distributed 1997.

Insulin: Guidelines to a Healthier You. Patient information. Bayer Inc. Healthcare Division, distributed 1997.

Is Your Insulin as Easy to Use as Humulin? Patient information. Eli Lilly of Canada Inc., distributed 1997.

It Takes Two: A Couple's Guide to Erectile Dysfunction. Patient information. Pharmacia and Upjohn, distributed 1997.

Jeffrey, Susan. "Uncooked Cornstarch Snacks Aid Diabetics." *The Medical Post* (November 12, 1996).

Jeffries, Glen Edward. "Preparing for Surgery." Retrieved on-line July 2001 from the Amputee Web Site www.amputee-online.com.

"A Jelly Bean Glucose Test." *American Baby* (April 1996): 6.

"Jelly Beans Offer Sweet Relief." *Diabetes Dialogue*, Vol. 44, No. 2 (Summer 1997): 52–53.

Jovanovic-Peterson, Lois, June Biermann and Barbara Toohey. *The Diabetic Woman: All Your Questions Answered.* New York: G.P. Putnam's Sons, 1996.

Joyce, Carol. "What's New in Type 2." *Diabetes Dialogue*, Vol. 43, No. 3 (Fall 1996): 32–36, 63.

Kalla, Timothy B. "Complications: Footcare and the Trouble with Ulcers." Retrieved on-line July 2001 from the Canadian Diabetes Association www.diabetes.ca.

Kaptchuk, Ted, and Micheal Croucher. *The Healing Arts: A Journey Through the Faces of Medicine.* London: The British Broadcasting Corporation, 1986.

Kea, David. "Herd Health: The Biggest Reward of Ecological Dairy Farming." *Cognition* 93 (Winter 1992): 26–27.

Keeping Well With Diabetes: Novolin Care. Patient information. Novo Nordisk Canada Inc., distributed 1996.

Kelly, Catherine. "Hormone Replacement Therapy." *Diabetes Dialogue*, Vol. 44, No. 2 (Summer 1997): 28–30.

Kenshole, Anne. "To Be or Not to Be Pregnant." *Diabetes Dialogue*, Vol. 44, No. 2 (Summer 1997): 6–8.

Kermode-Scott, Barbara. "NIDDM Affecting Huge Numbers, Says Expert." *Family Practice* (March 11, 1996): 21.

Ketone Testing: Guidelines to a Healthier You. Patient information. Bayer Inc. Healthcare Division, distributed 1997.

Kewayosh, Alethea. "The Way We Are: The Eye of the Storm—A First Nations Perspective on Diabetes." *Diabetes Dialogue* (Fall 1994): 56-57.

Khan, Gabriel M., and Henry J.L. Marriot. *Heart Trouble Encyclopedia.* Toronto: Stoddart, 1996.

Kidney Stones. Patient information. The Kidney Foundation of Canada, distributed 1995.

Kock, Henry. "Restoring Natural Vegetation as Part of the Farm." *Gardening without Chemicals '91.* Canadian Organic Growers Toronto Chapter, April 6, 1991.

Korytkowski, Mary. "Something Old, Something New." *Diabetes Spectrum*, Vol. 9 (November 4, 1996): 211–212.

Kra, J. Siegfried. *What Every Woman Must Know About Heart Disease.* New York: Warner Books, 1996.

Kuczmarski, R.J., et al. "Increasing Prevalence of Overweight Among U.S. Adults: The National Health and Nutrition Examination Surveys, 1960 to 1991." *Journal of the American Medical Association*, 272 (1994): 205–211.

Kumar, S., et al. "Troglitazone, an Insulin Action Enhancer, Improves Metabolic Control in NIDDM Patients." *Diabetologia*, Vol. 30, Issue 6 (June 1996): 701–709.

Kushi, Mishio. *The Cancer Prevention Guide.* New York: St. Martin's Press, 1993.

Lebovitz, Harold E. "Acarbose, an Alpha-glucosidase Inhibitor in the Treatment of NIDDM." *Diabetes Care*, 19, Suppl. 1 (1996): 554–561.

Leiter, Lawrence A. "Acarbose: New Treatment in NIDDM Patients." *New Drugs/ Drug News*, Vol. 14, No. 2 (1997). Ontario College of Pharmacists.

Levine, R.J. *Ethics and Regulation of Clinical Research.* New Haven: Yale University Press, 1988.

Lichtenstein, A.H., et al. "Hydrogenation Impairs the Hypolipidemic Effect of Corn Oil in Humans." *Arteriosclerosis and Thrombosis*, 13 (1993): 154–161.

Lichti, Janice C. "Mind Boosters." *Healing Arts Magazine* (March 1996): 14–15.

Liebman, Bonnie. "Syndrome X: The Risks of High Insulin." *Nutrition Action*, Vol. 27, No. 2 (March 2000): 3–8.

Linden, Ron. "Hyperbaric Medicine." *Diabetes Dialogue*, Vol. 43, No. 4 (Fall 1996): 24–26.

Lindesay, J.E. "Multiple Pain Complaints in Amputees." *Journal of Rehabilitation and Social Medicine*, Vol. 78 (1985): 452–455.

Little, Linda. "Vitamin E May Help Cut Diabetics' Risk of Heart Disease." *The Medical Post* (May 14, 1996): 5.

Little, Margaret. "Step Right Up." *Diabetes Dialogue*, Vol. 43, No. 3 (Fall 1996).

Living Well. Patient information. Canadian Diabetes Association, distributed 1997.

"Low Blood Sugars: Your Questions Answered." *Equilibrium*, Issue 1 (1996): 31–32.

Ludwig, Sora. "Gestational Diabetes." *Canadian Diabetes*, Vol. 10, No. 2 (June 1997): 1, 8.

Macdonald, Jeanette. "The Facts About Menopause." *Diabetes Dialogue*, Volume 44, No. 2 (Summer 1997): 24–26.

MacMillan, Harriet L., et al. "Aboriginal Health." *Canadian Medical Association Journal*, Vol. 155 (1996): 1569–1578.

Maltman, Grant. "Banting: Co-discoverer of Insulin and … Artist." *Diabetes Dialogue*, Vol. 41, No. 4 (Winter 1994): 41–42.

_____. "The Birth of an Idea." *Diabetes Dialogue*, Vol. 42, No. 4 (Winter 1995): 40–43.

Managing Your Diabetes with Humalog. Booklet. Eli Lilly and Company, distributed 1997.

Marliss, Errol B., and Rejeanne Gougeon, reviewers. "Focus on Women: Dieting as a Possible Risk Factor for Obesity." *The Lederle Letter*, Vol. 2. No. 4 (August 1993): 1–2. Lederle Consumer Health Products Department.

Marliss, Errol B., et al. reviewers. "Weight-Reducing Diets May Compromise Nutrition." *The Lederle Letter*, Vol. 1, No. 3 (August 1992): 1–2. Lederle Consumer Health Products Department.

Marshall, M., E. Helmes and A.B. Deathe. "A Comparison of Psychosocial Functioning and Personality in Amputee and Chronic Pain Patients." *Clinical Journal of Pain* 8 (1992): 351–357.

Martin, Cheryl. "Acarbose (Prandase)." *Communication* (March/April 1996): 38.

Mastroianni, Anna C., Ruth Faden and Daniel Federman, eds. *Women and Health Research: Ethical and Legal Issues of Including Women in Clinical Studies*, Vol. 1. Washington: National Academy Press, 1994.

Mature Lifestyles: High Blood Pressure. Patient information. Health Watch/Shoppers Drug Mart, distributed 1997.

McCarten, James. "Toxic or Not, Inuit Stand by Whale Meat." *The Edmonton Journal* (December 28, 1995).

MediSense Blood Glucose Sensor. Product monograph, 1995.

Micral-S Kidney Chek. Patient information. Eli Lilly of Canada/Boehringer Mannheim Canada Inc., distributed 1997.

Mihill, Chris. "New Fears Over Link Between Cow's Milk and Diabetes." *The Guardian* (October 4, 1996).

"Monitoring Your Blood Sugar." *Equilibrium*, Issue 1 (1996): 33.

Monoject: Diabetes Care Products. Patient information. Sherwood Medical Industries Canada Inc., distributed 1997.

Morrison, Bruce. R., and C. Roderick Williams. *Native Peoples Canadian Experience.* Toronto: McClelland & Stewart, Ltd., 1986.

Musgrove, Lorraine. "Ask the Professionals." *Diabetes Dialogue*, Vol. 44, No. 1 (Spring 1997): 60–61.

National Kidney Foundation. *Dialysis.* Booklet. Retrieved on-line from www.kidney.org, July 2001.

_____. *End Stage Renal Disease in the United States.* Booklet. Retrieved on-line July 2001 from www.kidney.org.

_____. "Microalbuninuria in Diabetic Kidney Disease." Retrieved on-line July 2001 from www.kidney.org.

_____. "Preventing Diabetic Kidney Disease." Retrieved on-line July 2001 from www.kidney.org.

Neergaard, Lauran. "Study Finds Low Hormone Levels May Encourage Weight Gain." Associated Press (May 14, 1997).

Neuschwander-Tetri, B.A., et al. "Troglitazone-Induced Hepatic Failure Leading to Liver Transplantation. A case report." *Annals of Internal Medicine*, Vol. 129 (July 1, 1998): 38–41.

"New Developments in the Management of Type II Diabetes." *The Diabetes Report*, Issue 2, Vol. 1 (1995): 1, 2.

"New Perspectives in the Management of NIDDM." *The Diabetes Report*, Issue 3, Vol. 1 (1996): 1, 3.

"New Tool Allows Early Prediction of Patient's Stroke Outcome." (June 28, 2001) Retrieved on-line from the National Institute Neurological Disorders and Stroke www.ninds.nih.gov.

Non-Insulin Dependent Diabetes Mellitus. Patient information. National Pharmacy Continuing Education Program and Bayer Inc., distributed February 1997.

Novolin ge Insulin, Human Biosynthetic Antidiabetic Agent. Product Monograph for Novo Nordisk Canada Inc., distributed 1997.

Novolin Product Monograph, 1997.

Nutrition for Diabetes. Patient information manual from Novo Nordisk Canada Inc., distributed 1996.

"Nutrition News." *Diabetes Dialogue*, Vol. 43, No. 4 (Winter 1996): 57.

"Nutrition News." *Diabetes Dialogue*, Vol. 44, No. 1 (Spring 1997): 56.

"Nutrition Principles for the Management of Diabetes and Related Complications (Technical Review)." *Diabetes Care*, Vol. 17 (1994): 490–518.

"Oats Are In." *Countdown USA: Countdown to a Healthy Heart.* Allegheny General Hospital and Voluntary Hospitals of America, Inc., 1990.

"Obese Children May Lack Antioxidants." Reuters Health Summary (April 22, 1997).

"Obesity Hormone May Prevent Diabetes." Reuters Health Summary (April 29, 1997).

"Olestra: Yes or No? Excerpt from The University of California at Berkeley Wellness Letter." *Diabetes Dialogue*, Vol. 43, No. 3 (Fall 1996): 44.

One Touch Profile: For Complete Diabetes Management. Patient information. LifeScan Canada Inc., distributed 1997.

Orbach, Susie. *Fat Is a Feminist Issue.* New York: Berkley Books, 1990.

Organ Donation: Have You Thought About It? Patient information. The Kidney Foundation of Canada, distributed 1995.

Orton, David. "Rethinking Environmental-First Nations Relationships." *Canadian Dimension*, Vol. 29, No. 1 (February-March 1995).

_____. "Some Limitations of a Left Critique and Deep Dilemmas in Environmental-First Nations Relationships." Learned Societies Conference on "The Environment and the Relations with First Nations," co-sponsored by the Society for Socialist Studies and the Environmental Studies Association of Canada, Montreal, June 5, 1995.

"Physical Activity." *Equilibrium*, Issue 1 (1996).

"Pills for Diabetes?" *Equilibrium*, Issue 1 (1996).

Pills for Treating Diabetes. Patient information. Canadian Diabetes Association, distributed March 1996.

Pocket Partner: A Guide to Healthy Food Choices. Booklet. Canadian Diabetes Association, distributed 1997.

Pocket Serving Sizer. Patient information. Canadian Diabetes Association, distributed 1997.

Poirier, Laurinda M., and Katharine M. Coburn. *Women and Diabetes: Life Planning for Health and Wellness.* New York: American Diabetes Association and Bantam Books, 1997.

"Position of the American Dietetic Association: Use of Nutritive and Nonnutritive Sweeteners." *Journal of the American Dietetic Association*, Vol. 93 (1993): 816–822.

Postl, B., et al. "Background Paper on the Health of Aboriginal Peoples in Canada." In *Bridging the Gap: Promoting Health and Healing for Aboriginal Peoples in Canada*. Ottawa: The Canadian Medical Association, 1994, 19–56.

Practical Advice for the Prandase Patient. Booklet. Bayer Inc. Healthcare Division, distributed 1996.

Prandase (Acarbose) Tablets. Product monograph. Bayer Inc. Healthcare Division, distributed April 14, 1997.

Prandase: A New Approach to NIDDM Therapy. Patient information booklet. Bayer Inc. Healthcare Division, distributed 1997.

Preventing the Complications of Diabetes: Guidelines to a Healthier You. Patient information. Bayer Inc. Healthcare Division, distributed 1997.

"Prevention and Treatment of Obesity: Application to Type 2 Diabetes (Technical Review)." *Diabetes Care*, Vol. 20 (1997): 1744–1766.

Prochaska, James O. "A Revolution in Diabetes Evaluation." Excerpted from the Canadian Diabetes Association Conference, 1995.

"Proper Knowledge of a Healthy Diet Makes Huge Difference." *The Globe and Mail* (November 1, 1996): 3.

PROSWEET: The Low Calorie Pure Sugar Taste Sweetener. Product information. PROSWEET Canada, distributed 1997.

"Protein Content of the Diabetic Diet (Technical Review)." *Diabetes Care*, Vol. 17 (1994): 1502–1513.

Purdy, Laura M. *Reproducing Persons: Issues in Feminist Bioethics.* Ithaca: Cornell University Press, 1996.

"Putting Fun Back into Food." International Food Information Council, 1100 Connecticut Avenue N.W., Suite 430, Washington D.C. 20036, 1997.

"Q & A About Fatty Acids and Dietary Fats." International Food Information Council, 1100 Connecticut Avenue N.W., Suite 430, Washington D.C. 20036, 1997.

"Q & A on Low-Calorie Sweeteners." *The Diabetes News*, Vol. 1, Issue 2 (Spring 1997): 3.

Real World Factors That Interfere with Blood-Glucose Meter Accuracy. Patient information. MediSense Canada Inc., distributed 1996.

The Receptor, Vol. 7, No. 3 (Fall/Winter 1996).

"Recovering After a Stroke." Retrieved on-line July 2001 from the Agency for Healthcare Research and Quality www.ahrq.gov.

Reddy, Sethu. "Smoking and Diabetes." *Diabetes Dialogue*, Vol. 42, No. 4 (Winter 1995): 33–35.

Reducing Your Risk of Diabetes Complications. Patient information. MediSense Canada Inc., distributed 1997.

"Report on the Second International Conference on Diabetes and Native Peoples." Prepared by the First Nations Health Commission, Assembly of First Nations, November 1993.

"Research, Improvement in Products Never Stops in Health Industry." *The Globe and Mail* (November 1, 1996).

Rifkin, Jeremy. "Playing God with the Genetic Code." *Health Naturally* (April/May 1995): 40–44.

Rosenthal, M. Sara. *Managing Diabetes for Women*. Toronto: Macmillan Canada, 1999.

_____. *The Breast Sourcebook*. Los Angeles: Lowell House, 1996, 1997.

_____. *The Breastfeeding Sourcebook,* 2nd ed. Los Angeles: Lowell House, 1998.

_____. *The Fertility Sourcebook,* 2nd ed. Los Angeles: Lowell House, 1998.

_____. *50 Ways to Manage Type 2 Diabetes*. Chicago: McGraw-Hill/ Contemporary, 2001.

_____. *The Gynecological Sourcebook,* 3rd ed. Los Angeles: Lowell House, 1999.

_____. *The Pregnancy Sourcebook,* 2nd ed. Los Angeles: Lowell House, 1997.

_____. *The Type 2 Diabetic Woman.* Chicago: NTC/Contemporary, 1999.

Rowlands, Liz, and Denis Peter. "Diabetes—Yukon Style." *Diabetes Dialogue*, Vol. 41, No. 3 (Fall 1994).

Rubin, Alan L. *Diabetes for Dummies.* Chicago: IDG Books, 1999.

Ruggiero, Laura. *Helping People with Diabetes Change: Practical Applications of the Stages of Change Model.* Professional information. LifeScan Education Institute, distributed 1997.

Ryan, David. "At the Controls." *Diabetes Dialogue*, Vol. 43, No. 3 (Fall 1996): 20–21.

Safety First. Patient information. Becton Dickinson and Co. Canada Inc., distributed 1997.

Schoepp, Glen. "What Is the Role of Acarbose (Prandase) in Diabetes Management?" *Pharmacy Practice*, Vol. 12, No. 4 (April 1996): 37–38.

Schwartz, Carol. "An Eye-Opener." *Diabetes Dialogue*, Vol. 43, No. 4 (Winter 1996): 20–22.

_____. "Complications: Your Eyes and Diabetic Retinopathy." Retrieved on-line July 2001 from the Canadian Diabetes Association www.diabetes.ca.

"Selected Vitamins and Minerals in Diabetes (Technical Review)." *Diabetes Care*, Vol. 17 (1994): 464–479.

Seto, Carol. "Nutrition Labelling—U.S. Style." *Diabetes Dialogue*, Vol. 42, No. 1 (Spring 1995): 32–34.

7 Key Factors for Real World Accuracy in the Real World. Patient information from MediSense Canada Inc., distributed 1997.

7 Key Steps to Control Your Diabetes. Patient information from MediSense Canada Inc., distributed 1997.

"Seven Tips for Your Sick Day Blues." *Equilibrium*, Issue 1 (1996): 38–41.

Sherwin, Susan. *Patient No Longer: Feminist Ethics and Health Care.* Philadelphia: Temple University Press, 1984.

Sinclair, A.J. "Rational Approaches to the Treatment of Patients with Non-insulin-Dependent Diabetes Mellitus." *Practical Diabetes Supplement*, Vol. 10, No. 6 (Nov./Dec. 1993): 515–520.

Society of Obstetricians and Gynecologists of Canada. *A Guide for Health Care Professionals Working with Aboriginal Peoples: A Policy Statement*, 1–15. Booklet. April 2001.

"Sorting Out the Facts About Fat." International Food Information Council, 1100 Connecticut Avenue N.W., Suite 430, Washington D.C. 20036, 1997.

Spicer, Kay. "Traditional Foods of Aboriginal Canadians." *Diabetes Dialogue*, Vol. 41, No. 3 (Fall 1994).

"Spring at Last!" *The Diabetes News,* prepared by the LifeScan Education Institute, Spring 1996.

Stehlin, Dori. "A Little Lite Reading" posted to FDA Web site www.fda.gov/fdac/foodlabel/diabetes.html.

"Study Finds That Teens Who Had Less Salt as Infants Have Lower Blood Pressure." Associated Press (April 8, 1997).

"Study Ranks Cities by Pudginess of Residents." The Associated Press (March 4, 1997).

"Study: You Can Lose Weight and Cigarettes." Reuters (June 19, 1997).

Sucralose Overview. Product information from Splenda (brand sweetener) Information Centre, distributed 1997.

Surestep. Patient information. LifeScan Canada Inc, distributed 1997.

"Sweet Promise from Sugar Substitute?" *The Medical Post* (July 2, 1996): 55.

Taking Care of Your Feet: Guidelines to a Healthier You. Patient information. Bayer Inc., Healthcare Division, distributed 1997.

"10 Tips to Healthy Eating." American Dietetic Association and National Center for Nutrition and Dietetics (NCND), April 1994.

Tetley, Deborah. "Fish Farmer Hopes to Tame Diabetes on Akwesasne." *The Toronto Star* (April 12, 1997).

Thompson, John Herd, with Allen Singer. *Canada 1922–1939: Decades of Discord.* Toronto: McClelland & Stewart, Ltd., 1985.

Todd, Robert. "The Sporting Life." *Diabetes Dialogue,* Vol. 43, No. 4 (Fall 1996): 28–29.

Tookenay, Vincent F. "Improving the Health Status of Aboriginal People in Canada: New Directions, New Responsibilities." *Canadian Medical Association Journal,* Vol. 155 (1996): 1581–1583.

"Trapped by Furs." Presentation at the Symposium *Conflicting Interests of Animal Welfare and Indigenous Peoples.* Erasmus University, Rotterdam, Finn Lynge, January 17, 1997.

Travelling with Diabetes. Booklet. Canadian Diabetes Association, distributed 1996.

Treating Kidney Failure. Patient information. The Kidney Foundation of Canada, distributed 1995.

Type II Diabetes. Shoppers Drug Mart Education Series NIDDM Vol. 95 (1996):11.

Understanding Type 2 Diabetes: Guidelines for a Healthier You. Patient information. Bayer Inc. Healthcare Division, distributed 1997.

Urinary Tract Infections. Patient information from The Kidney Foundation of Canada, distributed 1995.

Utiger, Robert. "Restoring Fertility in Women with PCOS." *The New England Journal of Medicine,* Vol. 335, No. 9 (August 29, 1996).

Veatch, R.M. "Abandoning Informed Consent." *HCR,* Vol. 25, No. 2 (1995): 5–12.

"VIP Conference on Elderly Attracts Canadian Media." *News from the VIP,* No. 2 (Fall 1995): 1–2. Vitamin Information Program, Fine Chemicals Division of Hoffman-La Roche Ltd.

Wanless, Melanie. "The Weight Debate." *Diabetes Dialogue,* Vol. 44, No. 1 (Spring 1997): 22–25.

Watch Your Step. Booklet. Norvo Nordisk Canada, Inc., distributed 1996.

"We're Winning: By Changing Lifestyles, We're Proving Every Day That Coronary Disease Can Be Beaten." *Countdown USA: Countdown to a Healthy Heart.* Allegheny General Hospital and Voluntary Hospitals of America, Inc., 1990.

"What Is Diabetes?" Canadian Diabetes Association (February 2, 1996). CDA Document ID: ADA037.

What Is Intensive Diabetes Management? Patient information. Diabetes Clinical Research Unit of Mount Sinai Hospital Toronto for Sherwood Medical Industries Canada Inc., distributed 1997.

"What You Should Know About Aspartame." International Food Information Council, 1100 Connecticut Avenue N.W., Suite 430, Washington D.C. 20036, November 4, 1996.

What You Should Know About Humulin. Booklet. Eli Lilly of Canada Inc., distributed 1997.

"What You Should Know About MSG." International Food Information Council, 1100 Connecticut Avenue N.W., Suite 430, Washington D.C. 20036, September 1991.

"What You Should Know About Sugars." International Food Information Council, 1100 Connecticut Avenue N.W., Suite 430, Washington D.C. 20036, May 1994.

"What's Your Type?" *News from the VIP*, No. 2 (Fall 1995): 1–2. Vitamin Information Program, Fine Chemicals Division of Hoffman-La Roche Ltd.

"When You Become an Amputee." Retrieved on-line July 2001 from the Amputee Web Site www.amputee-online.com.

Whitcomb, Randall. "The Key to Type 2." *Diabetes Dialogue*, Vol. 43, No. 4 (Winter 1996): 16–18.

White, John R., Jr. "The Pharmacologic Management of Patients with Type II Diabetes Mellitus in the Era of New Oral Agents and Insulin Analogs." *Diabetes Spectrum*, Vol. 9, No. 4 (1996): 227–234.

Willett, W.C., et al. "Intake of Trans Fatty Acids and Risk of Coronary Heart Disease Among Women." *Lancet*, Vol. 341 (1993): 581–585.

Williams, Michael. "Macleod: The Co-discoverer of Insulin." *Proceedings of the Royal College of Physicians of Edinburgh*, Vol. 23, No. 3 (July 1993).

Williamson, G.M., et al. "Social and Psychological Factors in Adjustment to Limb Amputation." *Journal of Social Behavior and Personality* 9 (1994): 249–268.

Williamson, Gail M. "Perceived Impact of Limb Amputation on Sexual Activity: A Study of Adult Amputees." *The Journal of Sex Research*, Vol. 33, No. 3 (1996): 221–230.

Worldwide Fund For Nature. *Caring for the Earth: A Strategy for Sustainable, Living IUCN—The World Conservation Union.* United Nations Environment Programme, Gland, Switzerland, 1991.

Wormworth, Janice. "Toxins and Tradition: The Impact of Food-Chain Contamination on the Inuit of Northern Quebec." *Canadian Medical Association Journal*, Vol. 152, No. 8 (April 15, 1995).

Yale, Jean-Francois. "Glucose Results: Plasma or Whole Blood?" *Monitor*, Vol. 1 No. 2 (1997): 1-4.

Yankova, Diliana. "Diabetes in Bulgaria." *Diabetes Dialogue*, Vol. 44, No. 1 (Spring 1997).

"You Are What You Eat." *Equilibrium*, Issue 1 (1996): 16–20.

You Have Diabetes ... Can You Have That? Booklet. Canadian Diabetes Association, distributed 1995.

Your Blood Sugar Level ... What Does It Tell You? Patient information. Eli Lilly of Canada Inc., distributed 1997.

Your Diabetes Healthcare Team. Equilibrium, Issue 1 (1996): 34–36.

Your Kidneys. Patient information. The Kidney Foundation of Canada, distributed 1993.

Zinman, Bernard. "Insulin Analogues." *Diabetes Dialogue*, Vol. 43, No. 4 (Winter 1996): 14–15.

INDEX

● ● ● ● ● ● ● ● ● ●